CURRENT TOPICS IN HYPOTHYROIDISM WITH FOCUS ON DEVELOPMENT

Edited by **Eliška Potluková**

Current Topics in Hypothyroidism with Focus on Development

http://dx.doi.org/10.5772/56084
Edited by Eliška Potluková

Contributors

Yardena Tenenbaum-Rakover, Ljiljana Saranac, Ashraf Soliman, Ferenc Péter, Ágota Muzsnai, Rózsa Gráf, Jandee Lee, Woong Youn Chung, Baha Zantour, Andrea Luigi Tranquilli, Piergiorgio Stortoni, Antonio Mancini, Eliska Potlukova, Jan Kratky, Jan Jiskra

Published by InTech

Janeza Trdine 9, 51000 Rijeka, Croatia

Publishing Process Manager Ana Pantar
Typesetting InTech DTP Team
Cover InTech Design Team

Additional hard copies can be obtained from orders@intechopen.com

Current Topics in Hypothyroidism with Focus on Development, Edited by Eliška Potluková
p. cm.
ISBN 978-953-51-0970-9

For EU product safety concerns:
IN TECH d.o.o., Prolaz Marije Krucifikse Kozulić 3, 51000 Rijeka, Croatia,
info@intechopen.com or visit our website at intechopen.com.

Meet the editor

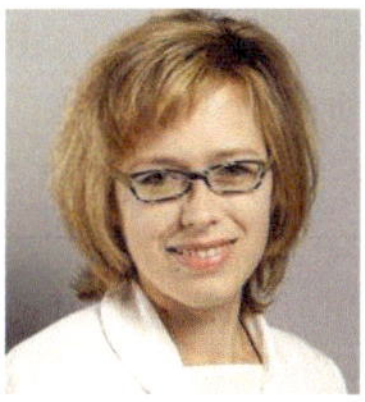

Eliska Potlukova graduated from the First Faculty of Medicine of the Charles University in Prague in 2001. During studies, she spent six months at the Yale School of Medicine (USA) working in a research lab. After graduation, she worked in the University Hospital Basel in Switzerland as a researcher in immunology and as a physician (internal medicine). She graduated from the Basel University in 2004. Since then, she has been working at the Third Department of Medicine of the General University Hospital in Prague as a physician (internal medicine, endocrinology), teacher and scientist. She is an author of a number of original articles published in well-regarded journals in the fields of endocrinology and immunology.

Contents

Preface

Dear Reader,

As a physician, you are aware of the ongoing need to update your knowledge on the latest research in the field of medicine that you are practicing. In endocrinology, we may not encounter such a large number of new medicaments as e.g. in cardiology. However, many interesting and mostly clinically oriented studies are ongoing also in our field. To be acquainted with them means to improve the care for our patients.

The more we worked on the book you are now reading, the more I got to like the idea of it. This book gives an opportunity to authors literally from all over the world to present their medical expertise and express their opinion on selected interesting topics in hypothyroidism. Individual chapters of this book represent the most up-to-date reviews of literature combined with the clinical experience of the authors.

Authors were asked to choose their own topic of interest concerning hypothyroidism. Interestingly, the majority chose to write on a theme connected with development: pregnancy, growth and hypothyroidism in childhood. Management of thyroid disorders in pregnancy seems to be a never-ending source of discussions and even disputes. Here we provide two comprehensive reviews on this controversial topic. Surprisingly for me as a non-paediatrician, the opinions on treatment of subclinical hypothyroidism in childhood may also differ quite substantially.

If you want to learn how to differentiate the conditions when watchful waiting is enough from situations when immediate levothyroxine substitution is crucial, our book might help you. Moreover, if you are thinking of performing thyroid ultrasound by yourself, or you do it already and maybe are not so sure about it, our last Chapter might be a practical guide for you in the visualisation of a hypothyroid gland.

Perhaps you will not agree with everything that is written in this book; and this was not our goal. Our book will help you form your own opinion. Our most important message is that whichever country we live in, we want to give the best treatment to our hypothyroid patients.

Eliška Potluková, MD, PhD
Third Department of Medicine, General University Hospital
And the First Faculty of Medicine, Charles University in Prague
Czech Republic

Section 1

Hypothyroidism in Pregnancy

Chapter 1

Hypothyroidism, Fertility and Pregnancy

Piergiorgio Stortoni and Andrea L. Tranquilli

Additional information is available at the end of the chapter

http://dx.doi.org/10.5772/54328

1. Introduction

Pregnancy has a profound effect on the thyroid gland and its function. In iodine-replete countries, the gland size has been found to increase by 10% during pregnancy, and in areas of iodine deficiency, the gland size increases by 20%–40%. The prevalence of hypothyroidism during pregnancy is estimated to be 0.3–0.5% for overt hypothyroidism and 2–3% for subclinical hypothyroidism. Worldwide, iodine deficiency remains one of the leading causes of both overt and subclinical hypothyroidism. However, there are many other causes of hypothyroidism during pregnancy, including autoimmune thyroiditis, the most common organic pathology [1]. Other causes include the following: thyroid radioiodine ablation (to treat hyperthyroidism or thyroid cancer), hypoplasia and/or agenesis of the thyroid gland, surgery (for thyroid tumors and, rarely, central hypothyroidism, including lymphocytic hypophysitis or ectopic thyroid) and some drugs, such as rifampin and phenytoin, which can alter thyroid metabolism [2].

It has long been recognized that iodine represents an essential element for fetal growth and development [3]. In fact, congenital hypothyroidism leads to cretinism, which is characterized by irreversible growth restriction and mental retardation. In mountain areas, such as the Himalayas, Alps and Andes, iodine depletion can be caused by glaciers and erosion [4], leading to the presence of cretinism in small sections of the population. Nonetheless, a significant proportion of the population is exposed to mild iodine deficiency, which is responsible for the clinical features of defined goiters, impaired cognition and hypothyroidism [5]. One way to escape the dangerous and hidden deficiency is to incorporate iodine into the daily diets of people all over the world [6]. Today, as a result of this strategy, there are no countries with endemic iodine deficiencies, and only approximately 32 countries in the world with a public problem of mild to moderate iodine deficiency [7]. Some meta-analyses have studied the intelligence quotient (IQ) reduction in children who suffered from iodine deficiency, but, due to confounding factors, it has not been well elucidated whether the IQ reduction depends on an "intra-" or "extra-" uterine iodine deficiency [8]. However, some studies have stressed that cognitive disorders that are linked to a mild-moderate iodine deficiency are a reversible clinical phenomenon [9-16]. These considerations are interesting because recent data have indicated the recurrence of iodine deficiency in developed countries, such as the United States, Australia, New Zealand, United Kingdom and, especially, in Europe [17,18].

Given that maternal iodine supplementation has a positive impact on the developmental quotient of children living in areas of iodine deficiency, the current WHO guidelines suggest that iodized salt provides sufficient iodine intake for pregnant women [19]. In particular, iodine supplementation is recommended beginning in early pregnancy to ensure adequate fetal brain development. A useful test to verify sufficient iodine intake is the assessment of urinary iodine concentration. Thresholds for median urinary iodine sufficiency have been identified for populations but not for individuals, given the significant day-to-day variation of iodine intake [20]. The cut-off for iodine sufficiency is a median urinary iodine concentration of 100–199 μg/L in adults and of 150–249 μg/L in pregnant women [21]. However, in some areas, iodine intake is sufficient in schoolchildren but not in pregnant women. This situation necessitates an additional strategy if iodized salt is already in use [22]. Some studies analyzing mildly iodine-deficient pregnant European women revealed that iodine supplementation is stopped before or at the moment of delivery [23]. In these patients, iodine supplementation was observed to increase maternal urinary iodine excretion and reduce thyroid volume. Additionally, no alterations in newborn thyroid volumes and no increased thyroglobulin maternal serum levels were present. However, these studies only demonstrate that iodine supplementation affects infant growth and development. Several studies [24-26] have attempted to analyze the relationship between iodine supplementation and fetal effects, but no significant effects on mental or motor development in the offspring were observed [8].

It is important to emphasize that following delivery, maternal iodine remains the only iodine source for breastfed infants; a breastfeeding woman excretes approximately 75–200 μg iodine daily in her breast milk [27,28]. Dietary iodine intake during lactation ranges from 250 to 290 μg/day, higher than the 150 μg/day recommended for non-pregnant women and adults. Adequate breast milk iodine levels are important for normal neurodevelopment in infants, and iodine supplements are essential for mothers living in iodine deficient areas, who are unable to meet the increased demands for iodine intake.

In cases of iodine deficiency, the safe upper limit of iodine intake during pregnancy remains controversial. If an individual is exposed to high iodine levels, the synthesis of T4 and T3 will be acutely inhibited by a process known as the acute Wolff–Chaikoff effect [29].

In summary, there are contrasting recommendations for the upper limit of iodine intake. The U.S. Institute of Medicine recommends an upper limit of 1100 μg dietary iodine daily in pregnancy, while the World Health Organization (WHO) recommends an upper limit of 500 μg per day [21,30].

2. Hypothyroidism and fertility

Thyroid function may be altered by serum thyroid antibodies, including serum anti-thyroglobulin antibodies (TgAb) and anti-thyroid peroxidase antibodies (TPOAb), particularly in older women [31].

Several studies [32-39] indicate that elevated levels of anti-thyroid antibodies are present in women three times more often than in men. This discordant predominance in thyroid autoimmunity could be associated with the X chromosome, which preserves some sex and immune-related genes responsible for immune tolerance [40]. Genetic defects of the X chromosome (monosomy or structural abnormalities) could be responsible for increased and altered immune-reactivity. In fact, patients with Turner's syndrome [41] and those with a higher rate of X chromosome monosomy in peripheral white blood cells [42] exhibit a higher incidence of thyroid autoimmunity than karyotypically normal individuals. Similarly, skewed X-chromosome inactivation leads to the escape of X-linked self-antigens from presentation in thymus and a subsequent loss of T-cell tolerance. The result is an associated higher risk of developing autoimmune thyroid diseases.

Self-tolerance is maintained by two mechanisms: central tolerance, which is performed by thymus deletion of auto-reactive T cells during fetal life, and peripheral tolerance, whereby those cells that escape central tolerance are inhibited to prevent them from triggering autoimmunity. It is well known that hormonal changes and trophoblastic immune-modulatory molecules enable the tolerance of the fetal semi-allograft during pregnancy. Both cell-mediated and humoral immune responses are attenuated, shifting the immune response toward the humoral with subsequent immune tolerance of the fetal tissues. It is for this reason that during pregnancy, both TPOAb and TgAb concentrations decrease, reaching the lowest values in the third trimester [43-48]. In puerperium, the immune response rapidly returns to the pre-pregnancy state, potentially promoting or aggravating autoimmune thyroid disease [43]. TPOAb concentrations rapidly increase and reach the maximum level at about 20 weeks after delivery [46-48]. Postpartum thyroiditis is a frequent complication, and 50% of females with positive TPOAbs (TPOAb+) in early pregnancy develop this condition. The clinical features of postpartum thyroiditis may arise within the first year after delivery as a transient thyrotoxicosis and/or a transient hypothyroidism, but permanent hypothyroidism develops in approximately one third of females [49].

Some analyses demonstrate that weakened immunosuppression in late pregnancy could contribute to postpartum thyroid dysfunction. In fact, females with postpartum thyroiditis exhibit increased secretion of IFN and IL-4 but lower median plasma cortisol concentrations in the 36th week of gestation than do euthyroid females [50].

In nature, there is a particular phenomenon, fetal microchimerism, that is responsible for the transfer of fetal cells to the maternal circulation during pregnancy. Several years after the delivery, the chimeric cells can be detected in different maternal districts, including the peripheral blood [51,52] and maternal tissues such as the thyroid, lung, skin, or lymph nodes [53]. In puerperium, immunotolerance decreases, and consequently, the activation of the fetal immune cells localized in the maternal thyroid gland can act as a trigger for autoimmune thyroid disease. In support of this, the presence of fetal microchimeric cells is significantly higher in autoimmune hypothyroidism than in the absence of autoimmune thyroid disease [54-57]. However, the data are contradictory. Some studies demonstrate that heterozygotic twins exhibit a significantly higher prevalence of Thyroid Antibodies (TAbs) compared to monozygotic twins [58] and that euthyroid females with a previous pregnancy more frequently exhibit positive TPOAb compared to nulliparous females [59]. However, large population-based studies have not confirmed the relationship between parity and autoimmune thyroid disease. Consequently, the contribution of fetal microchimerism to the pathogenesis of autoimmune thyroid disease remains to be elucidated [60-63].

Spontaneous pregnancy loss is an obstetrical complication occurring at less than 20 weeks of gestation and has a prevalence ranging between 17% and 31% of all gestations [64,65]. Recurrent pregnancy loss is defined as either two consecutive losses or three total spontaneous losses and may occur in up to 1% of all pregnant women [66]. The individual risk depends on several factors including maternal age, family history, environmental exposures [67], parental chromosomal anomalies, immunologic derangements, uterine pathology, endocrine dysfunction and medical co-morbidities [68]. Pregnancy loss may result in bleeding, infections, pain and surgical procedures. Obviously, patients are strongly emotionally involved in a negative pregnancy outcome. Endocrine disorders are important risk factors for spontaneous pregnancy loss; patients with poorly controlled diabetes mellitus may have up to a 50% risk of loss [69], and thyroid dysfunction has also been associated with elevated rates of pregnancy loss [70,71]. Stagnaro-Green and colleagues [72] published a prospective observational study indicating that patients positive for thyroid antibodies (TPO and Tg) had a two-fold increase in the risk of a pregnancy loss. Similarly, Iijima and colleagues [73] also reported an association between spontaneous pregnancy loss and the presence of anti-microsomal antibodies. In support of these studies, a meta-analysis [74] demonstrated a clear association between thyroid antibodies and spontaneous abortion. The study also reported that TAb+ women were slightly older and had slightly higher TSH levels than did antibody-negative women. Negro and colleagues [75-76] performed a prospective, randomized interventional trial of Levothyroxine (LT4) in euthyroid patients who were TPOAb+. The authors reported a significantly decreased rate of pregnancy loss in the treated group, but their analyses were limited because the mean estimated gestational age of the patients commencing LT4 therapy was 10 weeks, and all but one of the losses occurred at less than 11 weeks. In a case–control study of Iravani and colleagues [77] and in the study of Kutteh et al. [78], patients with primary recurrent pregnancy losses (three or more) had a higher prevalence of anti-thyroid antibody. In the prospective observational study of Esplin and colleagues [79], no difference in thyroid antibody positivity between patients with recurrent pregnancy loss and healthy controls was observed. Other authors reported a higher rate of subsequent pregnancy loss in patients with recurrent losses and thyroid antibody positivity [80]. In the clinical trial by Rushworth and colleagues [81], there was no significant difference in live birth rates between women with recurrent losses who were positive for anti-thyroid antibodies and those who were not.

Additionally, the coexistence of more elements may create a synergic effect. The study by De Carolis et al. demonstrated an apparent interaction between anti-phospholipid antibodies and thyroid antibodies in the risk of recurrent pregnancy loss [82].

The data for an association between thyroid antibodies and recurrent pregnancy loss are less robust than for sporadic loss. The results are also somewhat contradictory, and many trials did not consider other potential causes of recurrent losses.

Recently, Lazzarin et al. [83] performed TRH stimulation (200 μg) to evaluate thyroid function in patients with recurrent miscarriages and anti-thyroid antibodies. The authors determined that thyroid autoimmunity could be considered an indirect sign of mild thyroid dysfunction and that TRH stimulation could be a useful tool to detect subtle thyroid dysfunction.

Some authors have also established an 'iTSHa index' (TSH increase after TRH adjusted for the levels of basal TSH), determining TSH serum levels at time 0 and 20 min after TRH stimulation in women with two or more miscarriages within the first 10 weeks of pregnancy. This index is useful to identify women with recurrent miscarriages due to transient thyroid dysfunction of early pregnancy. If validated, the index could be used for those patients with no evidence of thyroid dysfunction and TSH levels within the low-normal reference range who may nonetheless be at risk for recurrent abortions [84].

Some authors tried to analyze the possible use of intravenous immunoglobulin (IVIG) to prevent recurrent pregnancy loss in women with anti-thyroid antibodies. Three small non-randomized case series have been published [85-87], and the live birth rates ranged from 80% to 95%. One study involved a comparison of a group of women who refused IVIG therapy (control group) with an IVG-treated group. A highly significant improvement in live births was reported in the IVIG-treated cohort [86]. In one study, a higher rate of term delivery was achieved by the LT4-treated group [87] compared to that of the IVIG group. In summary, all three studies had serious methodological problems (small sample size, heterogeneous patient populations, lack of or limited randomization, and differences in the timing of the treatment). These are the limitations of the intervention trials with IVIG or LT4 in TAb+ women with recurrent abortions.

In consideration of these findings, the Guidelines of the American Thyroid Association for the Diagnosis and Management of Thyroid Disease During Pregnancy and Postpartum [76] stress that there is insufficient evidence to recommend for or against screening all women for anti-thyroid antibodies in the first trimester of pregnancy (Level I). Additionally, it is stressed that, in euthyroid women with sporadic or recurrent abortions or in women undergoing in vitro fertilization (IVF), there is insufficient evidence to recommend for or against screening for anti-thyroid antibodies or treating in the first trimester of pregnancy with LT4 or IVIG (Level I). Similarly, in TAb+ euthyroid women during pregnancy, there is insufficient evidence to recommend for or against LT4 therapy (Level I).

Some authors [88] investigated the role of steroid pretreatment on the pregnancy rate and pregnancy outcomes in patients positive for anti-thyroid antibodies who were undergoing induction of ovulation and intrauterine insemination (IUI). The patients were divided into 3 groups: a control group of infertile women without anti-thyroid autoimmunity and two groups of infertile women with anti-thyroid autoimmunity, one treated with prednisone (administered orally for 4 weeks before IUI) and the other receiving placebo. Prophylactic therapy with steroids was associated with a significantly increased rate of pregnancy compared with placebo in infertile women with anti-thyroid antibodies undergoing induction of ovulation and IUI, although the miscarriage rate did not significantly differ among the groups.

Several studies reported an increased risk of pregnancy loss after assisted reproductive procedures in women who were positive for anti-thyroid antibodies [89-91], whereas other authors have detected no association [92,93]. Additionally, patients undergoing IVF in the presence of anti-thyroid antibodies exhibited an increased risk of pregnancy loss (meta-analysis of four trials) [94]. Negro et al. [95] performed a prospective placebo–controlled intervention trial. No difference in pregnancy loss was observed when LT4 was used to treat TPOAb+ women undergoing assisted reproduction technologies. The variable results highlight that there are a number of reasons for infertility or subfertility that may characterize patients undergoing assisted reproductive procedures for infertility.

The guidelines of the American Thyroid Association for the Diagnosis and Management of Thyroid Disease During Pregnancy and Postpartum [76] stress that in euthyroid TAb+ women undergoing assisted reproductive technologies, there is insufficient evidence to recommend for or against LT4 therapy (Level I).

Some studies have analyzed the role of selenium in diminishing the TPOAb titers [96-101], but at present, the risk to benefit comparison does not support routine selenium supplementation for TPOAb+ women during pregnancy [76] (Level C).

3. Hypothyroidism and pregnancy

Several physiological changes take place in a pregnant woman that could cause an increased incidence of hypothyroidism in the later stages of pregnancy in iodine-deficient women who were euthyroid in the first trimester.

In pregnancy, the production of thyroxin (T4) and triiodothyronin (T3) rapidly increases by 50% together with a subsequent 50% increase in the daily iodine requirement. The fetal thyroid begins to concentrate iodine to create triiodothyronin (T3) and thyroxin (T4) beginning at 10-12 weeks of gestation, while TSH (fetal pituitary thyroid stimulating hormone) begins to control thyroid function at approximately 20 weeks of gestation [102].

Maternal thyroxin crosses the placenta and maintains normal fetal thyroid function primarily in the early stages of gestation [103]. T3 is the active thyroid hormone produced after the deiodination of T4 in different tissues, and both are largely bound to thyroid hormone binding globulin (TBG). Rising maternal estradiol levels in early pregnancy causes increased liver sialyation and glycosylation of TBG [104,105] with a consequent decrease in the peripheral metabolism of TBG [106,107]. This change creates an increased need for T3-T4 production. During pregnancy, T4 and T3 are degraded at an increased rate to inactive iodothyronin (reverse T3) [108]. In addition, higher placental T4 transfer and hCG act as weak stimulators of T3-T4 secretion and suppressors of TSH levels [109].

Additionally, the increase in the maternal glomerular filtration rate enhances the iodine requirements in pregnancy. In fact, iodine is passively excreted by the kidney, and increased renal glomerular filtration results in increased losses of dietary iodine [110].

Under the influence of placental human chorionic gonadotropin (hCG), which also binds to and stimulates the thyroidal TSH receptor [111], the levels of thyrotrophin (TSH) are decreased throughout pregnancy, with the lower normal TSH level in the first trimester not well defined and an upper limit of 2.5 mIU/L.

High estrogen levels in pregnant women are responsible for a 1.5-fold increase in serum thyroxin binding globulin (TBG) concentrations. Therefore, there are higher levels of bound circulating total triiodothyronin (T3) and thyroxin (T4). In order to maintain free (or unbound) thyroid hormone levels, thyroid hormone gland production is enhanced [112].

Some studies have demonstrated that total body T4 concentrations must increase 20%–50% throughout gestation to maintain an euthyroid state [113,114], confirming that the increased requirement for T4 (or exogenous LT4) occurs as early as 4–6 weeks of pregnancy [114] and that such requirements gradually increase through 16–20 weeks of pregnancy with a subsequent plateau until the time of delivery.

Primary maternal hypothyroidism is defined as the presence of elevated TSH concentrations during gestation. There are rare exceptions to this definition, including a TSH-secreting pituitary tumor, thyroid hormone resistance, and a few cases of central hypothyroidism with biologically inactive TSH.

Pregnancy-specific reference ranges are necessary to define elevations in serum TSH during pregnancy. When maternal TSH is elevated, measurements of serum FT4 concentrations are necessary. The aim of such measurements is to classify the patient's diagnosis as either overt hypothyroidism (OH) or subclinical (SCH) hypothyroidism.

Patients exhibiting elevated TSH levels (>2.5 mIU/L) together with decreased FT4 concentrations and those with TSH levels of 10.0 mIU/L or above, irrespective of their FT4 levels, are considered to have overt hypothyroidism.

Patients with a serum TSH value between 2.5 and 10 mIU/L and with a normal FT4 concentration are affected by subclinical hypothyroidism. The clinical definition is dependent upon whether FT4 is within or below the trimester-specific FT4 reference range.

Data from a US population of iodine-sufficient women demonstrated that elevated serum TSH levels are present in at least 2%–3% of apparently healthy, non-pregnant women of childbearing age [115,116]. When thyroid function tests were performed, 0.3%–0.5% of those women were diagnosed with OH and 2%–2.5% were diagnosed with SCH.

When iodine intake is normal, Hashimoto's thyroiditis is the most frequent cause of hypothyroidism; more than 80% of patients with OH and 50% of pregnant women with SCH exhibit thyroid autoantibodies [116].

Maternal and fetal effects of hypothyroidism have been well studied, and the results allow for clinical recommendations for OH but not for SCH. There is a strict association between overt maternal hypothyroidism and adverse pregnancy outcomes, particularly if this condition arises early in pregnancy [116]. Some of these complications include preeclampsia, eclampsia, pregnancy-induced hypertension, low birth weight [117], preterm birth [118,119], breech delivery [120], placental abruption, infant respiratory distress syndrome, spontaneous abortion [115,121], perinatal death [122] and fetal neurocognitive development [123,124].

In reproductive aged women, the prevalence of subclinical hypothyroidism is about 0.5-5% [125]. It is well established that thyroid hormone is essential for fetal brain development and maturation, explaining why the maternal transfer of thyroid hormone is essential, especially during the first trimester of pregnancy. Children born to women who were inadequately treated for subclinical hypothyroidism exhibit impaired mental development compared to those born to women well-treated [123], but it is not well established whether the impaired mental development is due to the thyroid hormone deficiency itself or to the subsequent obstetric complications [126].

Although data regarding SCH are less complete than those regarding OH, Negro and colleagues [127] found that SCH increases the risk of pregnancy complications in anti-thyroid peroxidase antibody positive (TPOAb+) pregnant women. Their trial screened a low-risk pregnant population with SCH for TPOAb+ and TSH >2.5 mIU/ L. Half of the patients with this combination underwent LT4 treatment to normalize serum TSH, and the other half served as the control group. The results confirmed a significant reduction in the combined endpoint of pregnancy complications. Further, Negro et al. [128] noticed that TPOAb- (negative) women with TSH levels between 2.5 and 5.0 mIU/L exhibited a higher miscarriage rate compared with pregnant women with TSH levels below 2.5 mIU/L.

These prospective data are supported by previous retrospective data published by Casey and colleagues [115], who identified a two- to three-fold increased risk of pregnancy-related complications in untreated women with SCH. However, some published data reached conflicting conclusions; Cleary-Goldman et al. [129] reported no adverse effects in SCH pregnant women (detected in the first and second trimester). The limitation of this study is that the analysis was performed with only a selected subgroup of the entire study cohort, with a mean gestational age of screening between 10.5 and 14 weeks of gestation.

Recently, Ashoor et al. [130] evaluated TSH and FT4 levels in 202 singleton pregnancies at 11–13 weeks that subsequently resulted in miscarriage or fetal death. The results demonstrated that these patients had increased TSH levels above the 97.5th percentile and FT4 levels below the 2.5th percentile compared to the 4318 normal pregnancies of the control group. This trial suggests that SCH is associated with an increased risk of adverse pregnancy outcomes, although the detrimental effect of SCH on fetal neurocognitive development is less clear. The case-control study by Haddow et al. [123] demonstrated a reduction in the intelli-

http://dx.doi.org/10.5772/54328

gence quotient (IQ) among children born to untreated hypothyroid women when compared to the children of pregnant euthyroid controls. In summary, adverse fetal neurocognitive development is biologically plausible [131], though not clearly demonstrated, in SCH. For this reason, clinicians should consider these potential increased risks associated with SCH and could consider LT4 treatment for these patients.

The guidelines of the American Thyroid Association for the Diagnosis and Management of Thyroid Disease During Pregnancy and Postpartum [76] note that SCH has been associated with adverse maternal and fetal outcomes. However, due to the lack of randomized controlled trials, there is insufficient evidence to recommend for or against universal LT4 treatment in TAb- pregnant women with SCH (Level I). The aim of LT4 treatment is to normalize maternal serum TSH values within a trimester-specific pregnancy reference range (Level A).

Numerous retrospective and case-controlled studies confirm the detrimental effects of OH on pregnancy and fetal health, and the available data confirm the benefits of treating OH during pregnancy. This recommendation is useful for women with TSH concentrations above the trimester-specific reference interval and with decreased FT4 levels as well as for all women with TSH concentrations above 10.0 mIU/L, irrespective of FT4 levels (Level A). In addition, women positive for TPOAb and affected by SCH should be treated with LT4 (Level B).

The recommended treatment for maternal hypothyroidism is oral LT4. It is strongly recommended that other thyroid preparations, such as T3 or desiccated thyroid, not be used (Level A).

In the literature, the reference range for TSH is well established to be lower in pregnancy; both the lower and the upper limit of serum TSH are decreased by approximately 0.1–0.2 mIU/L and 1.0 mIU/L, respectively, compared to the usual TSH reference interval of 0.4–4.0 mIU/L in non-pregnant women. Serum TSH and its reference range gradually rise throughout the pregnancy, but this interval remains lower than in non-pregnant women [122,132]. Several confounding factors (e.g., diet), can influence TSH values in women with no thyroid pathologies.

In multiple pregnancies, the higher hCG level is responsible for lower TSH serum concentrations [133]. Therefore, some authors have suggested specific TSH ranges in pregnancy of 0.1-2.5 mUI/L for the first trimester, 0.2-0.3 mUI/L for the second trimester, and 0.3-3.0 for the third trimester [76,134].

As previously defined, overt hypothyroidism is characterized by elevated serum TSH levels with low serum FT4 levels, whereas subclinical hypothyroidism is characterized by elevated serum TSH levels with normal serum FT4 levels.

Isolated hypothyroxinemia is characterized by normal maternal TSH concentrations and FT4 concentrations in the lower 5th or 10th percentile of the reference range. It is controversial whether isolated hypothyroxinemia causes any adverse effects on the developing fetus. In the study of Pop and colleagues [135], psychomotor test scores among offspring born to women with normal serum TSH values and FT4 indices in the lowest 10th percentile were decreased compared to controls. In the analyses of Li et al. [124], mothers who experienced either hypothyroidism or isolated hypothyroxinemia during the first trimester gave birth to children with lower IQ scores. However, these studies have methodological limits.

In their prospective, Henrichs and colleagues conducted a prospective nonrandomized investigation on isolated maternal hypothyroxinemia [136] and reported that a 1.5- to 2-fold increased risk for adverse events (children at 3 years of age) in communication development was associated with maternal FT4 levels in the lower 5th and 10th percentiles. To date, there are no recommendations for isolated hypothyroxinemia, and consequently, isolated hypothyroxinemia should not be treated during pregnancy (Level C).

In the first trimester of pregnancy, approximately 10% to 20% of all pregnant women are TPO- or Tg-antibody positive and euthyroid. In addition, approximately 16% of the women who are euthyroid and positive for TPO or Tg antibodies in the first trimester will develop a TSH that exceeds 4.0 mIU/L by the third trimester, and approximately 33%–50% of women positive for TPO or Tg antibodies in the first trimester will develop postpartum thyroiditis. These data could be the result of a direct effect of the antibodies or an indirect marker of an autoimmune syndrome or the thyroid functional reserve [106].

Another important aspect to consider is the significant ethnic difference in serum TSH concentrations. In fact, pregnant women of Moroccan, Turkish, or Surinamese descent residing in The Netherlands exhibit TSH values 0.2–0.3 mIU/L lower than Dutch women throughout pregnancy [137]. Black and Asian women exhibit TSH values that are on average 0.4 mIU/L lower than those in white women; these differences persist during pregnancy [138,139].

There are different methods for the analysis of TSH levels, and TSH ranges vary slightly depending on the method used [140]. However, trimester-specific reference ranges for TSH should be applied (Level B). If they are not available in the laboratory, the following reference ranges are recommended: first trimester, 0.1–2.5 mIU/L; second trimester, 0.2–3.0 mIU/L; third trimester, 0.3–3.0 mIU/L (Level I).

Total T4-T3 values or the ratio of Total T4 to TBG are useful to calculate the normal ranges for the FT4 index, but there are not trimester-specific reference intervals for the FT4 index of a reference population. To assess serum FT4 during pregnancy, the optimal method is measurement of T4 in the dialysate or ultrafiltrate of serum samples employing on-line extraction/liquid chromatography/tandem mass spectrometry (LC/MS/ MS) (Level A). If not available, clinicians should use whichever measure or estimate of FT4 is available in their laboratory and should be aware of the limitations of each method. However, serum TSH remains the most accurate method to study thyroid status during pregnancy (Level A).

In the presence of high concentrations of bound T4, it is difficult to measure the levels of FT4 due to the abnormal binding-protein states such as pregnancy. Therefore, method-specific and trimester-specific reference ranges of serum FT4 are required (Level B).

The guidelines of the American Thyroid Association for the Diagnosis and Management of Thyroid Disease During Pregnancy and Postpartum [76] stress that, although not prospectively studied, the approach of not initially treating women with SCH in pregnancy should involve monitoring the women for possible progression to OH by measuring serum TSH and FT4 levels approximately every four weeks until 16– 20 weeks gestation and at least once between 26 and 32 weeks gestation (Level I).

These considerations are important to make the therapy adjustments in affected women once pregnant and to plan the follow-up intervals for TSH in treated patients. If necessary, LT4 adjustments should be made as soon as possible after pregnancy is confirmed; it is important to stress that between 50% and 85% [113,114,141] of hypothyroid women treated with exogenous LT4 require increased doses during pregnancy. This need for adjustment is related to the etiology of hypothyroidism itself.

The clinical recommendation is that treated hypothyroid patients (receiving LT4) and newly pregnant women should independently increase their dose of LT4 by 25%–30% upon a missed menstrual cycle or positive home pregnancy test. Pregnant women could accomplish this adjustment by increasing LT4 from once daily dosing to a total of nine doses per week (29% increase). (Level B)

Obviously, the aim of treatment is to optimize a woman's preconception thyroid status. Different studies have analyzed the possible TSH cutoff values for women planning a pregnancy, but other factors, like maternal estrogen levels, can influence the LT4 augmentation necessary to maintain a euthyroid state during pregnancy.

The guidelines of the American Thyroid Association for the Diagnosis and Management of Thyroid Disease During Pregnancy and Postpartum [76] indicate that preconception serum TSH values <2.5 mIU/L are an indirect marker of a good thyroid state in treated hypothyroid patients (receiving LT4) who are planning a pregnancy. Similarly, TSH values <1.5 mIU/L will likely further reduce the risk of mild hypothyroidism in early pregnancy by reducing the risk of TSH elevation during the first trimester. However, no differences in pregnancy outcomes have been demonstrated by this approach (Level B).

In these patients, maternal serum TSH levels should be monitored approximately every 4 weeks during the first half of pregnancy. Indeed, further LT4 dose adjustments are often required (Level B), and maternal TSH should be checked at least once between 26 and 32 weeks gestation (Level I).

Following delivery, LT4 should be reduced to the patient's preconception dose. Additional TSH testing should be performed at approximately 6 weeks postpartum (Level B).

However, women with Hashimoto's thyroiditis could need an increased LT4 dose in the postpartum period [142] compared to their prepartum dose.

Pregnant women treated and monitored appropriately should not require any additional tests; there are no other maternal and fetal recommended tests in the absence of other pregnancy complications (Level A).

Some studies [75,119] confirmed an increased requirement for thyroid hormone during gestation in women who are TAb+. Both OH and SCH may occur during the stress of pregnancy as a result of compromised thyroid function. This situation usually occurs later in gestation because in the first part of pregnancy, the residual thyroid function can act as a buffer.

Because the risk of hypothyroidism in women who are TAb+ is increased, a higher level of surveillance, by evaluating TSH levels approximately every 4–6 weeks during pregnancy, is required [114].

Fetal status in pregnant women under chronic therapy with levothyroxine has been studied by performing computerized FHR (fetal heart rate) analyses (cCTG). This is a sensible and reproducible method to identify pregnancies with a pathological neonatal outcome. Published data [143] suggest that maternal hypothyroidism and levothyroxine treatment have an important influence on FHR, and cCTG analyses are a sensible means of revealing and studying these conditions. In their analyses, the authors stressed that fetal reactivity, expressed by reduced baseline FHR and reduced fetal movements, remained suppressed in well-treated hypothyroid pregnant women who became euthyroid, suggesting that this suppression could be due to the influence of a chronic hypothyroid state.

4. Hypothyroidism and contraception

In the literature, there is little evidence about the influence of contraceptives on thyroid function. The study of Ågren et al. [144] analyzes the effects of two monophasic combined oral contraceptives (nomegestrol acetate/17 beta estradiol or levonorgestrel/ethinylestradiol) on androgen levels, endocrine function and sex hormone-binding globulin (SHBG) levels in 121 healthy women. The authors found that the levels of thyroxin-binding globulin (TBG), together with total cortisol and corticosteroid-binding globulin (CBG) levels, increased in both groups, with a significantly greater increase observed in the group with levonorgestrel/ethinylestradiol. Thyroid-stimulating hormone (TSH) and free thyroxin (T4) remained unaltered from their baseline values, and no difference was observed between the groups. If TBG rises, clearance of tri-iodothyronin (T3) and T4 is reduced, thereby increasing total T3 and T4 levels. However, as described, estroprogestin oral contraceptives have little or no effect on physiologically active free fractions of thyroid hormones. In fact, in the same study, no significant changes in free T4 or in TSH levels were observed in either group after six months of treatment, in agreement with other studies [145-147].

In summary, oral contraceptives can be responsible for increasing TBG without a significant influence on thyroid-stimulating hormone (TSH) and free thyroxin (T4) levels.

5. Conclusions

A euthyroid state is the goal for women affected by hypothyroidism; the normalization of thyroid markers is necessary for metabolic, endocrine and sexual improvement. Obviously, the presence of anti-thyroid antibodies signifies an underlying state of imbalanced patient-specific autoimmunity that can be addressed with effective treatments.

In pregnant women, treatment of hypothyroidism is not associated with adverse perinatal outcomes [148], and although it is not well known how levothyroxine treatment during pregnancy improves the neurological development of the offspring, clinical practice guidelines recommend this therapy [148, 149].

The choice of cut-off values for TSH in the three trimesters of pregnancy has important implications both for the interpretation of the literature and for the critical impact of the clinical diagnosis of hypothyroidism.

Overt hypothyroidism and overt hyperthyroidism have a deleterious impact on pregnancy. However, questions about hypothyroidism and pregnancy remain, including those regarding the impact of subclinical hypothyroidism on pregnancy; the impact of TAbs on miscarriage, preterm delivery and puerperal thyroiditis in euthyroid women; and if, when and who should be screened for anti-thyroid hormones during pregnancy. For this latter question, very recent papers addressed the problem with conflicting results: Lazarus et al. [150] conducted a randomized trial in which antenatal screening and maternal treatment for hypothyroidism did not result in improved cognitive function in three-year-old children (possible limitations of this study are that levothyroxine therapy was performed too late in gestation and that about 24% of the women were lost to follow-up) while Dosiou et al. [151] stressed that universal screening of pregnant women in the first trimester for autoimmune thyroid disease is cost-effective without the calculation of a possible decrease of the offspring cognitive function. The question remains open.

Acknowledgements

The strength of each recommendation was graded according to the United States Preventive Services Task Force (USPSTF) Guidelines [76]:

- Level A. The USPSTF strongly recommends that clinicians provide (the service) to eligible patients. The USPSTF found good evidence that (the service) improves important health outcomes and concludes that benefits substantially outweigh harms.
- Level B. The USPSTF recommends that clinicians provide (this service) to eligible patients. The USPSTF found at least fair evidence that (the service) improves important health outcomes and concludes that benefits outweigh harms.
- Level C. The USPSTF makes no recommendation for or against routine provision of (the service). The USPSTF found at least fair evidence that (the service) can improve health outcomes but concludes that the balance of benefits and harms is too close to justify a general recommendation.
- Level D. The USPSTF recommends against routinely providing (the service) to asymptomatic patients. The USPSTF found at least fair evidence that (the service) is ineffective or that harms outweigh benefits.

- Level I. The USPSTF concludes that evidence is insufficient to recommend for or against routinely providing (the service). Evidence that (the service) is effective is lacking, or poor quality, or conflicting, and the balance of benefits and harms cannot be determined.

Author details

Piergiorgio Stortoni and Andrea L. Tranquilli

*Address all correspondence to:

Department Clinical Sciences, Università Politecnica Marche, Ancona, Italy

References

[1] Klein RZ, Haddow JE, Faix JD, Brown RS, Hermos RJ, Pulkkinen A, et al. Prevalence of thyroid deficiency in pregnant women. Clin Endocrinol 1991;35:41–6.

[2] Say RK, Nagesh VR. Hypothyroidism in pregnancy. Indian J Endocrinol Metab. 2012; 16(3): 364–70.

[3] Hetzel BS. Iodine and neuropsychological development. J Nutr 2000;130:493S–5S.

[4] Koutras DA, Matovinovic J, Vought R. The ecology of iodine. In: Stanbury JB, Hetzel BS, editors. Endemic goiter and endemic cretinism. New York: John Wiley; 1980: p 185–95.

[5] Hetzel BS. Iodine Deficiency Disorders (IDD) and their eradication. Lancet 1983;2:1126–9.

[6] Zimmermann MB, Jooste PL, Pandav CS. Iodine deficiency disorders. Lancet 2008;372:1251–62.

[7] Andersson M, Karumbunathan V, Zimmermann MB. Global iodine status in 2011 and trends over the past decade. J Nutr 2012.

[8] Melse-Boonstra A, Gowachirapant S, Jaiswala N, Winichagoon P, Srinivasan K, Zimmermann MB. Iodine supplementation in pregnancy and its effect on child cognition. Journal of Trace Elements in Medicine and Biology 2012;26:134– 6.

[9] Conolly KJ, Pharoah POD, Hetzel BS. Fetal iodine deficiency and motor performance during childhood. Lancet 1979;2(8153):1149–51.

[10] Bautista A, Barker PA, Dunn JT, Sanchez M, Kaiser DL. The effects of oral iodized oil on intelligence, thyroid status, and somatic growth in school-age children from an area of endemic goiter. Am J Clin Nutr 1982;35:127–34.

[11] Shrestha RM. The effect of iodine and iron supplementation on physical, psychomotor and mental development in primary school children in Malawi. PhD thesis. Division of Human Nutrition, Wageningen University, the Netherlands; 1994.

[12] Van den Briel T, West CE, Bleichrodt N, van de Vijver FJ, Ategbo EA, Hautvast JG. Improved iodine status is associated with improved mental performance of schoolchildren in Benin. Am J Clin Nutr 2000;72(5):1179–85.

[13] Isa ZM, Alias IZ, Kadir KA, Ali O. Effect of iodized oil supplementation on thyroid hormone levels and mental performance among Orang Asli schoolchildren and pregnant mothers in an endemic goiter area in Peninsular Malaysia. Asia Pac J Clin Nutr 2000;9(4):274–81.

[14] Huda SN, Gratham-McGregor SM, Tomkins A. Cognitive and motor functions of iodine-deficient but euthyroid children in Bangladesh do not benefit from iodized poppy seed oil (Lipiodol). J Nutr 2001;131:72–7.

[15] Zimmermann MB, Connolly K, Bozo M, Bridson J, Rohner F, Grimci L. Iodine supplementation improves cognition in iodine-deficient schoolchildren in Albania: a randomized, controlled, double-blind study. Am J Clin Nutr 2006;83:108–14.

[16] Gordon RC, Rose MC, Skeaff SA, Gray AR, Morgan KMD, Ruffman T. Iodine supplementation improves cognition in mildly iodine-deficient children. Am J Clin Nutr 2009;90:1264–71.

[17] Vanderpump MPJ, Lazarus JH, Smyth PP, Laurberg P, Holder RL, Boelaert K, et al. Iodine status of UK schoolgirls: a cross-sectional survey. Lancet 2011;377:2007–12.

[18] Zimmermann MB. Iodine deficiency in industrialized countries. Clin Endocrinol 2011;75:287–8.

[19] WHO/UNICEF. Reaching optimal iodine nutrition in pregnant and lactating women and young children. Joint Statement by the World Health Organization and the United Nations Children Fund; 2007.

[20] Vejbjerg P, Knudsen N, Perrild H, Laurberg P, Andersen S, Rasmussen LB, et al. Estimation of iodine intake from various urinary iodine measurements in population studies. Thyroid 2009;19:1281–6.

[21] UNICEF, WHO and ICCIDD. Assessment of the iodine deficiency disorders and monitoring their elimination. 3rd ed. Geneva: World Health Organization; 2007.

[22] Gowachirapant S, Winichagoon P, Wyss L, Tong B, Baumgartner J, Melse-Boonstra A, et al. Urinary iodine concentrations indicate iodine deficiency in pregnant Thai women but iodine sufficiency in their school-aged children. J Nutr 2009;139:1169–72.

[23] Zimmermann MB, Delange F. Iodine supplementation of pregnant women in Europe: a review and recommendations. Eur J Clin Nutr 2004;58:979–84.

[24] Berbel P, Mestre JL, Santamaría A, Palazo I, Franco A, Graells M, et al. Delayed neurobehavioral development in children born to pregnant women with mild hypothyr-

oxinemia during the first month of gestation: the importance of early iodine supplementation. Thyroid 2009;19:511–9.

[25] Velasco I, Carreira M, Santiago P, Muela JA, García-Fuentes E, Sánchez-Mu˜noz B, et al. Effect of iodine prophylaxis during pregnancy on neurocognitive development of children during the first two years of life. J Clin Endocrinol Metab 2009;94(9):3234–41.

[26] Murcia M, Rebagliato M, I˜niguez C, Lopez-Espinosa MJ, Estarlich M, Plaza B, et al. Effect of iodine supplementation during pregnancy on infant neurodevelopment at 1 year of age. Am J Epidemiol 2011;173(7):804–12.

[27] Semba RD, Delange F. Iodine in human milk: perspectives for human health. Nutr Rev 2001;59:269–78.

[28] Dorea JG. Iodine nutrition and breast feeding. J Trace Elem Med Biol 2002;16:207–20.

[29] Wolff J, Chaikoff IL, et al. The temporary nature of the inhibitory action of excess iodine on organic iodine synthesis in the normal thyroid. Endocrinology 1949;45:504–13.

[30] Institute of Medicine Food and Nutrition Board. Dietary reference intakes. Washington, DC: National Academy Press; 2006.

[31] Gough SC. Polymorphism of the CTLA-4 gene is associated with autoimmune hypothyroidism in the United Kingdom. Thyroid 2002; 12: 3–6.

[32] Aghini-Lombardi F, Antonangeli L, Martino E, Vitti P, Maccherini D, Leoli F, Rago T, Grasso L, Valeriano R, Balestrieri A, Pinchera A. The spectrum of thyroid disorders in an iodine-deficient community: the Pescopagano survey. J Clin Endocrinol Metab 1999; 84: 561-6.

[33] Hollowell JG, Staehling NW, Flanders WD, Hannon WH, Gunter EW, Spencer CA, Braverman LE. Serum TSH, T(4), and thyroid antibodies in the United States population (1988 to 1994): National Health and Nutrition Examination Survey (NHANES III). J. Clin Endocrinol Metab 2002; 87: 489-99.

[34] Kasagi K, Takahashi N, Inoue G, Honda T, Kawachi Y, Izumi Y. Thyroid function in Japanese adults as assessed by a general health checkup system in relation with thyroid-related antibodies and other clinical parameters. Thyroid 2009;19: 937- 44.

[35] Spencer CA, Hollowell JG, Kazarosyan M, Braverman LE. National Health and Nutrition Examination Survey III thyroidstimulating hormone (TSH)-thyroperoxidase antibody relationships demonstrate that TSH upper reference limits may be skewed by occult thyroid dysfunction. J Clin Endocrinol Metab 2007; 92: 4236-40.

[36] Lucas A, Julián MT, Cantón A, Castell C, Casamitjana R, Martínez-Cáceres EM, Granada ML. Undiagnosed thyroid dysfunction, thyroid antibodies, and iodine excretion in a Mediterranean population. Endocrine 2010; 38: 391-6.

[37] Knudsen N, Jorgensen T, Rasmussen S, Christiansen E, Perrild H. The prevalence of thyroid dysfunction in a population with borderline iodine deficiency. Clin Endocrinol 1999; 51:361-7.

[38] Pedersen IB, Knudsen N, Jørgensen T, Perrild H, Ovesen L, Laurberg P. Thyroid peroxidase and thyroglobulin autoantibodies in a large survey of populations with mild and moderate iodine deficiency. Clin Endocrinol 2003; 58:36-42.

[39] Hoogendoorn EH, Hermus AR, de Vegt F, Ross HA, Verbeek AL, Kiemeney LA, Swinkels DW, Sweep FC, den Heijer M. Thyroid function and prevalence of anti-thyroperoxidase antibodies in a population with borderline sufficient iodine intake: influences of age and sex. Clin Chem 2006; 52:104-11.

[40] McCombe PA, Greer JM, Mackay IR. Sexual dimorphism in autoimmune disease. Curr Mol Med 2009; 9:1058-79.

[41] Larizza D, Calcaterra V, Martinetti M. Increased prevalence of autoimmunity in Turner syndrome--influence of age. J. Autoimmun 2009; 33: 25-30.

[42] Invernizzi P, Miozzo M, Selmi C, Persani L, Battezzati PM, Zuin M, Lucchi S, Meroni PL, Marasini B, Zeni S, Watnik M, Grati FR, Simoni G, Gershwin ME. Podda M. X chromosome monosomy: a common mechanism for autoimmune diseases. J Immunol 2005;175: 575-8.

[43] Weetman AP. Immunity, thyroid function and pregnancy: molecular mechanisms. Nat Rev Endocrinol 2010; 6: 311-8.

[44] Shevach EM. From vanilla to 28 flavours: multiple varieties of T regulatory cells. Immunity 2006; 25:195-201.

[45] Guerin LR, Prins JR, Robertson SA. Regulatory T-cells and immune tolerance in pregnancy: a new target for infertility treatment? Hum Reprod Update 2009; 15:517-35.

[46] Kämpe O, Jansson R, Karlsson FA. Effects of L-thyroxine and iodide on the development of autoimmune postpartum thyroiditis. J Clin Endocrinol Metab 1990; 70:1014-8.

[47] Kuijpens JL, Pop VJ, Vader HL, Drexhage HA, Wiersinga WM. Prediction of post partum thyroid dysfunction: can it be improved? Eur J Endocrinol 1998; 139:36-43.

[48] Smyth PP, Wijeyaratne CN, Kaluarachi WN, Smith DF, Premawardhana LD, Parkes AB, Jayasinghe A, de Silva D.G, Lazarus JH. Sequential studies on thyroid antibodies during pregnancy. Thyroid 2005; 15:474-7.

[49] Lazarus JH. The continuing saga of postpartum thyroiditis. J Clin Endocrinol Metab 2011; 96:614-6.

[50] Kokandi AA, Parkes AB, Premawardhana LD, John R, Lazarus JH. Association of postpartum thyroid dysfunction with antepartum hormonal and immunological changes. J Clin Endocrinol Metab 2003; 88:1126-32.

[51] Bianchi DW, Zickwolf GK, Weil GJ, Sylvester S, DeMaria MA. Male fetal progenitor cells persist in maternal blood for as long as 27 years postpartum. Proc Natl Acad Sci USA 1996; 93:705-8.

[52] Evans PC, Lambert N, Maloney S, Furst DE, Moore JM, Nelson JL. Long-term fetal microchimerism in peripheral blood mononuclear cell subsets in healthy women and women with scleroderma. Blood 1999; 93:2033-7.

[53] Koopmans M, Kremer Hovinga IC, Baelde HJ, Harvey MS, de Heer E, Bruijn JA, Bajema IM. Chimerism occurs in thyroid, lung, skin and lymph nodes of women with sons. J Reprod Immunol 2008; 78:68-75.

[54] Srivatsa B, Srivatsa S, Johnson KL, Samura O, Lee SL, Bianchi DW. Microchimerism of presumed fetal origin in thyroid specimens from women: a case-control study. Lancet 2001;358: 2034-8.

[55] Klintschar M, Schwaiger P, Mannweiler S, Regauer S, Kleiber M. Evidence of fetal microchimerism in Hashimoto's thyroiditis. J Clin Endocrinol Metab 2001; 86:2494-8.

[56] Renne C, Ramos Lopez E, Steimle-Grauer SA, Ziolkowski P, Pani MA, Luther C, Holzer K, Encke A, Wahl RA, Bechstein WO, Usadel KH, Hansmann ML, Badenhoop K. Thyroid fetal male microchimerisms in mothers with thyroid disorders: presence of Y-chromosomal immunofluorescence in thyroid-infiltrating lymphocytes is more prevalent in Hashimoto's thyroiditis and Graves' disease than in follicular adenomas. J Clin Endocrinol Metab 2004; 89:5810-4.

[57] Klintschar M, Immel UD, Kehlen A, Schwaiger P, Mustafa T, Mannweiler S, Regauer S, Kleiber M, Hoang-Vu C. Fetal microchimerism in Hashimoto's thyroiditis: a quantitative approach. Eur J Endocrinol 2006;154: 237-41.

[58] Brix TH, Hansen PS, Kyvik KO, Hegedüs L. Aggregation of thyroid autoantibodies in twins from opposite-sex pairs suggests that microchimerism may play a role in the early stages of thyroid autoimmunity. J Clin Endocrinol Metab 2009;94: 4439-43.

[59] Strieder TG, Prummel MF, Tijssen JG, Endert E, Wiersinga W.M. Risk factors for and prevalence of thyroid disorders in a cross-sectional study among healthy female relatives of patients with autoimmune thyroid disease. Clin Endocrinol (Oxf) 2003;59: 396-401.

[60] Walsh JP, Bremner AP, Bulsara MK, O'Leary P, Leedman PJ, Feddema P, Michelangeli V. Parity and the risk of autoimmune thyroid disease: a community-based study. J Clin Endocrinol Metab 2005; 90:5309-12.

[61] Bülow Pedersen I, Laurberg P, Knudsen N, Jørgensen T, Perrild H, Ovesen L, Rasmussen LB. Lack of association between thyroid autoantibodies and parity in a population study argues against microchimerism as a trigger of thyroid autoimmunity. Eur J Endocrinol 2006; 154:39-45.

[62] Friedrich N, Schwarz S, Thonack J, John U, Wallaschofski H, Völzke H. Association between parity and autoimmune thyroiditis in a general female population. Autoimmunity 2008; 4:174-80.

[63] Sgarbi JA, Kasamatsu TS, Matsumura LK, Maciel RM. Parity is not related to autoimmune thyroid disease in a population based study of Japanese-Brazilians. Thyroid 2010; 20:1151-6.

[64] Ellish NJ, Saboda K, O'Connor J, Nasca PC, Stanek EJ, Boyle C. A prospective study of early pregnancy loss.Hum Reprod 1996;11:406–12.

[65] Wilcox AJ, Weinberg CR, O'Connor JF, Baird DD, Schlatterer JP, Canfield RE, Armstrong EG, Nisula BC. Incidence of early loss of pregnancy. N Engl J Med 1988; 319:189–94.

[66] Lee RM, Silver RM. Recurrent pregnancy loss: summary and clinical recommendations. Semin Reprod Med 2000;18:433–40.

[67] Toth B, Jeschke U, Rogenhofer N, Scholz C, Wurfel W, Thaler CJ, Makrigiannakis A. Recurrent miscarriage: current concepts in diagnosis and treatment. J Reprod Immunol 2010;85:25–32.

[68] Baek KH, Lee EJ, Kim YS. Recurrent pregnancy loss: the key potential mechanisms. Trends Mol Med 2007 ;13:310–17.

[69] Dudley DJ. Diabetic-associated stillbirth: incidence, pathophysiology, and prevention. Clin Perinatol 2007;34:611–26.

[70] Casey BM, Dashe JS, Wells CE, McIntire DD, Leveno KJ, Cunningham FG. Subclinical hyperthyroidism and pregnancy outcomes. Obstet Gynecol 2006;107:337–41.

[71] De Vivo A, Mancuso A, Giacobbe A, Moleti M, Maggio Savasta L, De Dominici R, Priolo AM, Vermiglio F. Thyroid function in women found to have early pregnancy loss. Thyroid 2010; 20:633–7.

[72] Stagnaro-Green A, Roman SH, Cobin RH, el-Harazy E, Alvarez-Marfany M, Davies TF. Detection of at-risk pregnancy by means of highly sensitive assays for thyroid autoantibodies. JAMA1990; 264:1422–5.

[73] Iijima T, Tada H, Hidaka Y, Mitsuda N, Murata Y, Amino N. Effects of autoantibodies on the course of pregnancy and fetal growth. Obstet Gynecol 1997;90:364–9.

[74] Prummel MF, Wiersinga WM. Thyroid autoimmunity and miscarriage. Eur J Endocrinol 2004;150:751–5.

[75] Negro R, Formoso G, Mangieri T, Pezzarossa A, Dazzi D, Hassan H. Levothyroxine treatment in euthyroid pregnant women with autoimmune thyroid disease: effects on obstetrical complications. J Clin Endocrinol Metab 2006;91:2587–91.

[76] Stagnaro-Green A, Abalovich M, Alexander E, Azizi F, Mestman J, Negro R, et al. American Thyroid Association Taskforce on Thyroid Disease During Pregnancy and

Postpartum. Guidelines of the American Thyroid Association for the diagnosis and management of thyroid disease during pregnancy and postpartum. Thyroid 2011;21(10):1081–125.

[77] Iravani AT, Saeedi MM, Pakravesh J, Hamidi S, Abbasi M. Thyroid autoimmunity and recurrent spontaneous abortion in Iran: a case-control study. Endocr Pract 2008;14: 458–64.

[78] Kutteh WH, Yetman DL, Carr AC, Beck LA, Scott RT Jr. Increased prevalence of antithyroid antibodies identified in women with recurrent pregnancy loss but not in women undergoing assisted reproduction. Fertil Steril 1999;71:843–48.

[79] Esplin MS, Branch DW, Silver R, Stagnaro-Green A. Thyroid autoantibodies are not associated with recurrent pregnancy loss. Am J Obstet Gynecol 1998;179:1583–6.

[80] Pratt DE, Kaberlein G, Dudkiewicz A, Karande V, Gleicher N. The association of antithyroid antibodies in euthyroid nonpregnant women with recurrent first trimester abortions in the next pregnancy. Fertil Steril 1993;60:1001–5.

[81] Rushworth FH, Backos M, Rai R, Chilcott IT, Baxter N, Regan L. Prospective pregnancy outcome in untreated recurrent miscarriers with thyroid autoantibodies. Hum Reprod 2000;15:1637–9.

[82] De Carolis C, Greco E, Guarino MD, Perricone C, Dal Lago A, Giacomelli R, Fontana L, Perricone R. Anti-thyroid antibodies and antiphospholipid syndrome: evidence of reduced fecundity and of poor pregnancy outcome in recurrent spontaneous aborters. Am J Reprod Immunol 2004 ;52:263–6.

[83] Dal Lago A, Vaquero E, Pasqualetti P, Lazzarin N, De Carolis C, Perricone R, Moretti C. Prediction of early pregnancy maternal thyroid impairment in women affected with unexplained recurrent miscarriage. Hum Reprod 2011; 26(6):1324-30.

[84] Lazzarin N, Moretti C, De Felice G, Vaquero E, Manfellotto D. Further evidence on the role of thyroid autoimmunity in women with recurrent miscarriage. Int J Endocrinol 2012;2012:717185, 4 pages.

[85] Kiprov DD, Nachtigall RD, Weaver RC, Jacobson A, Main EK, Garovoy MR. The use of intravenous immunoglobulin in recurrent pregnancy loss associated with combined alloimmune and autoimmune abnormalities. Am J Reprod Immunol 1996;36:228–34.

[86] Stricker RB, Steinleitner A, Bookoff CN, Weckstein LN, Winger EE. Successful treatment of immunologic abortion with low-dose intravenous immunoglobulin. Fertil Steril 2000; 73:536–40.

[87] Vaquero E, Lazzarin N, De Carolis C, Valensise H, Moretti C, Romanini C. Mild thyroid abnormalities and recurrent spontaneous abortion: diagnostic and therapeutical approach. Am J Reprod Immunol 2000; 43:204–8.

[88] Turi A, Giannubilo SR, Zanconi S, Mascetti A, Tranquilli AL. Preconception steroid treatment in infertile women with antithyroid autoimmunity undergoing ovarian

stimulation and intrauterine insemination: a double-blind, randomized, prospective cohort study. Clin Ther 2010; 32(14):2415-21.

[89] Poppe K, Glinoer D, Tournaye H, Devroey P, van Steirteghem A, Kaufman L, Velkeniers B. Assisted reproduction and thyroid autoimmunity: an unfortunate combination? J Clin Endocrinol Metab 2003; 88:4149–52.

[90] Bussen S, Steck T, Dietl J. Increased prevalence of thyroid antibodies in euthyroid women with a history of recurrent in-vitro fertilization failure. Hum Reprod 2000;15: 545–48.

[91] Kim CH, Chae HD, Kang BM, Chang YS. Influence of antithyroid antibodies in euthyroid women on in vitro fertilization-embryo transfer outcome. Am J Reprod Immunol 1998 ;40:2–8.

[92] Negro R, Formoso G, Coppola L, Presicce G, Mangieri T, Pezzarossa A, Dazzi D. Euthyroid women with autoimmune disease undergoing assisted reproduction technologies: the role of autoimmunity and thyroid function. J Endocrinol Invest 2007;30:3–8.

[93] Kilic S, Tasdemir N, Yilmaz N, Yuksel B, Gul A, Batioglu S. The effect of anti-thyroid antibodies on endometrial volume, embryo grade and IVF outcome. Gynecol Endocrinol 2008;24:649–55.

[94] Toulis KA, Goulis DG, Venetis CA, Kolibianakis EM, Negro R, Tarlatzis BC, Papadimas I. Risk of spontaneous miscarriage in euthyroid women with thyroid autoimmunity undergoing IVF: a meta-analysis. Eur J Endocrinol 2010;162:643–52.

[95] Negro R, Mangieri T, Coppola L, Presicce G, Casavola EC, Gismondi R, Locorotondo G, Caroli P, Pezzarossa A, Dazzi D, Hassan H. Levothyroxine treatment in thyroid peroxidase antibody-positive women undergoing assisted reproduction technologies: a prospective study. Hum Reprod 2005;20:1529–33.

[96] Gartner R, Gasnier BC, Dietrich JW, Krebs B, Angstwurm MW. Selenium supplementation in patients with autoimmune thyroiditis decreases thyroid peroxidase antibodies concentrations. J Clin Endocrinol Metab 2002;87:1687–91.

[97] Duntas LH, Mantzou E, Koutras DA. Effects of a six month treatment with selenomethionine in patients with autoimmune thyroiditis. Eur J Endocrinol 2003;148:389–93.

[98] Mazokopakis EE, Papadakis JA, Papadomanolaki MG, Batistakis AG, Giannakopoulos TG, Protopapadakis EE, Ganotakis ES. Effects of 12 months treatment with Lselenomethionine on serum anti-TPO Levels in Patients with Hashimoto's thyroiditis. Thyroid 2007; 17:609–12.

[99] Karanikas G, Schuetz M, Kontur S, Duan H, Kommata S, Schoen R, Antoni A, Kletter K, Dudczak R, Willheim M. No immunological benefit of selenium in consecutive patients with autoimmune thyroiditis. Thyroid 2008;18:7–12.

[100] Negro R, Greco G, Mangieri T, Pezzarossa A, Dazzi D, Hassan H. The influence of selenium supplementation on postpartum thyroid status in pregnant women with thyroid peroxidase autoantibodies. J Clin Endocrinol Metab 2007; 92:1263–8.

[101] Stranges S, Marshall JR, Natarajan R, Donahue RP, Trevisan M, Combs GF, Cappuccio FP, Ceriello A, Reid ME. Effects of long-term selenium supplementation on the incidence of type 2 diabetes: a randomized trial. Ann Intern Med 2007;147:217–23.

[102] Brown RS. Minireview: developmental regulation of thyrotropin receptor gene expression in the fetal and newborn thyroid. Endocrinology 2004;145(9):4058–61.

[103] Fisher DA. Fetal thyroid function: diagnosis and management of fetal thyroid disorders. Clin Obstet Gynecol 1997;40(1):16–31.

[104] Ain KB, Mori Y, Refetoff S. Reduced clearance rate of thyroxine-binding globulin (TBG) with increased sialylation: a mechanism for estrogen-induced elevation of serum TBG concentration. J Clin Endocrinol Metab 1987; 65(4):689–96.

[105] Pittas AG, Lee SL. Evaluation of thyroid function. In: Hall JE, Niemann LK, editors. Handbook of diagnostic endocrinology. Totowa, New Jersey: Humana Press Inc 2003; p.112

[106] Glinoer D. The regulation of thyroid function in pregnancy: pathways of endocrine adaptation from physiology to pathology. Endocr Rev 1997;18(3):404–33.

[107] Mandel SJ, Spencer CA, Hollowell JG. Are detection and treatment of thyroid insufficiency in pregnancy feasible? Thyroid 2005;15(1):44–53.

[108] Roti E, Fang SL, Emerson CH, Braverman LE. Placental inner ring iodothyronine deiodination: a mechanism for decreased passage of T4 and T3 from mother to fetus. Trans Assoc Am Physicians 1981;94:183–9.

[109] Glinoer D, de Nayer P, Bourdoux P, Lemone M, Robyn C, van Steirteghem A, et al. Regulation of maternal thyroid during pregnancy. J Clin Endocrinol Metab 1990;71(2):276–87.

[110] Dafnis E, Sabatini S. The effect of pregnancy on renal function: physiology and pathophysiology. Am J Med Sci 1992; 303:184–205.

[111] Hershman JM. Physiological and pathological aspects of the effect of human chorionic gonadotropin on the thyroid. Best Pract Res Clin Endocrinol Metab 2004;18(2):249–65.

[112] Glinoer D. Pregnancy and iodine. Thyroid 2001;11:471–81.

[113] Mandel SJ, Larsen PR, Seely EW, Brent GA. Increased need for thyroxine during pregnancy in women with primary hypothyroidism. N Engl J Med 1990;323:91–6.

[114] Alexander EK, Marqusee E, Lawrence J, Jarolim P, Fischer GA, Larsen PR. Timing and magnitude of increases in levothyroxine requirements during pregnancy in women with hypothyroidism. N Engl J Med 2004;351:241–9.

[115] Casey BM, Dashe JS, Wells CE, McIntire DD, Byrd W, Leveno KJ, Cunningham FG. Subclinical hypothyroidism and pregnancy outcomes. Obstet Gynecol 2005;105:239–45.

[116] Allan WC, Haddow JE, Palomaki GE, Williams JR, Mitchell ML, Hermos RJ, Faix JD, Klein RZ. Maternal thyroid deficiency and pregnancy complications: implications for population screening. J Med Screen 2000; 7:127–30.

[117] Leung AS, Millar LK, Koonings PP, Montoro M, Mestman JH. Perinatal outcome in hypothyroid pregnancies. Obstet Gynecol 1993; 81(3):349–53.

[118] Stagnaro-Green A, Chen X, Bogden JD, Davies TF, Scholl TO. The thyroid and pregnancy: a novel risk factor for very preterm delivery. Thyroid 2005; 15(4):351–7.

[119] Glinoer D, Riahi M, Grun JP, Kinthaert J. Risk of subclinical hypothyroidism in pregnant women with asymptomatic autoimmune thyroid disorders. J Clin Endocrinol Metab 1994; 79:197–204.

[120] Kuppens SM, Kooistra L, Wijnen HA, Crawford S, Vader HL, Hasaart TH, et al. Maternal thyroid function during gestation is related to breech presentation at term. Clin Endocrinol (Oxf) 2010; 72:820–4.

[121] Wang S, Teng WP, Li JX, Wang WW, Shan ZY. Effects of maternal subclinical hypothyroidism on obstetrical outcomes during early pregnancy. J Endocrinol Invest (Epub ahead of print).

[122] Mannisto T, Vaarasmaki M, Pouta A, Hartikainen AL, Ruokonen A, Surcel HM, Bloigu A, Jarvelin MR, Suvanto-Luukkonen E. Perinatal outcome of children born to mothers with thyroid dysfunction or antibodies: a prospective population-based cohort study. J Clin Endocrinol Metab 2009; 94:772–9.

[123] Haddow JE, Palomaki GE, Allan WC, Williams JR, Knight GJ, Gagnon J, O'Heir CE, Mitchell ML, Hermos RJ, Waisbren SE, Faix JD, Klein RZ. Maternal thyroid deficiency during pregnancy and subsequent neuropsychological development of the child. N Engl J Med 1999; 341:549–555.

[124] Li Y, Shan Z, Teng W, Yu X, Li Y, Fan C, Teng X, Guo R, Wang H, Li J, Chen Y, Wang W, Chawinga M, Zhang L, Yang L, Zhao Y, Hua T. Abnormalities of maternal thyroid function during pregnancy affect neuropsychological development of their children at 25–30 months. Clin Endocrinol (Oxf) 2010; 72:825–9.

[125] Krassas GE, Poppe K, Glinoer D. Thyroid function and human reproductive health. Endocr Rev 2010; 31:702–55.

[126] David S Cooper, Bernadette Biondi. Subclinical thyroid disease. Lancet 2012; 379:1142–54.

[127] Negro R, Schwartz A, Gismondi R, Tinelli A, Mangieri T, Stagnaro-Green A. Universal screening versus case finding for detection and treatment of thyroid hormonal dysfunction during pregnancy. J Clin Endocrinol Metab 2010; 95:1699–1707.

[128] Negro R, Schwartz A, Gismondi R, Tinelli A, Mangieri T, Stagnaro-Green A. Increased pregnancy loss rate in thyroid antibody negative women with TSH levels between 2.5 and 5.0 in the first trimester of pregnancy. J Clin Endocrinol Metab 2010; 95:E44–8.

[129] Cleary-Goldman J, Malone FD, Lambert-Messerlian G, Sullivan L, Canick J, Porter TF, Luthy D, Gross S, Bianchi DW, D'Alton ME. Maternal thyroid hypofunction and pregnancy outcome. Obstet Gynecol 2008; 112:85–92.

[130] Ashoor G, Maiz N, Rotas M, Jawdat F, Nicolaides KH. Maternal thyroid function at 11 to 13 weeks of gestation and subsequent fetal death. Thyroid 2010; 20:989–93.

[131] de Escobar GM, Obregon MJ, del Rey FE. Maternal thyroid hormones early in pregnancy and fetal brain development. Best Pract Res Clin Endocrinol Metab 2004; 18:225–48.

[132] Haddow JE, Knight GJ, Palomaki GE, McClain MR, Pulkkinen AJ. The reference range and within-person variability of thyroid stimulating hormone during the first and second trimesters of pregnancy. J Med Screen 2004;11:170-74.

[133] Grun JP, Meuris S, De Nayer P, Glinoer D. The thyrotrophic role of human chorionic gonadotrophin (hCG) in the early stages of twin (versus single) pregnancies. Clin Endocrinol (Oxf) 1997;46(6):719–25.

[134] Mannisto T, Surcel HM, Ruokonen A, Vaarasmaki M, Pouta A, Bloigu A, et al. Early pregnancy reference intervals of thyroid hormone concentrations in a thyroid antibody-negative pregnant population. Thyroid 2011; 21(3):291–8.

[135] Pop VJ, Brouwers EP, Vader HL, Vulsma T, van Baar AL, de Vijlder JJ. Maternal hypothyroxinaemia during early pregnancy and subsequent child development: a 3-year follow-up study. Clin Endocrinol (Oxf) 2003; 59:282–8.

[136] Henrichs J, Bongers-Schokking JJ, Schenk JJ, Ghassabian A, Schmidt HG, Visser TJ, Hooijkaas H, de Muinck Keizer- Schrama SM, Hofman A, Jaddoe VV, Visser W, Steegers EA, Verhulst FC, de Rijke YB, Tiemeier H. Maternal thyroid function during early pregnancy and cognitive functioning in early childhood: the Generation R Study. J Clin Endocrinol Metab 2010; 95:4227–34.

[137] Benhadi N, Wiersinga WM, Reitsma JB, Vrijkotte TG, van der Wal MF, Bonsel GJ. Ethnic differences in TSH but not in free T4 concentrations or TPO antibodies during pregnancy. Clin Endocrinol (Oxf) 2007; 66:765–70.

[138] Price A, Obel O, Cresswell J, Catch I, Rutter S, Barik S, Heller SR, Weetman AP. Comparison of thyroid function in pregnant and non-pregnant Asian and western Caucasian women. Clin Chim Acta 2001; 308:91–98.

[139] Walker JA, Illions EH, Huddleston JF, Smallridge RC. Racial comparisons of thyroid function and autoimmunity during pregnancy and the postpartum period. Obstet Gynecol 2005; 106:1365–71.

[140] Thienpont LM, Van Uytfanghe K, Beastall G, Faix JD, Ieiri T, Miller WG, Nelson JC, Ronin C, Ross HA, Thijssen JH, Toussaint B, IFCC Working Group on Standardization of Thyroid Function Tests. Report of the IFCC Working Group for Standardization of Thyroid Function Tests; part 1: thyroid-stimulating hormone. Clin Chem 2010; 56:902–11.

[141] Abalovich M, Gutierrez S, Alcaraz G, Maccallini G, Garcia A, Levalle O. Overt and subclinical hypothyroidism complicating pregnancy. Thyroid 2002;12:63–8.

[142] Galofre JC, Haber RS, Mitchell AA, Pessah R, Davies TF. Increased postpartum thyroxine replacement in Hashimoto's thyroiditis. Thyroid 2010;20:901–8.

[143] Buscicchio G, Gentilucci L, Baldini E, Giannubilo SR, Tranquilli AL. Computerized analysis of heart rate in fetuses from mothers under levothyroxin treatment. Gynecological Endocrinology 2009; 25(10): 679-82.

[144] Ågren UM, Anttila M, Mäenpää –Liukko K, Rantala M, Rautiainen H, Sommer WP Mommers E. Effects of a monophasic combined oral contraceptive containing nomegestrol acetate and 17 β estradiol in comparison to one containing levonorgestrel and ethinylestradiol on markers of endocrine function. The European Journal of Contraception and Reproductive Health Care 2011; 16: 458–67.

[145] Wiegratz I, Kutschera E, Lee JH, et al. Effect of four oral contraceptives on thyroid hormones, adrenal and blood pressure parameters. Contraception 2003; 67:361 – 6.

[146] Sanger N, Stahlberg S, Manthey T, et al. Effects of an oral contraceptive containing 30 mcg ethinyl estradiol and 2 mg dienogest on thyroid hormones and androgen parameters: Conventional vs. extended-cycle use. Contraception 2008; 77:420 –5.

[147] Kuhl H, Gahn G, Romberg G, et al. A randomized crossover comparison of two low-dose oral contraceptives upon hormonal and metabolic serum parameters: II. Effects upon thyroid function, gastrin, STH, and glucose tolerance. Contraception 1985; 32:97 – 107.

[148] Stagnaro-Green A, Abalovich M, Alexander E, et al. Guidelines of The American Thyroid Association for the diagnosis and management of thyroid disease during pregnancy and the postpartum Thyroid 2011; 21:1–45.

[149] Abalovich M, Amino N, Barbour LA, et al. Management of thyroid dysfunction during pregnancy and postpartum: an Endocrine Society Clinical Practice Guideline. J Clin Endocrinol Metab 2007; 92 (suppl): S1–47.

[150] Lazarus JH, Bestwick JP, Channon S, Paradice R, Maina A, Rees R, Chiusano E, John R, Guaraldo V, George LM, Perona M; Dalla Amico D, Parkes AB, Joomun M, Wald NJ. Antenatal thyroid screening and childhood cognitive function. NEJM 2012; 366(6): 493-501.

[151] Dosiou C, Barnes J, Schwartz A, Negro R, Crapo L, Stagnaro-Green A. Cost-effectiveness of universal and risk-based screening for autoimmune thyroid disease in pregnant women. JCEM 2012; 97(5):1536-46.

Chapter 2

Hypothyroidism in Pregnancy

Baha Zantour, Wafa Alaya, Hela Marmouch and Wafa Chebbi

Additional information is available at the end of the chapter

http://dx.doi.org/10.5772/54745

1. Introduction

Changes in thyroid function tests occur during pregnancy as a result of physiologic alterations in several factors controlling thyroid homeostasis. Urinary iodine excretion increases along with the increase in thyroxine binding globulin (TBG) concentrations. Human chorionic gonadotrophin (hCG) having structural homology with thyroid stimulating hormone (TSH), stimulates thyroid cells. Thus, during pregnancy, functional activity and size of the thyroid gland are increased. Pregnancy is a stress test for the thyroid resulting in hypothyroidism in women with limited thyroidal reserve or iodine deficiency [1].

Thyroid dysfunction is common during gestation. The prevalence of hypothyroidism during pregnancy is estimated to be 0.3-0.5% for overt hypothyroidism (OH) and 2-3% for subclinical hypothyroidism (SCH). Thyroid antibodies are found in 8-14% of women in the childbearing age, and chronic autoimmune thyroiditis is the main cause of hypothyroidism during pregnancy, apart from iode deficiency [2,3].

Given the rapidity of advances in this field, it is not surprising that controversy surrounds optimal detection and management of thyroid disease in pregnant women. It is now well established that OH is associated with an increased risk of adverse pregnancy complications, as well as detrimental effects upon fetal neurocognitive development [4]. However, data regarding SCH are controversial [4,5]

In the past several years, there has been a debate about the universal screening of thyroid disorders. There is until now insufficient evidence to recommend for or against evaluating thyroid function in all pregnant women. OH should be treated in pregnancy. However, due to the lack of randomized controlled trials, there is no evidence to recommend universal treatment of SCH or isolated hypothyroxinemia [6,7]

Central hypothyroidism will not be discussed in this chapter

2. Physiology

Pregnancy profoundly influences thyroid function. This influence is due to many events which are specific to the pregnant state: the changes in thyroid hormone transport protein particularly in TBG, the effects of hCG on the maternal thyroid, the rise in the iodine requirement, the role of the placental deiodinase, and the modifications in the autoimmune regulation. These events occur at different time points during gestation, resulting in complex effects that may be seen only transiently or, by contrast, that persist until term [8]. Hence, pregnancy is a real test for thyroid gland.

2.1. Thyroid hormones transport proteins

Thyroid hormones (TH) circulate in plasma, mainly bounded to 3 transport proteins: TBG, albumin and prealbumin. Despite its smaller concentration compared with albumin and prealbumin, the TBG is the main transport protein of TH, because of its extremely high affinity to these hormones. In serum of normal subjects, TBG carries about two thirds of TH [9]. This bound hormone fraction is in equilibrium with a free unbound fraction, which is in contrast with its smaller amount (0.04% for T4 and 0.5% for T_3), represents the active fraction of TH [10].

In pregnant women, serum TBG rises sharply few weeks after the beginning of pregnancy, and reaches a plateau around midgestation, 2.5-fold higher than the initial value [11]. Subsequently, the TBG concentration remains stable until term (Figure 1) [12]. This increase in TBG level is due to the increase in estrogen concentration, resulting in a rise of TBG production and release by the liver, site of synthesis of the protein [11]. Furthermore, the circulating levels of both albumin and prealbumin remain stable, with only a discrete tendency to decrease near term, consequently to the hemodilution [13]. The respective affinities of the three binding proteins for TH are not significantly modified. Hence, the proportion of T4 carried by TBG reaches 75% during gestation [14].

In addition to its increased production, TBG has a longer half-life during gestation. Indeed, the TBG is more sialylated during pregnancy than in other conditions. This higher sialylation confers to the protein a longer half-life. However, the more sialylated fraction of TBG represents a small amount of the total circulating protein (10–15%), and can't explain alone the prolongation of the TBG half-life. This extension of half-life is promoted by the stabilization of the TBG due to the proportional increase in its binding to T4.

Thus, the major change for thyroid hormone-binding proteins involves TBG, with:

- An increase in its production and release by liver
- An extension of its half-life due to the increase in the degree of its scialylation and its stabilization consequently to the proportional increase in its binding to T4.

2.2. Thyroid hormones

2.2.1. Total thyroid hormones

In pregnancy, the total TH level increases consequently to the TBG increase. Since the affinity of TBG to T4 is 20 fold higher than that of TBG to T3, changes of total T4 level follow more closely changes of TBG, and the T3/T4 molar ratio remains unaltered during pregnancy. Total T4 level increases rapidly and markedly between the 6th and the 12th week of gestation and then progresses more slowly, until it stabilizes around midgestation when total T3 level increases more progressively [15].

2.2.2. Free thyroid hormones

Consequently to the increase of the bound fraction of TH, and to maintain free TH homeostasis, an increase in TH production is expected. This production enhancement is thought to be regulated primarily through the normal pituitary-thyroid feedback mechanisms; TSH stimulation of the thyroid gland. However, in healthy pregnant women, without thyroid autoimmunity or iodine deficiency, no increase in serum TSH is commonly observed [16], and free TH levels fluctuations differ in the early gestation than in its second half.

In the first trimester (as it will be discussed later), free T4 (FT4) level rises transiently in response to the peak of production of hCG. This increase in FT4 level is totally independent of the action of TSH which production decreases, in contrast, as a result of its down-regulation by high hCG levels during early pregnancy [17].

In the second half of gestation, longitudinal recent studies based on reliable methodology, carried out on large numbers of pregnant women without iodine deficiency, have showed that serum free TH levels are lower by an average of 10–15% at delivery, in comparison with nonpregnant female subjects, while remaining within reference range of these latters [18,19] (Figure 1). This decrease in free TH level during the second half of gestation in healthy pregnant women, considered euthyroid and without iodine deficiency, remains incompletely explained. Some authors suggest that high estrogen levels over a prolonged period of time may modify the regulation of both basal and TRH-stimulated TSH release by the pituitary gland [20]. Also, an increased nuclear binding capacity for TH in target cells may compensate for this decrease in free TH [21].

2.2.3. Peripheral metabolism of free thyroid hormones and role of placenta

Three enzymes catalyze the deiodination of thyroid hormones. Type I deiodinase, by deiodination of T4, is responsible for the production of most of the circulating T 3. Type II deiodinase, is expressed in certain tissues (pituitary gland, brain, brown adipose tissue) and also in the placenta. Its activity increases when the availability of T4 decreases. So, it ensures the maintenance of T3 production in the placenta as maternal T4 levels are reduced [22]. Placental type III deiodinase has an extremely high activity during fetal life. It converts T4 to reverse T3 and T3 to T2, and remarkably increases TH turn-over [23].

Thus, placenta is a selective barrier for the different constituents of thyroid metabolism: it regulates free TH transfer by deiodinases, allows the materno-fetal iodine transfer, and is impermeable to TSH. Placenta is also permeable to thyroid and TSH receptor antibodies and antithyroid drugs.

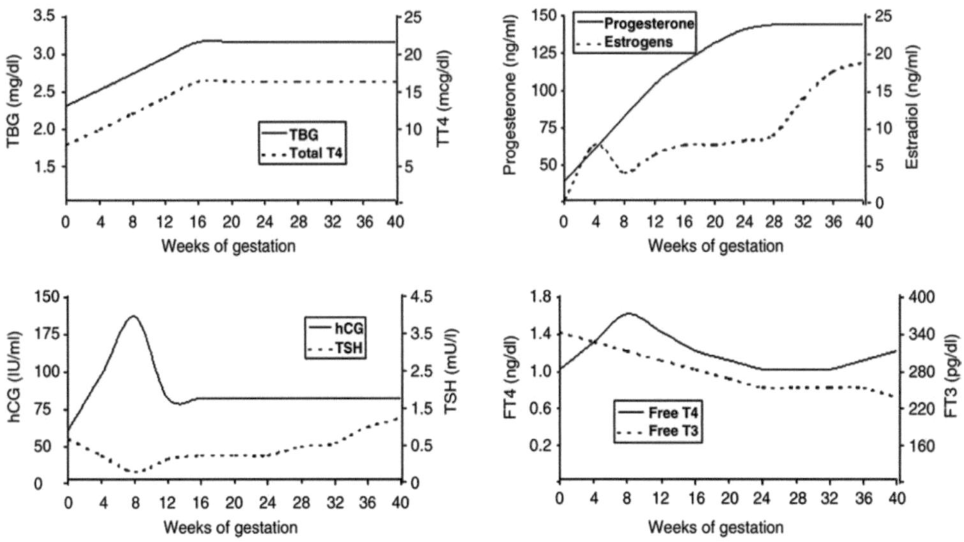

Figure 1. Variation in serum levels of thyroid function test and pregnancy-related hormones according to course of gestation. [19]

2.3. Hypothalamic-pituitary-thyroid axis in pregnancy and the effect of hCG

As it has been already mentioned, previous studies concluded that elevated estrogen levels in pregnancy may influence the hypothalamic-pituitary-thyroid axis (HPTA), perhaps by acting at different levels (and not yet clearly defined) in the thyroid gland feedback-regulatory mechanisms, resulting in a blunting of the TSH response. In normal pregnant women who have no evidence of thyroid autoimmunity and who reside in areas with a sufficient iodine supply, serum TSH remains stable and comparable to pregestation levels, after the transient fall due to high hCG in the first trimester. Conversely, when the iodine intake is restricted, an increase in serum TSH during late gestation (generally remaining within the reference range in normal pregnant women) reflects the stimulated thyroid state. Thus, iodine insufficiency is then revealed by pregnancy and explains the progressive increase in serum TSH observed after 16 weeks of gestation.

Concerning the effect of hCG on thyroid gland, it has been evoked from cases of thyrotoxicosis observed in pathological conditions accompanied by extremely high circulating hCG levels, such as molar pregnancy or other tropoblastic diseases [24]. Therefore, many studies have been carried out to better clarify the real effect of hCG on TH production and its consequences on TSH secretion. The results showed that the profiles of changes in serum TSH and hCG were clear mirror images, with a linear relationship between hCG and FT4 concentrations during early gestation (Figure 2). Thus, the lowering of TSH corresponds to a transient and partial blunting of the pituitary-thyroid axis associated with an increased hormonal output by the thyroid gland under hCG stimulation [18]. The thyrotropic action of hCG is explained by the structural homology between the hCG and TSH molecules, and between LH/hCG and TSH receptors. Thus, hCG is able to bind to the TSH receptor of thyroid follicular cells and exert its stimulatory effects [25]. However, it should be remembered that hCG behaves as a weak

http://dx.doi.org/10.5772/54745

thyroid stimulator *in vivo*. It is estimated that a 10,000 IU/liter increment in circulating hCG corresponds to a mean FT4 increment in serum of 0.6 pmol/liter (*i.e.* 0.1ng/dl) and, in turn, to a lowering of serum TSH of 0.1 mIU/liter. Hence, a transient increase in serum FT4 during the first trimester will only be observed when hCG levels reach or exceed 50,000 –75,000 IU/liter. Some studies assessed from a clinical stand point how often partial TSH suppression may occur in early pregnancy. In up to one fifth of normal pregnancies, serum TSH may be transiently suppressed in the first trimester to values below the lower limit of normal [26].

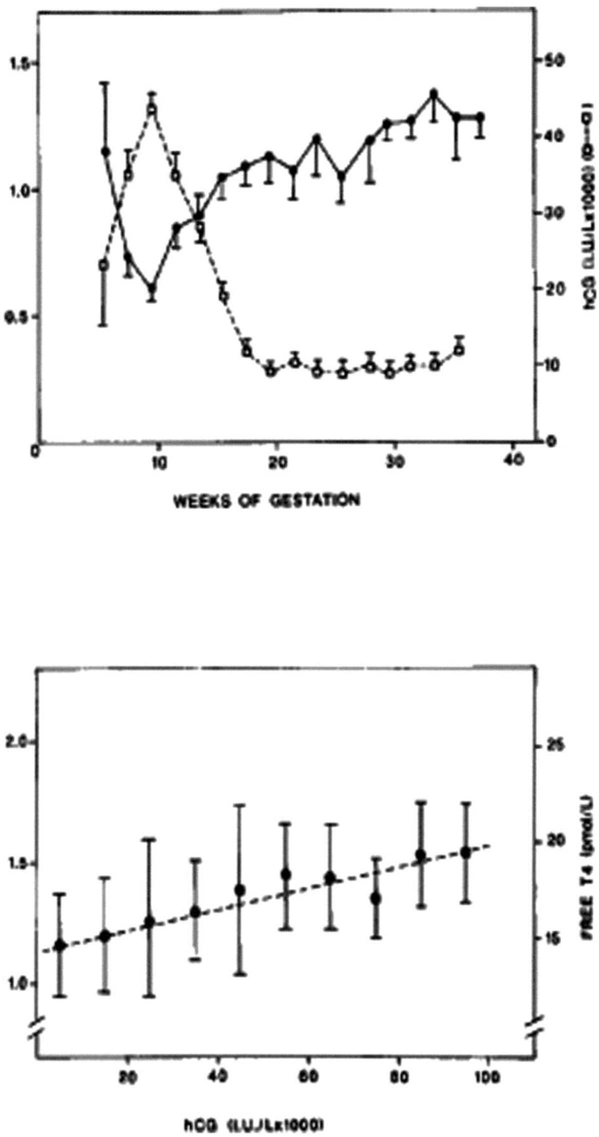

Figure 2. *Upper graph*, Serum TSH and hCG as a function of gestational age. *Lower graph*, Scattergram of free T levels in relation to hCG concentrations in the first half of gestation. [28]

In addition to the importance of the hCG peak amplitude on hCG effects on thyroid stimulation and TSH suppression, the duration of exposure to this peak is also important in modulating hCG effects. Thus, in twin pregnancies, where not only the peak hCG values are significantly higher than in single pregnancies (in fact, almost double), but also of much longer duration (6 weeks vs1 week), more profound and frequent lowering in serum TSH is observed. Among these cases, FT4 levels in the hyperthyroid range accompanied by clinical manifestation of thyrotoxicosis have even been described [27].

2.4. Iodine physiology during pregnancy

During pregnancy, dietary iodine requirements are higher than in nonpregnant women. Three main mechanisms explain this requirement increase: rise in TH production, increase in renal iodine filtration, and passage of a part of the available iodine from maternal circulation to the fetal-placental unit. Beginning in early pregnancy, the glomerular filtration rate of iodide increases by 30% to 50% [29], thus decreasing the circulating pool of plasma iodine. This induces in turn an increase in thyroidal iodine clearance, which reaches 60 ml/mn (versus 17 ml/mn behind pregnancy in sufficient iodine region) [30]. A comparison of pregnant women from various countries demonstrated that peak gestational urinary iodine levels vary, suggesting differences in renal excretion thresholds by regional dietary iodine intake [31]. In addition to the renal leakage of iodine, at midgestation, the fetal thyroid gland has already started to produce thyroid hormones, using iodine pumped in maternal circulation, which exacerbates mother iodine deprivation [32].

The consensus recommendation of the World Health Organization is that the iodine supply should be increased in pregnant and lactating women to at least 200 microg/day [33]. In pregnant women who reside in countries with an iodine sufficient environment (a daily iodine intake of more than 150 mg), iodine losses in the urine and from transfer to the fetus are probably of little importance. In iodine deficient regions, an increase in maternal TSH levels and consequently in thyroid size is observed. If iodine deficiency is severe, TSH increase is insufficient to ensure adequate TH production and hypothyroidism develops (Figure 3).

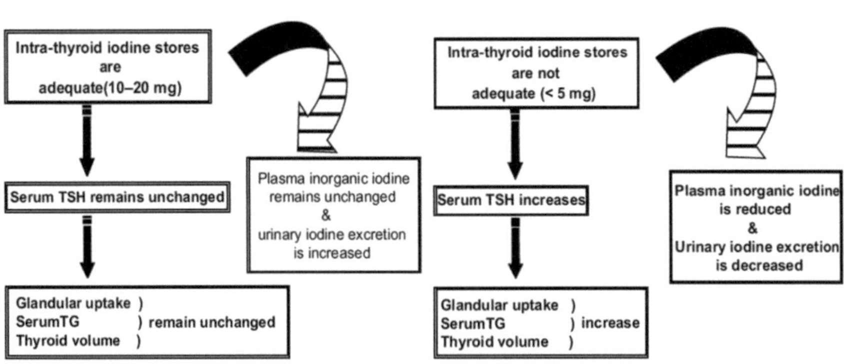

Figure 3. Conceptual models of adequate (*left panel*) and inadequate (*right panel*) iodine nutrition and thyroid function [34].

http://dx.doi.org/10.5772/54745

2.5. Gestational modifications of the autoimmune regulation

For a successful pregnancy outcome, the maternal immune system must tolerate the fetus. Therefore, placental trophoblast cells secrete a variety of cytokines and molecules having an immunomodulatory action (table 1). The result is an attenuation of immune responses with a general improvement in autoimmune diseases, including thyroid immune disease [35]

2.6. Fetal thyroid development

Fetal thyroid ontogeny begins at 10-12 weeks of gestation, and is not accomplished until delivery. T4 starts being secreted by 18-20th week of gestation [36]. Before this time, the fetus is dependent on a supply of maternal TH which is essential for early fetal development and, in particular, early central nervous system (CNS) development.

Place event	Adaptation	Result
Local	Trophoblast cells express several immune-modulating molecules (Fas-L, HLA-G and indoleamine 2,3-dioxygenase) as well as secreting a variety of cytokines	- Fas-L induces apoptosis on fetal antigen-reactive maternal lymphocytes -HLA-G inhibits both NK cell function and maturation of dendritic cells -Indoleamine 2,3-dioxigenase catalyzes triptophane in lymphocytes, which is critical in the maintenance of allogenic pregnancy
Systemic	T cell	-Decreased CD4, increased CD8 T cells and increasing activity of T regulatory cells -The immune response is turned from Th1 (cellular) to Th2 (humoral), with an increase in Th2 cytokine production
	B cell	Despite the shift to Th2, the relative B cell production and activity are downregulated, leading to a reduction in antibody production
	Hormonal changes	-Increase in plasma levels of estrogen, progesterone, and corticosteroids -Estrogen produces negative regulation of B cell activity -Progesterone generates variation in cytokine profiles -Corticosteroids induce immune cell apoptosis and immunosuppression
Postpartum	Recovery of prepregnancy immune function	-Increased titers of serum antibodies, reversed ratio CD4+/CD8+ T cells, and change in cytokine profiles favor Th1 responses

Fas-L, Fas-Ligand; HLA-G, Human leukocyte antigen-G; NK, natural killer; Th1, T helper cell 1; Th2, T helper cell 2

Table 1. Immune Adaptation to Pregnancy [19]

3. Epidemiology

In women of childbearing age, the prevalence of overt hypothyroidism is estimated at 0,3- 0,5% and that of subclinical hypothyroidism at 2-3%. Prevalence rates are similar during pregnancy [2,5]. Three large studies have assessed the prevalence of hypothyroidism in pregnant women. They have concerned respectively 1900, 2000 and 9403 pregnant women. The prevalence of hypothyroidism was similar in the three studies ranging from 2,2 to 2,4%. In the study carried out on 9403 pregnant women, subclinical hypothyroidism was detected in 0,4% of cases [37].

The prevalence of hypothyroidism in pregnancy is strongly linked to the TSH cut-off value used. In a Czech study on more than 5000 women, this prevalence reached 5.6 % if a cut-off at 3.67 mIU/l was used. However, using a cut-off at 2.5 mU/l, the proportion of pregnant women with TSH elevation increased to 16.7 % [38]. The large American study of Blatt et al. showed similar numbers [39].

Defining the true incidence of isolated maternal hypothyroxinemia is rather difficult, because of the differences in diagnostic criteria used to define the condition. In addition, the epidemiological data presently available are somewhat sparse. The issue of the epidemiological impact of isolated hypothyroxinemia was very recently reviewed by Krassas et al. [3], who estimated an overall incidence of approximately 2% in unselected pregnancies. However, there are wide differences among the studies, related mainly to differences in iodine nutrition status. Indeed, in regions where iodine intake is sufficient, as is the case in the United States, the prevalence of isolated hypothyroxinemia ranges between 1.3% [40] and 2.3% [41]. In contrast, in mildly to moderately iodine deficient regions, isolated hypothyroxinemia affects a much higher percentage of women, reaching values up to 25–30% [42,43]. Interestingly, in a very recent study by Henrichs et al.[44] carried out in The Netherlands on a cohort of 3659 women, the prevalence of mild hypothyroxinemia (FT4 < 10th percentile) was 8.5% and that of severe hypothyroxinemia (FT4 < 5th percentile) 4.3%. These figures are significantly higher than those reported in previous studies conducted in iodine sufficient regions [40,42].

4. Causes of hypothyroidism in pregnancy

Worldwide, particularly in mountainous regions and in Central Africa, South America and Northern Asia, the most common cause of hypothyroidism is iodine deficiency [45]. Because of increased thyroid hormone production, increased renal iodine excretion, and fetal iodine requirements, dietary iodine requirements are higher in pregnancy than they are for non pregnant adults [29]. Women with adequate iodine intake before and during pregnancy have adequate intra-thyroidal iodine stores and have no difficulty adapting to this increased demand. In these women, total body iodine levels remain stable throughout pregnancy [46]. However, in areas of even mild to moderate iodine deficiency, total body iodine stores, as reflected by urinary iodine values, decline gradually from the first to the third trimester of pregnancy [47].

It is difficult to determine the severity of iodine deficiency in pregnant women. The commonly used index for assessing iodine status in a population is the median urinary iodine concentration (MUIC) as determined from a casual or spot urine sample. A MUIC > 100 micog/l is indicative of adequate iodine status in children, men and non pregnant women. A MUIC of 50-99 microg/l, 20-49 microg/l and < 20 microg/l are indicative of mild, moderate and severe iodine deficiency respectively [48]. The World Health Organization estimates that about two billion people are iodine deficient [48].

In areas of iodine sufficiency, the most common cause of hypothyroidism in pregnant women is chronic autoimmune thyroiditis [49]. Anti-thyroid antibodies were found in 18% of Australian women in the late first trimester and were associated with subtle effects on thyroid function [50]. In a prospective population study of 9471 pregnant women in the United States in whom serum TSH was measured during the second trimester, hypothyroidism was diagnosed in 2.2% of the cohort, and autoimmune thyroiditis was present in 55% of women with SCH and more than 80% in women with OH [37].

Thyroidectomy, ablative iodine therapies or anti-thyroid drugs are other important causes of primary hypothyroidism [6].

5. Consequences of maternal hypothyroidism

Thyroid diseases are common in women of childbearing age and it is well known that untreated thyroid disturbances result in an increased rate of adverse events. Evaluation of thyroid status in pregnancy requires an understanding of pregnancy-associated changes in thyroid function tests and how they vary by trimester. The spectrum of hypothyroidism in pregnancy includes subclinical and overt hypothyroidism, and also isolated thyroid peroxidase antibody positivity and isolated hypothyroxinemia. These patterns, in some situations, may be related to iodine status, selenium status, or underlying thyroid disease.

5.1. Consequences of maternal hypothyroidism

Abnormal maternal thyroid parameters are associated with adverse pregnancy outcomes, with consequences for both mother and child. Although various studies evaluated maternal thyroid parameters during the first half of pregnancy, little is known about their relations with thyroid parameters of the child. There are correlations between maternal thyroid parameters and gestational age during the first half of pregnancy and a substantially increased risk of SCH in TPOAb-positive mothers [51]

5.1.1. Influence of maternal thyroid disease on fetal development

Any thyroid disease of the mother with disturbances in the functional state of the gland could induce an adverse influence on the course of pregnancy. Furthermore, it can be associated with adverse consequences on fetal development [37].

Enough evidence has been accumulated over the years about the role of T4 in normal development of the fetal brain. The presence of specific nuclear receptors of thyroid hormones in fetal brain at 8 weeks of gestation, the presence of FT4 in the coelomic and amniotic fluids and demonstration of the transfer of maternal thyroid hormones across the placenta, underline the role of thyroid hormones in fetal brain development. Complex interactions between the type II and type III iodothyronine deiodinases during gestation help to fine tune the supply of adequate amounts of T3 required for normal brain development [52].

Because thyroid hormones are crucial to fetal brain and nervous system development, uncontrolled hypothyroidism, especially during the first trimester, can affect the fetal's growth and brain development and can alter the neurocognitive development of the offspring [4].

Maintaining maternal euthyroidism during pregnancy is important for growth and development, in particular neurodevelopment of the fetus. Even subtle changes in thyroid function of the pregnant woman can cause detrimental effects for the fetus. In the first trimester, the foetus relies solely on the thyroid hormones T4 and T3 and iodine from the mother. Later in pregnancy and during lactation, maternal TH still contribute significantly to fetal thyroid homeostasis [32]. The impact of overt maternal hypothyroidism on pregnancy is profound. The severity, timing of onset and duration, as well as postnatal management, all influence fetal and neonatal brain development. It is now believed than even mild maternal hypothyroidism (from mild iodine deficiency, thyroid autoimmunity, or thyroid under-replacement) may affect fetal brain development [5,6]

Adequate thyroid hormone is critical for cerebellar development. Developmental hypothyroidism induced by iodine deficiency during the perinatal period results in permanent impairments of cerebellar development with an unclear mechanism [52].

Hypothyroidism during pregnancy has been also associated with impaired cognitive development and increased fetal mortality [37].

5.1.2. b-Obstetrical complications of maternal hypothyroidism

Women with hypothyroidism have decreased fertility; even if they conceive, risk of abortion is increased, and risk of gestational hypertension, anemia, abruption placenta and postpartum hemorrhage is increased [49]

The association between overt maternal hypothyroidism, particularly in early pregnancy, and adverse obstetric outcomes is well-established. In a study of women during the second trimester of pregnancy, the prevalence of fetal death was over 4-fold higher in mothers with a TSH concentration ≥6 mIU/L, compared to those whose mothers had a TSH <6 mIU/L (3.8% vs. 0.9%) [37]

Untreated hypothyroidism is associated with increased risk of preeclampsia, low birth weight, placental abruption, miscarriage, and perinatal mortality [53,54]. In addition to an increased risk of low birth weight, hypothyroidism (as defined by increased serum TSH) early and late in pregnancy may also increase the rate of caesarean section [55].

Raised maternal serum TSH in the second trimester is also associated with an increased rate of fetal death after 16 weeks' gestation [37]. Other studies have found that although women treated for hypothyroidism may have higher rates of preeclampsia and caesarean section than euthyroid women, they are not at any higher risk for adverse outcomes such as fetal anomalies, fetal demise, or preterm birth. In hypothyroidism there are placental hypoxic changes. This may be responsible for thick meconium, stained liquor and/or fetal distress [37].

5.1.3. Neonatal and long-term complications of maternal hypothyroidism

In addition to adverse obstetrical outcomes, maternal hypothyroidism is associated with adverse neonatal outcomes. As the fetus does not begin to produce its own TH until approximately 12 weeks' gestation, it is solely dependent on maternal T4 during early gestation [56,57]. After 12 weeks, thyroid hormone in the fetus continues to be partly supplied by the mother [58].

Untreated maternal hypothyroidism can lead to preterm birth, low birth weight, and respiratory distress in the neonate.

Many studies [4,59] have conclusively proved that children born to mothers with hypothyroidism had a significantly increased risk of impairment in IQ scores, neuropsychological developmental indices and learning abilities. This risk applies to children born not only of untreated women, but also women with suboptimal supplementation.

Children born to uncontrolled hypothyroid mothers are at increased risk of psychomotor development alterations and diminished school performance, reaching recognition and IQ scores [60]

5.1.4. Subclinical hypothyroidism

The risk of pregnancy complications is greater in women with overt, rather than subclinical hypothyroidism [49].

Wang et al. reported an association between SCH and increased risk of spontaneous abortions, but not with gestational hypertension, premature delivery, anemia, postpartum hemorrhage, low APGAR scores, and low birth weight [61].

During pregnancy, TSH levels higher than 4.5 mIU/l have been related to impaired fetal neurological and psychomotor development and an increased risk of premature labor, preeclampsia, and abruption placenta [53,59]

Although the majority of large-scale, well-designed studies depict a consistent adverse impact from mild to moderate to moderate maternel hypothyroidism, some studies are contradictory [49,62]

5.2. Thyroid auto-immunity

Multiple observational studies [63,64,65] and 2 meta-analyses [66,67] have confirmed a 2-4 fold risk of miscarriage among euthyroid TPO antibody-positive women, compared to euthyroid

TPO antibody-negative women. Some studies [68,69] but not all [70,71], have also found associations between thyroid autoimmunity and increased rates of recurrent miscarriage.

The presence of maternal thyroid antibodies has also been associated with a 3-fold risk for premature delivery before 37 weeks gestation [72], postpartum thyroiditis [73], thyroiditis after pregnancy loss [74], and placental abruption. Moreover, the positivity for thyroid autoantibodies in euthyroid pregnant women affects neuropsychological development of the offspring per se [75]

The reasons for the associations between anti-thyroid antibodies and obstetric complications remain unclear. They may be related to a direct effect of the anti-thyroid antibodies, or the anti-thyroid antibodies may serve as a marker for other causative autoimmune syndromes. Alternatively, anti-thyroid antibodies may simply indicate limited thyroid functional reserve [1], suggesting that the association between TPO antibody positivity and obstetric complications may be confounded by even mild hypothyroidism obtained during pregnancy.

Although positive association exists between the presence of thyroid antibodies and pregnancy loss, universal screening for antithyroid antibodies and possible treatment cannot be recommended at this time. However, women with elevated anti-TPO antibodies are at increased risk for miscarriage, preterm delivery and progression of hypothyroidism. Therefore, if identified, such women should be screened for serum TSH abnormalities before pregnancy, as well as during the first and second trimesters of pregnancy.

5.3. Isolated maternal hypothyroxinemia

Isolated maternal hypothyroxinemia is defined as a low FT4 and normal TSH, which can be found in approximately 1% to 2% of pregnancies. In some studies, infants and toddlers whose mothers had isolated maternal hypothyroxinemia during gestation (12 to 20 weeks) had lower mean intelligence, psychomotor, or behavioral scores compared with children born to women with normal thyroid function during gestation [60].

In another study, risks of adverse pregnancy outcomes were not increased in over 200 pregnant women with isolated hypothyroxinemia [40].

However, till date, no study has shown benefit from levothyroxine treatment of isolated hypothyroxinemia during pregnancy, on pregnancy outcome or subsequent infant development.

6. Diagnosis

Clinical semiology of hypothyroidism may be confused or changed by signs of the pregnancy. Tachycardia and cardiovascular erethism, so frequent during pregnancy can mask some signs of pregnancy. On the contrary, other common symptoms during pregnancy can be mistaken for signs of hypothyroidism: fatigue, fluid retention, muscle cramps, constipation, dry skin and hair. Obvious signs such as bradycardia, cold sensitivity, hyporeflexia, paresthesia of extremities, are present in frank hypothyroidism where fertility rate is so small that the possibility of pregnancy is quite unlikely [76].

Because many women may remain asymptomatic, particular attention is required from obstetrical care providers for this condition to be diagnosed and to evaluate more systematically thyroid function when women attend the prenatal clinic for the first time. Only thyroid function tests confirm the diagnosis [77]. Their results differ in healthy pregnant women from those of healthy non pregnant women. This calls for pregnancy-specific and ideally trimester-specific reference intervals for all thyroid function tests but in particular for the most widely applied tests, TSH and FT4 [78]. If a non pregnant reference range is used, many maternal thyroid diseases could be potentially misclassified [79]. Some researchers have established trimester-specific reference intervals for a local population (table 2)

1st author [reference]	1st trimester	2nd trimester	3rd trimester
Stricker R [79]	1.04 (0.09–2.83)	1.02 (0.20–2.79)	1.14 (0.31–2.90)
Haddow JE [80]	0.94 (0.08–2.73)	1.29 (0.39–2.70)	-
Panesar NS [81]	0.80 (0.03–2.30)	1.10 (0.03–3.10)	1.30 (0.13–3.50)
Soldin OP [82]	0.98 (0.24–2.99)	1.09 (0.46–2.95)	1.20 (0.43–2.78)
Bocos-Terraz JP [83]	0.92 (0.03–2.65)	1.12 (0.12–2.64)	1.29 (0.23–3.56)
Marwaha RK [84]	2.10 (0.60–5.00)	2.40 (0.43–5.78)	2.10 (0.74–5.70)
Wang QW [85]**	1.00 (0.02-3.65)	1.26 (0.36-3.46)	1.50 (0.44-5.04)

*Median TSH in mIU/l, with parenthetical data indicating 5th and 95th percentiles [80,81,84] or 2.5th and 97.5th percentiles [79,82,83,85]. **Self-sequential longitudinal reference intervals

Table 2. Sample trimester-specific reference intervals for serum TSH*

The reference range for TSH is lower throughout pregnancy; both the lower normal limit and the upper normal limit of serum TSH are decreased by about 0.1-0.2 mIU/l and 1 mIU/l respectively, compared with the customary TSH reference interval of 0.4-4 mIU/l of non pregnant women. Serum TSH and its reference range rise gradually in the second and third trimesters, except for the study of Marwaha et al. [84], but it is noteworthy that the TSH reference interval remains lower than in non pregnant women [80,81,85].

There are slight but significant ethnic differences in serum TSH concentrations. Black and Asian women have TSH values that are on average 0.4 mIU/l lower than in white women, these differences persist during pregnancy [86]. Pregnant women of Moroccan, Turkish or Surinamese descent residing in the Netherlands have TSH values 0.2-0.3 mIU/l lower than Dutch non pregnant women [87]. TSH concentrations are lower in multiple pregnancies since hCG concentrations are higher [88].

A serum TSH elevation suggests primary hypothyroidism, and serum T4 levels further distinguish between SCH and OH. Only 0.03% of serum total T4 (TT4) content is unbound to serum proteins and is the free T4 available for tissue uptake. Measuring FT4 in the presence of high concentrations of bound T4 has proved challenging especially in abnormal binding-protein states such as pregnancy [78]. According to the recommendations of the American Thyroid Association [78], the optimal method to assess serum FT4 during pregnancy is the measurement of T4 in the dialysate or ultrafiltrate of serum samples employing on-line extraction/liquid chromatography/tandem mass spectrometry (LC/MS/MS). If this method is not available, the free T4 index (adjusted T4) appears to be a reliable assay during pregnancy [77]. The normal ranges for FT4 index are calculated by TT4xT3 uptake or a ratio of TT4 and TBG, but trimester-specific reference intervals for FT4 index have not been established in a reference population [78]. Reference ranges provided by the manufacturers of most T4 measurement kits have been established using pools of non pregnant normal sera [2] and such reference ranges are not valid during pregnancy. The Endocrine Society in 2012 recommended caution in the interpretation of serum FT4 levels during pregnancy and that each laboratory establishes trimester-specific reference ranges for pregnant women [77]. The non pregnant TT4 range (5-12 microg/dl or 50-150 nmol/l) can be adapted in the second and third trimesters by multiplying this range by one and a half-fold [77].

A TSH of 2.5 mIU/l is now accepted as the upper limit of normal for TSH in the first trimester [77]. OH is defined as an elevated TSH (>2.5 mIU/l) in conjunction with a decreased FT4 concentration. Women with TSH levels of 10.0 mIU/l or above, irrespective of their FT4 levels are also considered to have OH. SCH is defined as a serum TSH between 2.5 and 10.0 mIU/l with a normal FT4 concentration. Isolated hypothyroxinemia is defined as a normal maternal TSH concentration in conjunction with FT4 concentrations in the lower 5th or 10th percentile of the reference range [78].

7. Specific interventions

Over the last decade there has been enhanced awareness of the appreciable morbidity of thyroid dysfunction, particularly thyroid deficiency.

Well controlled hypothyroidism does not usually pose major problems in pregnancy and there may be good evidence that the benefits of appropriate interventions largely outweigh the potential risks associated with treatment. Uncertainty exists about the benefits of treatment of women with subclinical hypothyroidism. The overall lack of evidence precluded a recommendation for universal screening [77].

We present here main interventional studies, that compared an intervention for hypothyroidism and/or subclinical hypothyroidism in pregnancy with another intervention, no treatment or placebo, and those that evaluated effects of iodine supplementation during pregnancy, and their effects on maternal and fetal outcomes (Table 3)

7.1. Interventions using Levothyroxine (LT4)

Levothyroxine was compared to no treatment or to no change in treatment during the pregnancy in four randomized controlled trials studies:

- *Negro Ret al*, in a study published in 2006 [72] evaluated 984 pregnant women for autoimmune thyroid disease. Were excluded pregnant women with pre-existing thyroid dysfunction. 11.7% (115 participants) were TPO antibody positive (TPOAb+). They were divided into two groups. Group A (n:57) was treated with LT4, and group B (n:58) was not treated.

http://dx.doi.org/10.5772/54745

The 869 TPOAb- patients (group C) served as a control group. The dosage of LT4varied dependly on TSH and TPOAb titers. The rates of obstetrical complications including gestational hypertension, pre-eclampsia, placental abruption, miscarriage, and preterm birth as well as serum TSH and FT4 were measured. Other outcomes included clinical characteristics of new borns (weight, height, cranial perimeter, Apgar score).

At baseline, TPOAb+ women had higher TSH compared with TPOAb- throughout gestation, FT4 values were lower and TSH higher in group B compared with groups A and C. Groups A and C showed a similar miscarriage rate which was lower than group B. Rate of premature deliveries was higher in group B than groups A and C. Substitutive treatment with LT4 was than able to lower significantly the chance of premature delivery with a trend to a reduced risk miscarriage. Main limitations of this study were the absence of placebo group, the blinding of the outcome assessor was unclear.

- *Rotondi M et al.* [89] in a study published in 2004 conducted a prospective parallel randomized trial. 25 patients with compensated hypothyroidism of different etiology (thyroidectomized and Hashimoto's thyroiditis) and anticipating pregnancy were assigned into two groups. In group 1 (modified n:14), the LT4 dose was adjusted to maintain low-normal TSH levels. Group 2 (unmodified n:11) continued the same treatment. Thyroid function tests were performed pre-conception (at least 60 days from the LT4 increase for the group 1 participants) and at the first post-conception endocrinological visit.

Pre-conception thyroid function evaluation demonstrated significantly higher FT4 and lower TSH in group 1. At the first post-conception thyroid function evaluation, all women in group 1 showed adequate serum FT4 levels while in group 2, three patients had low-normal FT4 levels and one had low FT4 level. The difference was statistically significant between the two groups. None of the Hashimoto's affected patients showed low or low-normal FT4 levels. This study suggests that in hypothyroid women anticipating pregnancy, the pre-conception adjustment of LT4 doses may result in adequate maternal thyroid function up to the first post-conception evaluation. The main limitation of this study was the absence of blinding of the participants, the blinding of the clinicians and outcome assessors was unclear.

- *Negro R et al* [7] in a trial published in 2010 randomly assigned 4562 women in the first trimester to the universal screening or case finding group. Women in both groups were stratified as high risk or low risk based on risk factors for thyroid disease. All women in the universal screening group (n:2280)and high risk women (n:454) in the case-finding group (n:2282) were immediately tested for FT4, TSH and TPO Ab. Low risk women in the case-finding group had their sera tested post-partum. Women with TSH above 2.5 mIU/l and TPOAb+ were given LT4. Women with undetectable TSH and elevated FT4 were given anti-thyroid medication. The rates of obstetrical complications and neonatal outcomes were evaluated.

No significant differences were seen in adverse outcomes between the case-finding and universal screening groups. However, low-risk women in the universal screening group had fewer overall adverse outcomes than low-risk women in the case-finding group. Moreover, more low risk women in the universal screening group with abnormal thyroid function (so treated) avoided adverse outcomes more often than low risk women in the case finding group with abnormal thyroid function (who were not detected and therefore not treated). Main limitation of the study was the lack of direct comparison of treatment and of treatment and non-treatment among the high risk women, and that a power analysis was not performed to determine the sample size

- *Lazarus JH et al.* [90] in a study published in 2012 conducted a randomized trial of antenatal hypothyroidism screening with selective treatment, and assessment of childhood cognitive function. 21846 pregnant women at a median gestational age of 12 weeks 3 days, provided blood samples for measurement of TSH and FT4. Women were assigned to a screening group (n:10924), in which measurements were obtained immediately, or a control group (n: 10922) in which serum was stored and measurements were obtained shortly after delivery. Women with TSH levels >97.5th centile and/or FT4 levels <2.5th centile were designated positive and women in the screening group were prescribed LT4. The primary outcome was IQ at 3 years of age in children of women with positive results, as measured by psychologists who were unaware of the group assignments.

The proportions of women classified as having positive screening results were 4.6% in the screening group and 5% in the control group. 19% of women required LT adjustment. There were no significant difference between IQ scores in the screening and control positive groups, by intension-to-treat analysis. There were no differences between the proportions of children with IQ of less than 85 between the screening and control group. An on-treatment analysis showed no significant difference.

In this study, antenatal screening and treatment for hypothyroidism from about 12 weeks of pregnancy showed no benefit in childhood cognitive function assessed at age three.

Main limitations of this study were: about 24% of the women were lost to follow-up with similar proportions, but 19 women from the screening and 41 from the control group declined to have their child assessed, screening was performed too late in gestation to have a major influence on brain development, childhood cognitive assessment was performed early, and IQ is not sufficient to evaluate cognitive function

7.2. Interventions using selenium

Negro R et al. [91] in his placebo controlled trial published in 2007, examined whether selenium supplementation during and after pregnancy reduces the rate of postpartum thyroiditis and permanent hypothyroidism. Of the 2143 euthyroid pregnant women studied, 7.9% were TPOAB+. During pregnancy and the postpartum period, 77 TPOAb+ women received Selenomethionine 200 microg/d (group S1), 74 TPOAb+ women received placebo (group S0) and 81 TPO Ab- age-matched women were the control group (group C). All the women were advised to use iodized salt. Thyroid function tests were performed at 20 and 30 weeks, at delivery and months 1-2, 5,9 and 12 postpartum. Selenium concentrations were measured at the first visit (mean 9.4 ± 2.7 gestation), at 20 and 30 weeks' gestation, at delivery and 6 and 12 months postpartum. Participants also underwent thyroid ultrasound scanning to assess for thyroiditis at the first visit, at delivery and at 12 months postpartum. Postpartum thyroiditis and permanent hypothyroidism were significantly lower in group S1 compared with S0 (p<0.01).

Main limitation was the loss to follow-up data; in the selenium group 8/85 and in the placebo group 10/84.

7.3. Interventions using iodine

- In severe iodine deficiency areas

Cao XY et al. [92] in a study published in 1994 examined the effect of iodized oil given during pregnancy on neurological outcomes in a severely iodine-deficient area of China (n = 295). Babies were followed for two years. Three independent measures of neural development were used: the results of neurologic examination, the head circumference and indexes of cognitive and motor development. Children of mothers given iodine earlier in pregnancy had improved all neurologic outcomes compared to mothers given iodine later in pregnancy. Treatment later in pregnancy may improve brain growth and developmental achievement slightly, but it does not improve neurologic status.

O'Donnell KJ et al. [93] in their study published in 2002 evaluated growth and development of 689 children (range 4 to 7.3 years whose mothers received iodine during pregnancy, and children who received iodine first in their 2nd year) in a part of China's Province which has the lowest levels of iodine in water and soil ever recorded. Head circumference but not height was improved for those whose mothers received iodine during pregnancy (compared with those receiving iodine at age 2) and for those supplemented before the end of the 2nd trimester (relative to those supplemented during the 3rd trimester). Iodine before the 3rd trimester predicted higher psychomotor test scores for children relative to those provided iodine later in pregnancy or at 2 years. Results from the test for cognitive development resulted in trend only differences between those children supplemented during pregnancy versus later.

- In moderate to mild iodine deficiency areas

In 2009, two randomized trials were published investigating the effect of iodine supplementation in moderately iodine deficient pregnant women on neurodevelopment of their children. *Berbel P et al.* [94] recruited three groups of pregnant women living in Spain at different phases of gestation; the first group of women had T4 concentrations >20th percentile at recruitment (>0.92 ng/dL at 4–6 weeks gestation), while the second and third groups of women had T4 concentrations <10th percentile (<0.83 ng/dL) at 12–14 weeks gestation and near term, respectively. All three groups of women were supplemented with 200 μg of iodine until the end of lactation. When the children were 18 months old, the development quotient of children in mothers supplemented in the first group was significantly higher than that of children whose mothers received supplements from 12–14 weeks gestation and near term. A limitation of this study was the small numbers of children tested, with less than 20 children in each of the three groups. Furthermore, the women supplemented later in pregnancy or at term were specifically selected because they had low FT4 in pregnancy, while the women supplemented earlier in pregnancy had a higher FT4, thus a difference in FT4 rather than the iodine supplementation may account for the findings. A second Spanish study conducted in an area of moderate iodine deficiency by *Velasco I et al.* [95], evaluated the psychological development of infants aged 3 to 18 months whose mothers (n:133) had received 300 microg of potassium iodide during the first trimester of their pregnancy and compared with infants whose mothers had received no iodine supplements (n:61). Were evaluated the neuropsychological status of the children and levels of TSH, FT3, FT4, and urinary iodine. Those children whose mothers had received iodine supplement had a more favorable psychometric assessment than those of the other group of mothers. A limitation of this study was that children were tested at different ages in this study (5.5 months *vs.* 12.4 months), and the possible presence of confounding variables not controlled for in this study. Finally, both studies were not randomized, double-blind, placebo-controlled trials, and although they suggest that neurodevelopment in the child may be adversely affected by moderate iodine deficiency, they are certainly not definitive

Author (year)	Country	n	Methods	Outcome measures
Negro R (2006) [72]	Italy	984	Pregnant women TPOAb+ randomized to levothyroxine vs no treatment	Miscarriage, gestational hypertension, pre-eclampsia, preterm birth, placental abruption
Rotondi M (2004) [89]	Italy	25	Women with overt hypothyroidism anticipating pregnancy randomized to adjusted dose of LT4 to have TSH low-normal or unmodified treatment	FT4, FT3, TSH
Negro R (2010) [7]	Italy	4562	Women in first trimester pregnancy randomized to universal screening group or case-finding group. LT4 was given if TSH"/ >2.5 mIU/l and TPOAb+	Obstetrical complications (miscarriage, gestational hypertension, preeclampsia..) and neonatal outcomes (weight, preterm delivery, Apgar score…)
Lazarus JH (2012) [90]	United Kingdom, Italy	21846	Pregnant women at 15weeks 6days or less provided blood samples for TSH and FT4, randomized to screening group or control group. Women with TSH"/>97.5 and/or FT4<2.5th centile in the screening group were given LT4	IQ of children at age 3 years
Negro R (2007) [91]	Italy	2143	Euthyroid pregnant women studied. TPOAb+ randomized to receive selenomthionine 200 microg/d or placebo	Thyroid function tests, thyroid antibodies, thyroid ultrasound
Cao XY (1994) [92]	China	295	Pregnant women in severely iodine deficient area given iodized oil	Neurologic examination, head circumference, indexes of cognitive and motor development
O'Donnel KJ (2002) [93]	USA	689	A group of pregnant women received iodine during pregnancy and a group of children received iodine during their 2nd year	Head circumference, height, psychomotor and cognitive development
Berbel P (2009) [94]	Spain	96	Women 4–6 weeks gestation with FT4 "/> 20th percentile (Group1) *vs.* women with FT4 < 10th percentile at 12–14 weeks (Group 2) or at 37–40 weeks (Group3) given iodine 200 microg /d until end of lactation.	Brunet-Lezine developmental quotient
Velasco I (2009 [95]	Spain	191	Women <10 weeks gestation (Group 1) *vs.* last month of pregnancy (Group 2) given iodine 300 microg /d until end of lactation	Bayley Psychomotor Development Index

Table 3. Interventional studies for clinical and subclinical hypothyroidism in pregnancy

8. Screening

In the past several years, there has been considerable discussion about whether all pregnant women should be screened in order to identify and treat thyroid dysfunction. Screening is defined as 'the presumptive identification of unrecognized disease or defect by the application of tests, examinations, or other procedures which can be applied rapidly. Screening tests sort out apparently well persons who probably have a disease from those who probably do not' [96]. Ideally all the following criteria should be met: The Condition should be an important health problem, its epidemiology and natural history should be well known. The test should be a simple, safe, precise and validated with agreed reference range. The treatment should be effective, there should be agreed evidence based policies covering which subjects need treatment and the appropriate treatment to be offered. The Screening Program should be effective in reducing mortality or morbidity (evidence from high quality Randomized Controlled Trials); should be clinically, socially and ethically acceptable to health professionals and the public. The benefit from the screening program should outweigh the physical and psychological harm (caused by the test, diagnostic procedures and treatment). The opportunity cost of the screening program should be economically balanced in relation to expenditure on medical care as a whole (cost benefit and/or cost effectiveness analyses) [97].

In the case for thyroid screening in pregnancy, most of the above points are satisfied. Both OH and SCH are prevalent. Serum TSH is relatively inexpensive, widely available and is a reliable test in pregnancy, assuming that trimester-specific reference ranges are applied [78]. The adverse maternal and fetal effects associated with OH have been clearly demonstrated. The problem is still represented by the halo of uncertainty that surrounds clinical entities such as SCH and isolated hypothyroxinemia. The lack of high quality randomized controlled trials in these two conditions had led to mixed viewpoints among members of the American Thyroid Association [78] and the Endocrine Society [77]. Both agree that there are not enough data for or against universal screening but also acknowledge that lack of evidence of benefit doesn't mean that there is no benefit.

In their recent guidelines, the American Thyroid Association [78], and the Endocrine Society [77] recommend prenatal measurement of serum TSH in women at high risk for thyroid illness on the basis of their medical history, physical exam, or prior chemical data. (Table 4)

There is insufficient evidence to recommend for or against screening all women for thyroid antibodies in the first trimester of pregnancy [78]. Universal screening for the presence of anti-TPO antibodies either before or during pregnancy is therefore not recommended [77]. However, women with elevated anti-TPO antibodies are at increased risk for miscarriage, preterm delivery, progression of hypothyroidism, and postpartum thyroiditis. Therefore, if identified, such women should be screened for serum TSH abnormalities before pregnancy, as well as during the first and second trimesters of pregnancy.

Women over age 30 years
Women with a family history or autoimmune thyroid disease or hypothyroidism
Women with a goiter
Women with thyroid antibodies, primarily thyroid peroxidase antibodies
Women with symptoms or clinical signs suggestive of thyroid hypofunction
Women with type 1 diabetes mellitus, or other autoimmune disorders
Women with infertility
Women with a prior history of miscarriage and preterm delivery
Women with prior therapeutic head or neck irradiation or prior thyroid surgery
Women currently receiving levothyroxine replacement
Women living in a region presumed with iodine deficiency

Table 4. Recommended patient profiles for targeted thyroid disease case finding in women seeking pregnancy, or newly pregnant [77]

9. Management

Hypothyroidism is treated with synthetic thyroid hormone called Levothyroxine (LT4), a medication which is identical to the T_4 made by the thyroid. Synthetic thyroxine is safe and necessary for the well-being of the fetus if the mother has hypothyroidism. It is strongly recommended not to use other preparations such as T3 or desiccated thyroid [78]. There are a variety of approaches to the management of thyroxine replacement in known hypothyroid women at the time of pregnancy that are all effective for maintaining a normal range during pregnancy. Women with preexisting hypothyroidism will need to increase their prepregnancy dose of thyroxine to maintain a normal thyroid function.

Thyroid function should be checked every 6 to 8 weeks during pregnancy.

9.1. Overt hypothyroidism and pregnancy

9.1.1. Pre-pregnancy

Physicians should consider diagnosis of hypothyroidism in patients with infertility or menstrual disorders, medical therapy should be optimized and pregnancy delayed until good control is achieved [98].

9.1.2. *Pregnancy*

In a newly diagnosed hypothyroid patient, a full replacement thyroxine dose should be instituted immediately, assuming there are no abnormalities in cardiac function.

Thyroxine requirement increases in pregnant patients as early as fifth week of pregnancy [98].Hypothyroid women who are already on thyroxine prior to pregnancy need to increase their daily dosage, on an average, by 30-50% above preconception dosage as soon as pregnancy is diagnosed [77]. The adjustment is based on results of thyroid function tests. Thyroxine replacement should be given at a dose that insures a serum FT4 level at the upper end of normal range for each trimester of pregnancy and a serum TSH level < 2.5 mIU/L in the first trimester or 3 mIU/l in the second and third trimesters. In women who have had a thyroidectomy for thyroid cancer, it is necessary to suppress TSH secretion [77].

Treatment should be initiated at a dose of 100–150 microgm/day or titrated according to body weight (2.0–2.4 micrograms/kg body weight/day). In diagnosed cases, as thyroxine requirements increase, dosage adjustments are required. Suggested mechanisms for this increased requirement include an elevated extrathyroidal pool of T4; the need to saturate large quantities of TBG; increased degradation of T4; reduced absorption of T4, especially if taken with iron supplements; and increased transfer of T4 from mother to fetus. Because a similar increased requirement is seen in hypothyroid post menopausal women who are given estrogen replacement, this increased demand in pregnancy may be caused by increased estrogen production [99].

Dose of thyroxine also depends on the etiology of hypothyroidism. In disorders with very little residual tissue, like radioiodine ablation or extensive thyroid surgery, increment in thyroxine dosage is greater than women with Hashimoto's thyroiditis, who usually have some residual thyroid tissue. Women should be followed up every 4–6 weeks with serum TSH value, till delivery, to facilitate periodic adjustment of LT4 supplementation. [77]

Thyroxine absorption is decreased by certain drugs including iron and calcium supplement. Thyroxine is best taken on an empty stomach and four hours apart from iron supplements or soy products. [32].

When adequate control is achieved, no specific measures are needed for labour and delivery. However, when large goiter causes respiratory compromise, anesthetic or surgical advice may be required [100].

c-After delivery, hypothyroid women need to decrease the LT4 dosage they received during pregnancy to prepregnancy dose and have their serum TSH level re-evaluated after 6 weeks [77].

9.1.3. *Post-partum follow-up: At post-partum, two patterns of thyroid dysfunction can be discerned*

- Postpartum thyroiditis characterized by transient hyperthyroidism or transient hyperthyroidism followed by transient or rarely permanent hypothyroidism,
- Postpartum exacerbation of chronic Hashimoto's thyroiditis leading to transient or permanent hypothyroidism.

The hyperthyroid phase of postpartum thyroiditis is treated with a beta-adrenergic antagonist drugs. Transient hypothyroidism is treated with LT4, which may be continued till six months and then tapered to determine if the hypothyroidism is permanent. Thyroid function tests should be monitored for at least 6 months after delivery [78].

9.2. Subclinical hypothyroidism and pregnancy

Since maternal morbidity as well as prenatal morbidity and consequences on the neuropsychological development of the child have been reported in subclinical hypothyroidism, most guidelines recommend thyroxine replacement in women with subclinical hypothyroidism. Association studies have yielded conflicting results regarding outcomes such as miscarriage, hypertension, placental abruption, and preterm delivery, and to date, one single center has demonstrated a significant reduction in obstetrical and neonatal complications when subclinically hypothyroid women are treated from the first trimester [3,7].

The endocrine guidelines 2012 confirm the suggestion of treating subclinical autoimmune hypothyroidism with LT4 because the potential benefits from treatment outweigh the risk of potential adverse events [77]. The panel also recommends treating antibody-negative women who have subclinical hypothyroidism. Despite the absence of relevant single center, this recommendation seems reasonable given that independent of thyroid autoimmunity, an increased TSH level is associated with a miscarriage risk, and an elevated TSH at the beginning of pregnancy may predispose the mother to further impairment of thyroid function in the following months [77].

9.3. Isolated hypothyroxinemia

Its management is controversial and requires further study. “Partial replacement therapy” with LT4 may be initiated at the discretion of the physician, with continued monitoring [77]. This recommendation directly leads to another point examined in the guidelines: awareness about the possible inaccuracy of serum FT4 measurement in pregnancy.

The absence of a universally accepted trimester-specific reference range (and the common absence of each single laboratory-specific reference range) is an issue that makes defining cutoff values difficult and complicates clear identification of isolated hypothyroxinemia as a clinical entity. [77]

9.4. Iodine intake during pregnancy

Iodine is an essential nutrient required for thyroid hormone production and is primarily derived from the diet and from vitamin/mineral preparations. The Institute of Medicine recommended dietary allowances to be used as goals for individual total daily iodine intake (dietary and supplement) are 150 microg/d for women planning a pregnancy, 220 microg/d for pregnant women, and 290 microg/d for women who are breastfeeding [101]. WHO recommends 250 microg/d for pregnant women and for lactating women [102]. Iodine intake during pregnancy should not exceed twice the daily recommended nutrient intake for iodine, *i.e.* 500 microg iodine per day [77]. To reach the daily recommended nutrient intake for iodine, multiple means must be considered, tailored to the iodine intake level in a given population.

Different situations must therefore be distinguished:

1. Countries with iodine sufficiency and/or with a well-established universal salt iodization (USI) program;

2. Countries without a USI program or with an established USI program where the coverage is known to be only partial

3. Remote areas with no accessible USI program and difficult socioeconomic conditions.

The Endocrine Society recommend once-daily prenatal vitamins containing 150–200 microg iodine, in the form of potassium iodide or iodate, the content of which is verified to ensure that all pregnant women taking prenatal vitamins are protected from iodine deficiency. Ideally, supplementation should be started before conception.

10. Conclusion

Thyroid hormone production increases in pregnancy and requires increased iodine intake. Serum TSH concentrations should be interpreted in the context of pregnancy physiology. Thyroid function and thyroid antibody screening during pregnancy is controversial. Further research is needed to determine whether mild maternal hypothyroidism or positive thyroid antibodies are associated with obstetric complications.

Maternal hypothyroidism is a disorder with great potential to adversely affect maternal and fetal outcomes. If the condition is detected early, it is easy to treat, with very little detriment to the mother and the fetus. Hence, this condition needs early detection, prompt initiation of treatment, adequate follow-up and most importantly, sufficient education of the doctors and the patients regarding these objectives, the importance of this condition and the ease and advantages of prompt management.

Author details

Baha Zantour[1*], Wafa Alaya[1], Hela Marmouch[2] and Wafa Chebbi[1]

*Address all correspondence to: bahazantour@yahoo.fr

1 Department of Endocrinology, Tahar Sfar Hospital, Mahdia, Tunisia

2 Department of Endocrinology, Fattouma Bourguiba Hospital, Monastir, Tunisia

References

[1] Glinoer D. The regulation of thyroid function in pregnancy: pathways of endocrine adaptation from physiology to pathology. Endocrine Reviews 1997; 18(3): 404-433. http://edrv.endojournals.org/content/18/3/404.full.pdf+html

[2] Abalovich M, Amino N, Barbour LA, Cobin RH, Degroot LJ, Glinoer D, Mandel SJ, Stagnaro-Green A. Management of thyroid dysfunction during pregnancy and postpartum: an Endocrine Society Clinical Practice Guideline. Journal of Clinical Endocrinology and Metabolism 2007; 92 (8 suppl): S1-47. http://www.ncbi.nlm.nih.gov/pubmed/17948378

[3] Krassas GE, Popper K, Glinoer D. Thyroid function and human reproductive health. Endocrine Reviews 2010; 31(5): 702-755. http://edrv.endojournals.org/content/31/5/702.full.pdf+html

[4] Haddow JE, Palomaki GE, Allan WC, Williams JR, Knight GJ, Gagnon J, O'Heir CE, Mitchell ML, Hermos RJ, Waisbren SE, Faix JD, Klein RZ. Maternal thyroid deficiency during pregnancy and subsequent neuropsychological development of the child. New England Journal of Medicine 1999; 341(8): 549-555. http://www.nejm.org/doi/pdf/10.1056/NEJM199908193410801

[5] Casey BM, Dashe JS, Wells CE, McIntire DD, Byrd W, Leveno KJ, Cunningham FG. Subclinical hypothyroidism and pregnancy outcomes. Obstetrical Gynecology 2005; 105(2): 239-215. http://www.ncbi.nlm.nih.gov/pubmed/15684146

[6] Reid SM, Middleton P, Cossich MC, Crowther CA. Interventions for clinical and subclinical hypothyroidism in pregnancy. Cochrane Database of systematic reviews 2010, Issue 7. Art. N°: CD007752. DOI: 10.1002/14651858. CD007752.pub2. http://onlinelibrary.wiley.com/doi/10.1002/14651858.CD007752.pub2/pdf

[7] Negro R, Schwartz A, Gismoudi R, Tinelli A, Mangieri T, Stagnaro-Green A. Universal screening versus case finding for detection and treatment of thyroid hormonal dysfunction during pregnancy. Journal of Clinical Endocrinology and Metabolism 2010; 95(4): 1699-1707. http://jcem.endojournals.org/content/95/4/1699.full.pdf+html

[8] Glinoer D, De Nayer P. Thyroid and its diseases in pregnancy. In: Monaco F, Satta MA, Shapiro B, Troncone L. Thyroid Diseases: Clinical Fundamentals and Therapy 1993; 517–527.

[9] Robbins J. Thyroid hormone transport proteins and the physiology of hormone binding. In: Braverman LE, Utiger RD. The Thyroid, JB Lippincott, Philadelphia, 1996,96–111

[10] Robbins J. Thyroxine transport and the free hormone hypothesis. Endocrinology 1992; 131(2):546 –547. http://www.ncbi.nlm.nih.gov/pubmed/1639006

[11] Glinoer D, McGuire RA, Gershengorn MC, Robbins J, Berman M. Effects of estrogen on thyroxine-binding globulin metabolism in Rhesus monkeys. Endocrinology1977;100(1): 9–17. http://www.ncbi.nlm.nih.gov/pubmed/401485

[12] Sparre LS, Brundin J, Carlstro° m K, Carlstro°m A. Oestrogen and thyroxine-binding globulin levels in early normal pregnancy. Acta Endocrinologica (Copenh) 1987;114(2): 298 –304. http://www.ncbi.nlm.nih.gov/pubmed/3103363

[13] Robbins J, Nelson JH. Thyroxine-binding by serum proteins in pregnancy and in the newborn. The journal of clinical Investigation 1958; 37(2):153–159. http://www.ncbi.nlm.nih.gov/pmc/articles/PMC293071/pdf/jcinvest00323-0029.pdf

[14] Robbins J, Cheng S-Y, Gershengorn M, Glinoer D, Cahnmann HJ, Edelhoch H. Thyroxine transport proteins of plasma: molecular properties and biosynthesis. Recent Progress in Hormon Research 1978; 34:477–519. http://www.ncbi.nlm.nih.gov/pubmed/216060

[15] Hotelling DR, Sherwood LM. The effects of pregnancy on circulating triiodothyronine. The journal of clinical endocrinology and metabolism 1971;33(5):783–786. http://www.ncbi.nlm.nih.gov/pubmed/5001493

[16] Glinoer D. Thyroid regulation during pregnancy. In: Iodine Deficiency in Europe: A Continuing Concern. NATO ASI Series (Vol 241). Plenum Press, New York, 1993; 181–190

[17] Ballabio M, Poshyachinda M, Ekins RP. Pregnancy-induced changes in thyroid function: role of human chorionic gonadotropin as putative regulator of maternal thyroid. Journal of Clinical Endocrinology and Metabolism 1991;73(4):824 –831. http://www.ncbi.nlm.nih.gov/pubmed?term=Pregnancy-induced%20changes%20in%20thyroid%20function%3A%20role%20of%20human%20chorionic%20gonadotropin%20as%20putative%20regulator%20of%20maternal%20thyroid

[18] Ball R, Freedman DB, Holmes JC, Midgley JE, Sheehan CP. Low-normal concentrations of free thyroxin in serum in late pregnancy: physiological fact, not technical artefact. Clinical Chemistry 1989;35(9): 1891–1896. http://www.clinchem.org/content/35/9/1891.long

[19] Juan C. Galofre, Terry F. Davies. Autoimmune Thyroid Disease in Pregnancy: A Review. Journal of women's health 2009;18(11):1847-1856 http://www.ncbi.nlm.nih.gov/pmc/articles/PMC2828163/pdf/jwh.2008.1234.pdf

[20] Ylikorkala O, Kivinen S, Reinila M. Serial prolactin and thyrotropin responses to thyrotropin-releasing hormone throughout normal human pregnancy. Journal of Clinical Endocrinology and Metabolism 1979;48(2): 288 –292. http://jcem.endojournals.org/content/48/2/288.long

[21] Kvetny J, Poulsen HK. Nuclear thyroxine and 3,5,39-triiodothyronine receptors in human mononuclear blood cells during pregnancy. Acta Endocrinologica (Copenh) 1984;105(1):19 –23. http://www.ncbi.nlm.nih.gov/pubmed?term=Nuclear%20thyro-

xine%20and%203%2C5%2C39-triiodothyronine%20receptors%20in%20human %20mononuclear%20blood%20cells%20during%20pregnancy

[22] Hidal JT, Kaplan MM. Characteristics of thyroxine 59-deiodination in cultured human placental cells: regulation by iodothyronines. The journal of clinical investigation 1985;76(3):947–955. http://www.ncbi.nlm.nih.gov/pmc/articles/PMC423958/pdf/jcinvest00123-0061.pdf

[23] Roti E, Fang SL, Emerson CH, Braverman LE. Human placenta is an active site of thyroxine and 3, 39, 5-triiodothyronine tyrosyl ring deiodination. Journal of Clinical Endocrinology and Metabolism 1981;53(3):498 –501. http://www.ncbi.nlm.nih.gov/pubmed?term=Human%20placenta%20is%20an%20active%20site%20of%20thyroxine%20and%203%2C%2039%2C%205-triiodothyronine%20tyrosyl%20ring%20deiodination

[24] Lemon M, Bevan BR, Li TC, Pennington GW. Thyroid function in trophoblastic disease. British Journal of Obstetrics and Gynaecology 1987;94(11):1084 –1088. http://www.ncbi.nlm.nih.gov/pubmed?term=Thyroid%20function%20in%20trophoblastic %20disease%20British%20Journal%20of%20Obstetrics%20and%20Gynaecology

[25] Kosugi S, Mori T. TSH receptor and LH receptor. Endocrine Journal 1995;42(5):587–606. https://www.jstage.jst.go.jp/article/endocrj1993/42/5/42_5_587/_pdf

[26] Glinoer D, De Nayer P, Robyn C, Lejeune B, Kinthaert J, Meuris S. Serum levels of intact human chorionic gonadotropin (hCG) and its free a and b subunits, in relation to maternal thyroid 3 stimulation during normal pregnancy. Journal of Clinical Investigation 1993;16(11):881–888. http://www.ncbi.nlm.nih.gov/pubmed?term=Serum %20levels%20of%20intact%20human%20chorionic%20gonadotropin%20(hCG) %20and%20its%20free%20a%20and%20b%20subunits%2C%20in%20relation%20to %20maternal%20thyroid%203%20stimulation%20during%20normal%20pregnancy.

[27] Grün JP, Meuris S, De Nayer P, Glinoer D, The thyrotropic role of human chorionic gonadotropin (hCG) in the early stages of twin (vs. single) pregnancy. Clinical Endocrinology (Oxf) 1997; 46(6):719-725. http://www.ncbi.nlm.nih.gov/pubmed?term=The %20thyrotropic%20role%20of%20human%20chorionic%20gonadotropin%20(hCG) %20in%20the%20early%20stages%20of%20twin%20(vs.%20single)%20pregnancy

[28] Glinoer D, De Nayer P, Bourdoux P, Lemone M, Robyn C, Van Steirteghem A, Kinthaert J, Lejeune B. Regulation of maternal thyroid during pregnancy. Journal of Clinical Endocrinology and Metabolism 1990;71(2):276 –287. http://www.ncbi.nlm.nih.gov/pubmed/2116437

[29] Glinoer D. The importance of iodine nutrition during pregnancy. Public Health Nutrition 2007;10(12A):1542–1546. http://journals.cambridge.org/abstract_S1368980007360886

[30] Pochin EE. The iodine uptake of the human thyroid throughout the menstrual cycle and in pregnancy. Clinical Science1952;11(4):441– 445.

[31] Smyth PP. Variation in iodine handling during normal pregnancy. Thyroid 1999;9(7): 637–42. http://www.ncbi.nlm.nih.gov/pubmed?term=Variation%20in%20iodine%20handling%20during%20normal%20pregnancy

[32] Ballabio M, Nicolini U, Jowett T, Ruiz de Elvira MC, Ekins RP, Rodeck CH. Maturation of thyroid function in normal human foetuses. Clinical Endocrinology (Oxf) 1989;31(5): 565–571. http://www.ncbi.nlm.nih.gov/pubmed/2516787

[33] Delange F, Dunn JT, Glinoer D. General comments, conclusions and final recommendations. In: Delange F, Dunn JT, Glinoer D. Iodine Deficiency in Europe: A Continuing Concern. NATO ASI Series. Plenum Press, New York, 1993;241: 473–478.

[34] Leung AM, Pearce EN, Braverman LE. Iodine Nutrition in pregnancy and Lactation. Endocrinology and Metabolism Clinics of North America 2011;40(4): 765–777. http://www.ncbi.nlm.nih.gov/pubmed?term=Endocrinology%20and%20Metabolism%20Clinics%20of%20North%20America.%202011%3B%2040(4)%3A%20765%E2%80%93777

[35] Skjo° ldebrand L, Brundin J, Carlstro° m A, Pettersson T. Thyroid associated components in serum during normal pregnancy. Acta Endocrinologica (Copenh) 1982;100(4): 504 –511. http://www.ncbi.nlm.nih.gov/pubmed/6812340

[36] Burrow GN, Fisher DA, Larsen PR. Maternal and fetal thyroid function. New England journal of Medicine 1994;331:1072–1078. http://www.nejm.org/doi/pdf/10.1056/NEJM199503023320919

[37] Allan WC, Haddow JE, Palomaki GE, Williams JR, Mitchell ML, Hermos RJ, Faix JD, Klein RZ. Maternal thyroid deficiency and pregnancy complications: implications for population screening. Journal of medical Screening 2000;7(3):127-130. http://jms.rsmjournals.com/content/7/3/127.full.pdf

[38] Potlukova E, Potluka O, Jiskra J, Limanova Z, Telicka Z, Bartakova J, Springer D. Is age a risk factor for hypothyroidism in pregnancy? An analysis of 5223 pregnant women. Journal of Clinical Endocrinology and Metabolism 2012; 97(6):1945-1952. http://www.ncbi.nlm.nih.gov/pubmed?term=Potlukova%20JCEM%202012

[39] Blatt AJ, Nakamoto JM, Kaufman HW. National status of testing for hypothyroidism during pregnancy and postpartum. Journal of Clinical Endocrinology and Metabolism 2012;97(3):777-784. http://www.ncbi.nlm.nih.gov/pubmed?term=Blatt%20JCEM%202011

[40] Casey BM, Dashe JS, Spong CY, McIntire DD, Leveno KJ, Cunningham GF. Perinatal significance of isolated maternal hypothyroxinemia identified in the first half of pregnancy. Obstetrical Gynecology 2007; 109(5):1129-1135. http://www.ncbi.nlm.nih.gov/pubmed/17470594

[41] Cleary-Goldman J, Malone FD, Lambert-Messerlian G, Sullivan L, Canick J, Porter TF, Luthy D, Gross S, Bianchi DW, D'Alton ME. Maternal thyroid hypofunction and

pregnancy outcome. Obstetrical Gynecology 2008; 112(1):85-92. http://www.ncbi.nlm.nih.gov/pubmed/18591312

[42] Berbel P, Mestre JL, Santamaría A, Palazón I, Franco A, Graells M, González-Torga A, de Escobar GM. Delayed neurobehavioral development in children born to pregnant women with mild hypothyroxinemia during the first month of gestation: the importance of early iodine supplementation. Thyroid 2009; 19(5):511-519. http://www.ncbi.nlm.nih.gov/pubmed/19348584

[43] Moleti M, Lo Presti VP, Mattina F, Mancuso A, De Vivo A, Giorgianni G, Di Bella B, Trimarchi F, Vermiglio F. Gestational thyroid function abnormalities in conditions of mild iodine deficiency: early screening versus continuous monitoring of maternal thyroid status. European Journal of Endocrinology 2009; 160(4): 611-617. http://www.ncbi.nlm.nih.gov/pubmed/19179457

[44] Henrichs J, Bongers-Schokking JJ, Schenk JJ, Ghassabian A, Schmidt HG, Visser TJ, Hooijkaas H, de Muinck Keizer-Schrama SM, Hofman A, Jaddoe VV, Visser W, Steegers EA, Verhulst FC, de Rijke YB, Tiemeier H. Maternal thyroid function during early pregnancy and cognitive functioning in early childhood: the generation R study. Journal of Clinical Endocrinology and Metabolism 2010; 95(9):4227-4234. http://www.ncbi.nlm.nih.gov/pubmed/20534757

[45] Jameson JL, Weetman AP. Disorders of the thyroid gland. Harrison's principles of internal medicine. 17th Edition. USA: Blackwell publishing; 2008: 2224-2247

[46] Liberman CS, Pino SC, Fang SL, Baverman LE, Emerson CH. Circulating iodide concentrations during and after pregnancy. Journal of Clinical Endocrinology and Metabolism 1998; 83(10): 3545-3549. http://jcem.endojournals.org/content/83/10/3545.full.pdf+html

[47] Brander L, Als C, Buess H, Haldimann F, Harder M, Hanggi W, Herrmann U, Lauber K, Niederer U, Zurcher T, Burgi U, Gerber H. Urinary iodine concentrations during pregnancy in an area of unstable dietary iodine intake in Switzerland. Journal of Endocrinological Investigations 2003; 26(5): 389-396. http://www.jendocrinolinvest.it/jei/en/abstract.cfm?articolo_id=5638

[48] 48-WHO, UNICEF, ICCIDD. Assessment of iodine deficiency disorders and monitoring their elimination. A guide for programme managers. Third edition. World Health Organization, Geneva, Switzerland, 2007

[49] Abalovich M, Gutierrez S, Alcaraz G, Maccallini G, Garcia A, Levalle O. Overt and subclinical hypothyroidism complicating pregnancy. Thyroid 2002; 12(1): 63-68. http://online.liebertpub.com/doi/pdf/10.1089/105072502753451986

[50] McElduff A, Morris J. Thyroid function tests and thyroid antibodies in an unselected population of women undergoing first trimester screening for aneuploidy. Australian and New Zealand Journal of Obstetrics and Gynecology 2008; 48(5): 478-480. http://onlinelibrary.wiley.com/doi/10.1111/j.1479-828X.2008.00903.x/abstract

[51] Medici M, de Rijke YB, Peeters RP, Visser W, de Muinck Keizer-Schrama SM, Jaddoe VV, Hofman A, Hooijkaas H, Steegers EA, Tiemeier H, Bongers-Schokking JJ, Visser TJ. Maternal early pregnancy and newborn thyroid hormone parameters: the Generation R study. Journal of Clinical Endocrinology and Metabolism 2012; 97(2):646-652. http://jcem.endojournals.org/content/97/2/646.long

[52] Wang Y, Zhong J, Xu H, Wei W, Dong J, Yu F, Wang Y, Gong J, Shan Z, Teng W, Chen J. Perinatal iodine deficiency and hypothyroidism increase cell apoptosis and alter doublecortin and reelin protein expressions in rat cerebellum. Archives of medical research 2012; 43(4): 255-264. http://www.arcmedres.com/article/S0188-4409(12)00127-0/abstract

[53] LaFranchi SH, Haddow JE, Hollowell JG. Is thyroid inadequacy during gestation a risk factor for adverse pregnancy and developmental outcomes? Thyroid 2005;15(1):60–71. http://online.liebertpub.com/doi/abs/10.1089/thy.2005.15.60

[54] Montoro MN. Management of hypothyroidism during pregnancy. Clinical Obstetrics Gynecology 1997;40(1):65–80. http://www.ncbi.nlm.nih.gov/pubmed?term=LaFranchi%20SH%2C%20Haddow%20JE%2C%20Hollowell%20JG.%20Is%20thyroid%20inadequacy%20during%20gestation%20a%20risk%20factor%20for%20adverse%20pregnancy%20and%20developmental%20outcomes%3F%20Thyroid%202005%3B15(1)%3A60%E2%80%9371.

[55] Idris I, Srinivasan R, Simm A, Page RC. Maternal hypothyroidism in early and late gestation: effects on neonatal and obstetric outcome. Clinical Endocrinology (Oxf) 2005; 63(5):560–565. http://onlinelibrary.wiley.com/doi/10.1111/j.13652265.2005.02382.x/abstract;jsessionid=571F2AA67A189EBC2DD6E7004DCF0BDB.d04t03

[56] Contempre B, Jauniaux E, Calvo R, Jurkovic D, Campbell S, de Escobar GM. Detection of thyroid hormones in human embryonic cavities during the first trimester of pregnancy. Journal of Clinical Endocrinology and Metabolism 1993;77(6):1719-1722. http://jcem.endojournals.org/content/77/6/1719.long

[57] Morreale de EG, Obregon MJ, Escobar del RF. Role of thyroid hormone during early brain development. European Journal of Endocrinology 2004;151(Suppl 3): U25-U37. http://eje-online.org/content/151/Suppl_3/U25.long

[58] Utiger RD. Maternal hypothyroidism and fetal development. New England Journal of Medecine 1999; 341(8):601-602. http://www.nejm.org/doi/full/10.1056/NEJM199908193410809

[59] Pop VJ, Kuijpens JL, van Baar AL, Verkerk G, van Son MM, de Vijlder JJ, Vulsma T, Wiersinga WM, Drexhage HA, Vader HL. Low maternal free thyroxine concentrations during early pregnancy are associated with impaired psychomotor development in infancy. Clinical Endocrinology (Oxf) 1999;50(2): 149–155. http://onlinelibrary.wiley.com/doi/10.1046/j.1365-2265.1999.00639.x/abstract

[60] Vermiglio F, Lo Presti VP, Moleti M, Sidoti M, Tortorella G, Scaffidi G, Castagna MG, Mattina F, Violi MA, Crisà A, Artemisia A, Trimarchi F. Attention deficit and hyper-

activity disorders in the offspring of mothers exposed to mild-moderate iodine deficiency: A possible novel iodine deficiency disorder in developed countries. Journal of Clinical Endocrinology and Metabolism 2004;89(12): 6054–6060. http://jcem.endojournals.org/content/89/12/6054.long

[61] Wang S, Teng WP, Li JX, Wang WW, Shan ZY. Effects of maternal subclinical hypothyroidism on obstetrical outcomes during early pregnancy. Journal of Endocrinology Investication 2012; 35(3):322-325. http://www.jendocrinolinvest.it/jei/en/abstract.cfm?articolo_id=7772

[62] Männistö T, Vääräsmäki M, Pouta A, Hartikainen AL, Ruokonen A, Surcel HM, Bloigu A, Järvelin MR, Suvanto-Luukkonen E Perinatal outcome of children born to mothers with thyroid dysfunction or antibodies: a prospective population-based cohort study. Jounal of Clinical Endocrinolology and Metabolism 2009; 94(3):772–779. http://www.ncbi.nlm.nih.gov/pubmed/19106271

[63] Abbassi-Ghanavati M, Casey BM, Spong CY, McIntire DD, Halvorson LM, Cunningham FG. Pregnancy outcomes in women with thyroid peroxidase antibodies. Obstetrics Gynecology 2010; 116(2 Pt 1): 381–386. http://www.ncbi.nlm.nih.gov/pubmed?term=Pregnancy%20outcomes%20in%20women%20with%20thyroid%20peroxidase%20antibodies.%20Obstetrics%20Gynecology%202010%3B116(2%20Pt%201)%3A381%E2%80%936.

[64] Bagis T, Gokcel A, Saygili ES. Autoimmune thyroid disease in pregnancy and the postpartum period: relationship to spontaneous abortion. Thyroid 2001;11(11):1049–1053. http://www.ncbi.nlm.nih.gov/pubmed?term=Autoimmune%20thyroid%20disease%20in%20pregnancy%20and%20the%20postpartum%20period%3A%20relationship%20to%20spontaneous%20abortion.%20Thyroid%202001%3B11(11)%3A1049%E2%80%9353.

[65] Glinoer D, Soto MF, Bourdoux P, Lejeune B, Delange F, Lemone M, Kinthaert J, Robijn C, Grun JP, de Nayer P. Pregnancy in patients with mild thyroid abnormalities: maternal and neonatal repercussions. Journal of Clinical Endocrinology and Metabolism 1991;73(2):421–427. http://jcem.endojournals.org/content/73/2/421.long

[66] Thangaratinam S, Tan A, Knox E, Kilby MD, Franklyn J, Coomarasamy A. Association between thyroid autoantibodies and miscarriage and preterm birth: meta-analysis of evidence. British Medical Journal 2011;342:d2616. http://www.bmj.com/content/342/bmj.d2616?view=long&pmid=21558126

[67] Prummel MF, Wiersinga WM. Thyroid autoimmunity and miscarriage. European Journal of Endocrinology 2004;150(6):751–755. http://www.ncbi.nlm.nih.gov/pubmed?term=Thyroid%20autoimmunity%20and%20miscarriage.%20Eur%20J%20Endocrinol%202004%3B150(6)%3A751%E2%80%935.

[68] De Carolis C, Greco E, Guarino MD, Perricone C, Dal Lago A, Giacomelli R, Fontana L, Perricone R. Anti-thyroid antibodies and antiphospholipid syndrome: evidence of reduced fecundity and of poor pregnancy outcome in recurrent spontaneous aborters.

American Journal Reproduction Immunology 2004;52(4):263–266. http://onlinelibrary.wiley.com/doi/10.1111/j.1600-0897.2004.00215.x/abstract

[69] Bussen S, Steck T. Thyroid autoantibodies in euthyroid non-pregnant women with recurrent spontaneous abortions. Human Reproduction 1995;10(11): 2938-2940.http://humrep.oxfordjournals.org/content/10/11/2938.long

[70] Rushworth FH, Backos M, Rai R, Chilcott IT, Baxter N, Regan L. Prospective pregnancy outcome in untreated recurrent miscarriers with thyroid autoantibodies. Human Reproduction 2000; 15(7):1637–1639. http://humrep.oxfordjournals.org/content/15/7/1637.long

[71] Esplin MS, Branch DW, Silver R, Stagnaro-Green A. Thyroid autoantibodies are not associated with recurrent pregnancy loss. American Journal of Obstetrics Gynecology 1998;179(6Pt 1):1583–1586. http://www.ncbi.nlm.nih.gov/pubmed?term=Thyroid%20autoantibodies%20are%20not%20associated%20with%20recurrent%20pregnancy%20loss.%20American%20Journal%20of%20Obstetrics%20Gynecology%201998%3B179(6Pt%201)%3A1583%E2%80%936.

[72] Negro R, Formoso G, Mangieri T, Pezzarossa A, Dazzi D, Hassan H. Levothyroxine treatment in euthyroid pregnant women with autoimmune thyroid disease: effects on obstetrical complications. Journal Clinical Endocrinology Metabolism 2006;91(7):2587–2591. http://jcem.endojournals.org/content/91/7/2587.long

[73] Pearce EN, Farwell AP, Braverman LE. Thyroiditis. New England Journal of Medicine 2003; 348(26):2646–2655. http://www.nejm.org/doi/full/10.1056/NEJMra021194

[74] Marqusee E, Hill JA, Mandel SJ. Thyroiditis after pregnancy loss. Journal of Clinical Endocrinology and Metabolism 1997;82(8):2455-2457. http://jcem.endojournals.org/content/82/8/2455.long

[75] Li Y, Shan Z, Teng W, Yu X, Li Y, Fan C, Teng X, Guo R, Wang H, Li J, Chen Y, Wang W, Chawinga M, Zhang L, Yang L, Zhao Y, Hua T. Abnormalities of maternal thyroid function during pregnancy affect neuropsychological development of their children at 25-30 months. Clinical Endocrinology (Oxf) 2010;72(6):825-829. http://www.ncbi.nlm.nih.gov/pubmed/19878506

[76] Schlienger JL. Hypothyroidie et grossesse. In: Leclère J, Orgiazzi J, Rousset B, Schlienger JL, Wémeau JL. (Ed.). La thyroide. 2nd edition. France: Elsevier; 2001: 503-506

[77] De Groot L, Abalovich M, Alexander EK, Amino N, Barbour L, Cobin R, Eastman C, Lazarus J, Luton D, Mandel S, Mestman J, Rovet J, Sullivan S. Management of thyroid dysfunction during pregnancy and postpartum: An Endocrine Society Clinical Practice Guideline. Journal of Clinical Endocrinology and Metabolism 2012; 97(8): 2543-2565. http://jcem.endojournals.org/content/97/8/2543.long

[78] Stagnaro-Green A, Abalovich M, Alexander E, Azizi F, Mestman J, Negro R, Nixon A, Pearce EN, Soldin OP, Sullivan S, Wiersing W. Guidelines of the American Thyroid Association for the diagnosis and management of thyroid disease during pregnancy

and postpartum. Thyroid 2011; 21(10): 1081-1125. http://online.liebertpub.com/doi/pdf/10.1089/thy.2011.0087

[79] Stricker R, Echenard M, Eberhart R, Chevailler MC, Perez V, Quinn FA, Stricker R. Evaluation of maternal thyroid function during pregnancy: The importance of using gestational age-specific reference intervals. European Journal of Endocrinology 2007; 157(4): 509-514. http://eje-online.org/lookup/pmid?view=long&pmid=17893266

[80] Haddow JE, Knight GJ, Palomaki GE, McClain MR, Pulk-Kinen AJ. The reference range and within-person variability of thyroid stimulating hormone during the first and second trimesters of pregnancy. Journal of Medical Screening 2004;11(4): 170-174. http://jms.rsmjournals.com/content/11/4/170.long

[81] Panesar NS, Li SY, Rogers MS. Reference intervals for thyroid hormones in pregnant chineese women. Annals of Clinical Biochemistry 2001; 38(Pt4): 329-332. http://acb.rsmjournals.com/content/38/4/329.long

[82] Soldin OP, Soldin D, Sastoque M. Gestation-specific thyroxine and thyroid stimulating hormone levels in the United States and worldwide. Therapeutic Drug Monitoring 2007; 29(5); 553-559. http://journals.lww.com/drug-monitoring/pages/articleviewer.aspx?year=2007&issue=10000&article=00001&type=abstract

[83] Bocos-Terraz JP, Izquierdo-Alvarez S, Bancalero-Flores JL, Alvarez-Lahuerta R, Aznar-Sauca A, Real-Lopez E, Ibanez-Marco R, Bocanegra-Garcia V, Rivera-Sanchez G. Thyroid hormones according to gestational age in pregnant Spanish women. BMC Research Notes 2009; 2: 237. http://www.ncbi.nlm.nih.gov/pmc/articles/PMC2788578/pdf/1756-0500-2-237.pdf

[84] Marwaha RK, Chopra S, Gopalakrishnan S, Sharma B, Kanwar RS, Sastry A, Singh S. Establishment of reference range for thyroid hormones in normal pregnant Indian women. BJOG 2008;115(5): 602-606. http://onlinelibrary.wiley.com/doi/10.1111/j.1471-0528.2008.01673.x/pdf

[85] Wang QW, Yu B, Huang RP, Cao F, Zhu Z-q, Sun D-c, Zhou H. Assessment of thyroid function during pregnancy: The advantage of self-sequential longitudinal reference intervals. Archives of Medical Sciences 2011;7(4): 679-684. http://www.ncbi.nlm.nih.gov/pmc/articles/PMC3258790/pdf/AMS-7-4-679.pdf

[86] Walker JA, Illions EH, Huddleston JF, Smallridge RC. Racial comparisons of thyroid function and autoimmunity during pregnancy and the postpartum period. Obstetrical Gynecology 2005;106(6): 1365-1371. http://www.ncbi.nlm.nih.gov/pubmed?term=Racial%20comparisons%20of%20thyroid%20function%20and%20autoimmunity%20during%20pregnancy%20and%20the%20postpartum%20period.

[87] Benhadi N, Wiersing WM, Reitsma JB, Vrijkotte TG, Vanderwal MF, Bousel GJ. Ethnic differences in TSH but not in free T4 concentrations or TPO antibodies during pregnancy. Clinical Endocrinology (Oxford) 2007; 66(6): 765-770. http://www.ncbi.nlm.nih.gov/pubmed/17466012

[88] Dashe JS, Casey BM, Wells CE, McIntira DD, Byrd EW, Leveno KJ, Cunnigham FG. Thyroid stimulating hormone in singleton and twin pregnancy: importance of gestational age specific reference ranges. Obstetrical Gynecology 2005;106(4): 753-757. http://www.ncbi.nlm.nih.gov/pubmed/16199632

[89] Rotondi M, Mazziotti G, Sorvillo F, Piscopo M, Cioffi M, Amato G, Carella C. Effects of increased thyroxine dosage pre-conception on thyroid function during early pregnancy. European Journal of Endocrinology 2004;151(6): 695-700. http://eje-online.org/content/151/6/695.full.pdf

[90] Lazarus JH, Bestwick JP, Channon S, Paradice R, Maina A, Rees R, Chiusano E, John R, Guaraldo V, Chem MS, George LM, Perona M, Chen MS, Dall'Amico D, Parkes AB, Joomum M, Wald NP. Antenatal thyroid screening and childhood cognitive function. New England Journal of Medicine 2012;366(6): 493-501. http://www.nejm.org/doi/pdf/10.1056/NEJMoa1106104

[91] Negro R, Greco G, Mangieri T, Pezzarossa A, Dazzi D, Hassan H. The influence of selenium supplementation on post-partum thyroid status in pregnant women with thyroid peroxidase autoantibodies. Journal of Clinical Endocrinology and Metabolism 2007; 92(4): 1263-1268. http://jcem.endojournals.org/content/92/4/1263.full.pdf+html

[92] Cao XY, Jiang XM, Dou ZH, Rakeman MA, Zhang ML, O'Donnell KJ, Ma T Amette K, DeLong, N, DeLong R. Timing of vulnerability of the brain to iodine deficiency in endemic cretinism. New England Journal of Medecine 1994;331(26): 1739–1744. http://www.nejm.org/doi/pdf/10.1056/NEJM199412293312603

[93] O'Donnell KJ, Rakeman MA, Zhi-Hong D, Xue-Yi C, Mei ZY, DeLong N, Brenner G, Tai M, Dong W, DeLong GR. Effects of iodine supplementation during pregnancy on child growth and development at school age. Developmental Medicine and Child Neurology 2002;44(2):76-81. http://onlinelibrary.wiley.com/doi/10.1111/j.1469-8749.2002.tb00291.x/abstract

[94] Berbel P, Mestre JL, Santamaria A, Palazon I, Franco A, Graells M, Gonzalez-Torga A, de Escobar GM. Delayed neurobehavioral development in children born to pregnant women with mild hypothyroxinemia during the first month of gestation: the importance of early iodine supplementation. Thyroid 2009;19(5): 511–519. http://online.liebertpub.com/doi/abs/10.1089/thy.2008.0341

[95] Velasco I, Carreira M, Santiago P, Muela JA, Garcia-Fuentes E, Sanchez-Munoz B, Garriga MJ, Gonzalez-Fernandez MC, Rodriguez A, Caballero FF, Machado A, Gonzalez-Romero S, Anarte MT, Soriguer F. Effect of iodine prophylaxis during pregnancy on neurocognitive development of children during the first two years of life. Journal of Clinical Endocrinology and Metabolism 2009; 94(9): 3234–3241. http://jcem.endojournals.org/content/94/9/3234.full.pdf+html

[96] Last JM. A dictionary of epidemiology (4th edition). Oxford university press. Oxford 2001. http://books.google.tn/books?hl=fr&lr=&id=RPa-QY8cG4N4C&oi=fnd&pg=PR5&dq=Last+JM.+A+dictionary+of+epidemiology+(4th

+edition).+Oxford+university+press.+Oxford+2001.&ots=GdtDy3k1N8&sig=edwX-BoW6-HXPQ7WKJ7X8Wo5DkXw&redir_esc=y#v=onepage&q&f=false

[97] UK National Screening Committee criteria. www.nhs.uk/whatscreening/what-screen_ind.htm

[98] Erik K, Marqusee E, Laurens J, Jarolin P, Fischer GA, Larsen PR. Timing and magnitude of increases in Levothyroxine requirements during pregnancy in women with hypothyroidism. New England Journal of Medecine 2004; 351: 241-249. http://www.nejm.org/doi/full/10.1056/NEJMoa040079

[99] Arafah BM. Increased need for thyroxine in women with hypothyroidism during estrogen therapy. New England Journal of Medecine 2001; 344: 1743. http://www.nejm.org/doi/full/10.1056/NEJM200106073442302

[100] Negro R, Mestman JH. Thyroid disease in pregnancy. Best Practice and Research Clinical Endocrinology and Metabolism 2011;25(6):927-43. http://www.ncbi.nlm.nih.gov/pubmed/22115167

[101] Trumbo P, Yates AA, Schlicker S, Poos. Dietary reference intakes: vitamin A, vitamin K, arsenic, boron, chromium, copper, iodine, iron, manganese, molybdenum, nickel, silicon, vanadium, and zinc. Journal of the American Dietitic Association 2001; 101(3): 294–301. http://www.ncbi.nlm.nih.gov/pubmed?term=Dietary%20reference%20intakes%3A%20vitamin%20A%2C%20vitamin%20K%2C%20arsenic%2C%20boron%2C%20chromium%2C%20copper%2C%20iodine%2C%20iron%2C%20manganese%2C%20molybdenum%2C%20nickel%2C%20silicon%2C%20vanadium%2C%20and%20zinc

[102] Berghout A, Wiersinga W. Thyroid size and thyroid function during pregnancy: an analysis. European Journal of Endocrinology 1998: 138(5):536–542. http://eje-online.org/cgi/pmidlookup?view=long&pmid=9625365

Section 2

Hypothyroidism in Childhood

Chapter 3

Congenital Hypothyroidism

Ferenc Péter, Ágota Muzsnai and Rózsa Gráf

Additional information is available at the end of the chapter

http://dx.doi.org/10.5772/54660

1. Introduction

Congenital hypothyroidism is the most frequent congenital endocrine disorder and preventable cause of mental retardation. The remarkable irreversible mental damage can be avoided by the replacement therapy introduced before the age of 3 weeks. Therefore a screening program implemented in the early seventies to pick up the affected babies on the first weeks of life [1,2]. After pilot studies started in 1977 a national neonatal TSH screening program was introduced in Hungary in 1982 [3]. It has continued in two centers from 1984 covering the whole country (50-50 % of the expected newborns were assigned to one lab). Patients screened and confirmed as CH were followed-up at the endocrine outpatient clinics. Replacement was adjusted according to the laboratory results and somatic-mental development of the child. The authors (two pediatric endocrinologists and one psychologist) have worked together in this project throughout 26 years in one of these centers. They present their experiences with the screening program and the endocrine/psychological follow-up gained during this period discussing the results with literature data.

The widely known incidence data on congenital hypothyroidism before the introduction of neonatal screening originate from the North European countries: 1 to 6000-10000 [4-6]. Nowadays when the usage of the national language is increasingly accepted in authentic translation at the international forums the Hungarian contribution may be interesting. The Thyroid Work Group of Hungarian Pediatric Institute collected five years incidence data (1966-70) from the pediatricians all over the country and "... 40/year new hypothyroid children were reported". The birthrate was 160.000/year that time, so the incidence was calculated 1:4000, published in Hungarian in 1972 [7]. This numerical value almost corresponds to the data experienced by the neonatal screening.

According to the recent data the incidence of congenital hypothyroidism varies from 1:1000 to 1:3500 life births depending on the iodine sufficiency, demographic and other unknown factors as well as on laboratory methods and screening practice. Several work groups noted a progressively rise since the early 1990s both in America and Europe [8-16], however the question was raised with reason: "Was this increasing incidence real ... or was ... an artifact, explained by modifications of screening programs such as a change in test cutoffs?" (LaFranchi 2011; [13]. According to a convincing Canadian study the incidence of thyroid dysgenesis, which form is more than 80 % within the CH, has remained relatively stable over the last decades [9,15]. Demographic factors were "suspected" to be responsible for this phenomenon [8] but it was not confirmed as a complete explanation [9]. The changes in test cutoffs [13,14] or simply the used different laboratory and screening methods in certain centres [17] might be also the first candidates behind the increasing incidence rate in some screening programs. These data "highlight the need for consensus development regarding the diagnosis and treatment of congenital hypothyroidism" according to Rapaport's commentary [18] to one of these reports [12]. And indeed, recently (November 2011) recommendations were prepared at the ESPE consensus meeting (complete version is in press) for orientation relating to the screening, investigation, treatment, long terms outcomes and genetic/antenatal diagnosis in CH [19].

In Hungary the screening program is based on primary TSH determination and the overall incidence of CH is 1:3316, namely 413 cases were diagnosed out of 1,369.503 newborns screened between 1982 and 2007 in our Screening Center. The annual incidence is relatively constant (Figure 1.). Opposite to primary T_4/FT_4 measurement with backup TSH determination it was not necessary to change the cutoff levels of TSH for increasing the sensitivity and other conflicting factors could be avoided, namely the low FT4 levels of preterm babies and obtaining the blood specimens remarkably earlier.

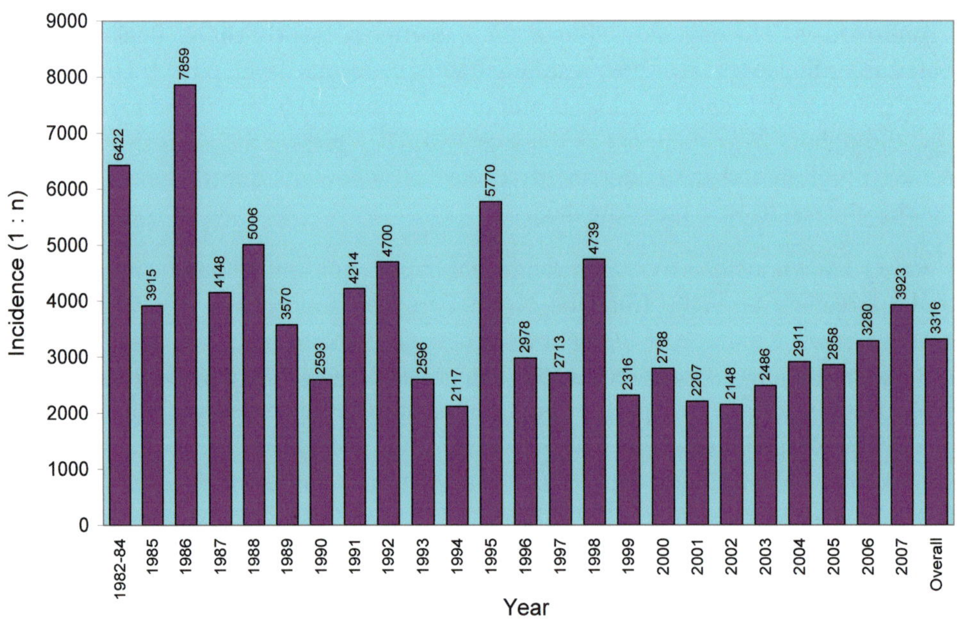

Figure 1. Annual incidence of congenital hypothyroidism

Most of the cases detected in newborn age have permanent hypothyroidism caused by abnormal thyroid gland development (dysgenesis) or that of inborn error of thyroid hormonogenesis (dyshormonogenesis). Thyroxine-binding globulin (TBG) deficiency occurs in 1 to 9000 life births, while congenital central hypothyroidism (TSH and/or TRH deficiency) occurs in less than 1:20000-100000. Transient hypothyroidism may occur because of delay in maturation of the hypothalamic-pituitary-thyroid axis, both iodine deficiency and excess, dysfunction of the mother-placenta-fetal unit or the effect of medication used on the intensive care unit. Both monoallelic and biallelic mutations in DUOX2 gene result transient CH reported recently [20,21]. Permanent CH patients need a life-long treatment while transient cases can quit of replacement after recovery of thyroid function.

As the postnatal development of the nervous system is thyroid hormone dependent up to 2-3 years none of the patient were put on higher risk by suspend the therapy to early therefore the revision of the neonatal diagnosis was postponed above the age of 2-3 years. Classifying the disorder as permanent or transient was obtained on abnormal or normal hormone levels after withdrawal of levothyroxine replacement. Before 2 years of age the following course of the disease was suspicious for transient dysfunction of the thyroid. Shortly after the introduction of replacement therapy TSH normalized and never increased above the upper limit parallel with decreasing demand of levothyroxine to keep T4/FT4 in the reference range. In 21 patients out of 291 substituted infants we could simply withdraw the replacement and the TSH remained normal.

Above the age of 3 years a T3 withdrawal test was performed in 197 children to reconsider the diagnosis of CH. We applied the same method for all patients: L-T4 was shifted to L-T3 for 3 weeks, which has a shorter half-life. After one week L-T3 was also stopped, patients were off-treatment altogether for one week. At the end of the 4th week presenting a normal thyroid function test is considered to be a transient hypothyroid case. Five out of 197 patients tested have proven transient CH. The total number of children reached 3 years of age and who were old enough for T3 withdrawal test were 310, which give the overall transient CH rate as 8.4 % (21+5/310).

2. Methodology

From the very beginning up to the end of 2007 we used a primary TSH screen and a secondary serum thyroid hormone measurement to confirm the abnormal TSH results. A drop of whole blood was obtained and dried on filter paper between the ages of 3-5 days. Samples were sent to the assigned screening laboratory via mail. Measurement of TSH was performed after an elution process using a home-developed RIA until 1993 [21,22]. Cessation of the cheap antibody supply forced us to buy commercial kits changing for DELFIA, LIA, IRMA and ELISA methods. All tests offered narrower measuring ranges and cutoff values became more precise. The algorithm for selection of specimen for further evaluation was very simple. Samples below the cutoff level (25 μU/ml later on 20 μU/ml) were considered as normal, between the range 25(later on 20)-50 as suspected positive and above 50μU/ml as true positive. Technical errors were ruled out by repeated measurement from the blood spot and only samples above the cutoff limit were recognized and infants were called to visit us immediately. Physical examination and blood sample were taken for peripheral thyroid hormones and TSH measurement from the serum. The diagnosis of CH was confirmed by low T4/FT4, T3/FT3 levels and elevated TSH.

2.1. Etiology

Almost 95% of cases born with CH have primary hypothyroidism reflecting peripheral defects and less than 5% has secondary/tertiary hypothyroidism results from lack of TSH and/or TRH production. Both the presentation and the sequel of the congenital central hypothyroidism are less severe although most commonly it is part of a disorder causing congenital hypopituitarism. Several imaging methods are suitable to describe the position and size of the thyroid. Localization or absence of the gland helps to differentiate dysgenesis and dyshormonogenesis in CH patients.

I^{123} scan is optimal to test the newborn babies for possible developmental defect of the thyroid gland before replacing them but it was not available for us. During replacement therapy the background of thyroid dysfunction was tested using different imaging techniques. Ultrasonography is a non-invasive method but requires a baby-head for apparent description of a tiny or absent gland. Thyroid scintigraphy is a more precise but invasive method requiring an unreplaced situation. Scintigraphy was performed in 182 cases combined with T3-withdrawal test. Thyroid dysgenesis occurred in 84% (agenetic: 47%, ectopic lingual: 28%, hypoplastic: 9%), an enlarged thyroid was seen in 6% and a normal-sized eutopic gland – so-called "thyroid in situ" [12,13] – in 10%.

Further distinction of etiology is offered by molecular genetics. Several genes involved in thyroid ontogenesis and in normal function of it. An abnormal expression of the thyroid specific genes can be manifested in different phenotype, which is summarized in Table 1.

Gene	Chromosome region	Role of gene in organogenesis/ protein function	Phenotype (by morphology or function)	Associated disorders
		DYSGENESIS		
TITF1/NKX2.1	14q13	*Development of both follicular and C-cells*	Aplasia or Hemiagenesis or Hypoplasia (with or without ectopy)	Choreoathetosis, RDS, pulmonary disease
PAX8	2q12-q14	*Thyroid follicular cell development*		Renal agenesis
TITF2/FOXE1	9q22	*Migration of thyroid precursor cells*		Cleft palate, choanal atresia, bifid epiglottis, spiky hair (Bamforth-Lazarus sy.)
GNAS1	20q13.2	Signalling protein	*Resistance to thyrotropin*	Osteodystrophy (hereditary Albright sy.)

http://dx.doi.org/10.5772/54660

Gene	Chromosome region	Role of gene in organogenesis/ protein function	Phenotype (by morphology or function)	Associated disorders
TSHR	14q31	*Thyroid differentiation* Thyrotropin receptor	Hypoplasia (without ectopy) *Resistance to thyrotropin*	-
		INBORN ERROR OF THYROID HORMONOGENESIS		
TITF1, PAX8, TITF2/ FOXE1	See above	During later stages*: Regulation of thyroid specific gene expression*	Enlarged thyroid gland	-
TPO	2p25	*Thyroid differentiation* Iodide organification		-
TG	8q24.2-q24.3	*Thyroid differentiation* Structural prohormone		-
NIS	19p13.2-p12	Iodide transport from the blood into thyroid cell (basal membrane)		-
PDS	7q31	Iodide transport from thyroid cell to follicular lumen (apical membrane)		Sensorineural deafness (Pendred sy.)
DUOX1/THOX1 DUOX2/THOX2	15q15.3	Thyroidal H_2O_2 generation		-
DUOXA2	15q21.1			
IYD/DEHAL1	6q24-q25	Deiodination for iodide recycling		-
		THYROID HORMONE TRANSPORTER DEFECT		
MCT8	Xq13.2	Transmembrane T_4, T_3, rT_3, T_2 transport	*Thyroid hormone resistance*	Severe neurological abnormalities (Allan-Herndon-Dudley sy.)
THRB	3p24.3	Nuclear thyroid hormone receptor		Hyperactivity, learning disability
SBP2	9q22.2	Synthesis of selenoproteins	*Abnormal TFT*	Delayed puberty (?)
		IMPAIRED HYPOTHALAMIC-PITUITARY-THYROID AXIS		
LHX3	9q34.3	*Early pituitary development*	*Secondary/tertiary hypothyroidism*	CPHD, pituitary mass, rigid cervical spine
LHX4	1q25			CPHD, sella turcica defect
PROP1	5q	*Expression of all pituitary cell lineage*		CPHD, pituitary mass

Gene	Chromosome region	Role of gene in organogenesis/ protein function	Phenotype (by morphology or function)	Associated disorders
POU1F1	3p11	*Generation and cell-type specification*		GH, PRL deficiency
HESX1, PHF6	3p21.2-p21.1	*Forebrain, midline and pituitary development*		Septo-optic dysplasia, CPHD, epilepsy
TRHR	8q23	TRH receptor		-
TSHB	1p13	TSH β subunit		-
OTHER				
DUOX2/THOX2 DUOX/DUOXA	15q15.3	Partial defect in H_2O_2 production	*Transient CH*	-

CH= Congenital hypothyroidism, CPHD = Combined pituitary hormone deficiency, GH = Growth hormone, PRL = Prolactine, RDS = Respiratory distress sy, TFT = Thyroid function test

Table 1. Thyroid specific genes involved in congenital hypothyroidism [23-39]

A cohort of 58 patients was analyzed for PAX8 (exon2 and exon3) mutation. Genetic screening did not reveal any mutation on the PAX8 gene in children with thyroid dysgenesis. It supports the recent notion that non-syndromic thyroid dysgenesis is rather a heterogeneous disease than a monogenetic one. Up to now the exact etiology of CH remained unknown for the great majority of the cases. More candidate genes have been verified in syndromic CH patients as distinct gene loci can be connected to distinct clinical feature. Analyzing our cohort congenital malformations were found in 45 cases (Table 2.) and concomitant disorders in 46 cases out of 210 CH patients (Table 3) [40]. Phenotypes specific gene on selected CH patients with associated disorders should be analyzed to gain more information on fetal thyroid development. Recently Park and Chatterjee proposed an algorithm for investigating the genetic basis of congenital hypothyroidism [41].

Malformations, syndromes	Male	Female	Cytogenetic location
Congenital heart disease	6	3	
Renal malformation		5	
Urogenital malformation	11	2	
Musculoskeletal malformation		3	
Scoliosis	2	1	
CNS malformation	1	1	
Dysmorphic auricle/face	2	2	
Pulmonary fibrosis		1	

Malformations, syndromes	Male	Female	Cytogenetic location
DiGeorge sy.	1		22q11
Kabuki make-up sy.		1	8p22-23.1
Marfan sy.		1	15q21.1
Mayer-Rokitansky-Küster-Hauser sy.		2	1p35

CNS = central nervous system

Table 2. Congenital malformations found in CH patients (45/210)

Impaired function	Male	Female
Delayed speech development	3	4
Stammer	2	
Behavioral problem	3	4
Delayed motor development	1	1
Disturbed motor coordination	2	2
Nocturnal enuresis		7
Strabismus	3	1
Congenital nystagmus		1
GORD	1	2
Epilepsy	1	
Malignancy		2
Serious infection	2	
T1DM	1	
Angioedema		1

GORD = gastro-oesophageal reflux disease, T1DM = type 1 diabetes mellitus

Table 3. Concomitant disorders found in CH patients (46/210)

2.2. Clinical signs

The classical picture of CH with characteristic clinical features develops by the age of three months with irreversible neurological damage. Non-specific signs and symptoms can be noticed during the first weeks of life, which help to set the diagnosis of CH in screened but not confirmed newborns. During the first 10 years of screening program all newborns identified by an abnormal TSH were admitted to the hospital and were assessed by history and complete physical examination. More than 10 unspecific symptoms and history data recorded of 87 suspected babies were analysed to identify any factors that could predict congenital hypothyroidism. Based on confirmatory laboratory results 67 babies out of 87 proved to have CH (true positive or CH group) and 20 was false positive (reference group). Between the two groups 8 parameters (opened posterior fontanel, umbilical hernia, dry skin, enlarged tongue, constipation, laziness, wide nasal bridge, and prolonged jaundice) were found to have significant differences by linear discriminant analysis that were ranked and weighted for scoring. An additional score was calculated from the blood-spot TSH namely the quotient of measured TSH and the cutoff limit for normal thyrotropin. Figures above 6 were correct for predicting CH in 99% of cases. This score system developed (Table 4.) advises the clinicians to pick up and replace the affected babies earlier than 3 weeks of age [22,42].

Clinical sign	Score	Clinical sign	Score
Opened posterior fontanel	2	Constipation	1
Umbilical hernia	2	Laziness	1
Dry skin	2	Wide nasal bridge	1
Enlarged tongue	1	Prolonged jaundice	1
Blood spot TSH: Quotient of measured and cutoff limit for normal			1
Cutoff value for predicting CH			"/> 6

Table 4. Score system for predicting congenital hypothyroidism using primary TSH measurement

2.3. Endocrine and psychological care

2.3.1. Thyroid hormone replacement

The timing of T_4-level's normalization is crucial to the neuropsychological development therefore the first aim of the neonatal screening programs is to reach the earliest start of the hormone replacement. At the beginning the intervals between the birth and start of T_4 replacement were reduced in length as follows: in 1985: 25 ± 5 days, in 1987: 20 ± 9 and in 1990 18 ± 9 days. This length of time improved to ≤ 14 days on average after the introduction of one-day TSH assays and successful education of the personnel involved.

Concerning the dosage and the formulation of thyroid hormone replacement let us call to mind some of our former results, namely in the 1980s both lower and higher thyroxin doses were applied [43–49]. In our early study [22,50] the higher L-T_4 dose was found to be more effective than the lower one (Table 5). It was confirmed recently also by the Glasgow-group recommending the 50 μg initial dose on the basis of their results in 314 children with CH [51]. In our program 10-15 μg/kg as an initial dose is used since the middle eighties [22,42].

At the beginning of our TSH-screening pilot studies (in the early seventies) the synthetic L-T_4 preparations were not available in Hungary, therefore the thyroid hormone replacement was started with oral administration of thyroid extract (thyreoidea sicca: Thyranon, Organon). Later on we changed to the L-T_4 monotherapy and according to our first impressions the

http://dx.doi.org/10.5772/54660

Number of children		**22**		**13**	
Dose of L-T_4		**25 µg**	**6,6 µg/kg**	**50 µg**	**13,4 µg/kg**
Starting values	T_4 (µg/dl)	3,3 ± 2,9		3,6 ± 3,5	
	T_3 (ng/ml)	1,14 ± 0,77		1,34 ± 0,59	
	TSH (mIU/L)	75,1 ± 16,3		74,9 ± 10,4	
Values at first visit	T_4 (µg/dl)	13,2 ± 3,9		18,9 ± 3,6	
	T_3 (ng/ml)	2,2 ± 0,65		2,09 ± 0,33	
	TSH (mIU/L)	**29,1 ± 31,4**		**1,0 ± 0,9**	
Interval (days)		28 ± 35		19 ± 7	

Normal values: T_4: 9,0-15,0 (newborn: -20,0) µg/dl; T_3: 1,5-3,5 (newborn: -4,0) ng/ml;
TSH: 0,5-5,0 (newborn: -20,0) mIU/L

Table 5. Correlation between starting L-T_4 dose and changes of thyroid parameters during hormone replacement

Thyranon proved to be more effective at least regarding the decrease of TSH level [22,50]. It was confirmed in our systematic study but the increase of T_3 level was also detectable (Table 6.)

	T_4 (µg/dl)		**T_3 (ng/ml)**		**TSH (mIU/L)**	
	at start	at control	at start	at control	at start	at control
Thyranon (T_3+T_4) n = 21	3,0 ± 2,6	11,3 ± 4,2	1,15 ± 0,51	3,07 ± 1,70	73,84 ± 10,49	**13,16** ± 26,35
L-Thyroxin (T_4) n= 22	3,3 ± 2,9	13,0 ± 3,9	1,3 ± 0,77	2,2 ± 0,65	75,19 ± 16,30	**29,10** ± 31,41
	before	after	before	after	before	after
Thyranon⇒L-T_4 n = 19			change of replacement			
	10,4 ± 3,2	11,9 ± 2,4	2,63 ± 0,96	2,03 ± 0,66	13,75 ± 22,21	14,13 ± 16,79

Normal values: T_4: 9,0-15,0 (newborn: -20,0) µg/dl; T_3: 1,5-3,5 (newborn: -4,0) ng/ml;
TSH: 0,5-5,0 (newborn: -20,0) mIU/L

Table 6. Changes of thyroid parameters on T_4 or T_4 + T_3 replacement

At that time our conclusion was: "these results confirm the suggestion that T_3 may play a more important role than T_4 in regulating the serum TSH concentration" [50].

One of the main goals of thyroid hormone replacement in congenital hypothyroidism is to restitute the biochemical euthyroidism (the TSH and thyroid hormone levels into the reference ranges) to avoid the prolonged hyperthyroxinemia and the permanent overproduction (or suppression) of thyrotropin. The most important period to monitor the adequate thyroid hormone replacement is the first three years of life to ensure optimal somatic and psycho-neurological development. Our practice harmonize the recent recommendation: follow-up every 1-2 months in the first 6 months, every 2-3 months between 6 months and 3 yrs of age and every 6-12 months later in childhood [52,53].

There are warning data on the importance of well-organized care of children with CH. According to a new American publication based on health insurance claims data of 704 children with presumed CH 38 % (!) discontinued replacement of thyroid hormone within the first 3 yrs of life [54]. In another smaller cohort (140 children) 48,6 % were lost to follow-up (!); of the 72 patients who were re-evaluated at age 3 yrs, treatment had been stopped without medical supervision in 15 [55]. The puberty and adolescence are the most critical periods regarding the compliance in our experience.

In our practice another unexpected alteration has been occurred during the long and continuous follow-up. In a few cases with stable FT_4/TSH relation for many years under gradually increased L-T_4 dose according to the somatic development and TSH-FT_4 values, later we measured elevated TSH despite high FT_4 levels almost regularly. On the basis of our good experience with Thyranon (L-T_4 + L-T_3) replacement therapy in the 1970s, we tried to normalize both serum TSH and FT_4 level administered combined L-T_4 and L-T_3 treatment in these patients. Applying an L-T_4/L-T_3 dose ratio between 13:1 and 18:1 by weight, this modification of therapy mostly proved to be successful (one exemplar on Table 7). The dose of L-T_4 was reducible in some other patients. Unfortunately once-daily slow-release formulation of L-T_3 [56] was not available for us.

Age (year)	TSH (mIU/L)	FT_4 (pmol/L)	FT_3 (pmol/L)	L-T_4 µg/day	L-T_3 µg/day
12	**13,24**	19,43	5,1	125	-
14,5	**11,25**	18,7	5,4	150	-
15	**6,59**	**22,26**	5,5	150	-
15,5	**9,35**	20.18	5,8	150	-
16,5	2,25	11,24	5,8	100	**20**
16,75	3,30	12,80	**9,0**	125	**10**
17	**6,05**	16,14	5,8	150	**10**
17,25	*2,20*	*19,96*	*6,9*	*150*	**10**

Table 7. Some data from the last six years of an adolescent boy

Recently the use of L-T_4 + L-T_3 in the treatment of hypothyroidism is one of the "hot topics" in thyroidology (see excellent papers [57,58] and "2012 ETA guidelines" [59]), however our observation is different from those. These children and adolescents do not have hypothyroid symptoms comparing to the adults (5-10 %) and do have elevated TSH (and FT_4) level. The congenital form of hypothyroidism – as an entity – is not included in the ETA guidelines at all [59]); it is restricted on adults with autoimmune hypothyroidism or caused by definitive therapy (radioiodine, surgery). Now we are analysing the data of our patients in this small cohort.

2.3.2. *Evaluation of the somatic development*

The aim of thyroid hormone replacement is to ensure optimal somatic and neuropsychological development. The evaluation of somatic and psychological parameters is also necessary to control the quality of compliance, what may be disturbed, – as was mentioned before – especially in the adolescent period. The hormone parameters are relative "quick variable". The state of thyroid hormone supply at the less and less frequent outpatient visits is well reflected in the somatic development, as "slow variable".

Somatic development was analyzed using the height and bone age data of 83 prepubertal children. *Height* was measured regularly by Harpenden stadiometer and evaluated by Hungarian reference data [60]. *Bone age* was also determined repeatedly up to the disappearance of bone age retardation using the Greulich-Pyle atlas [61]. *Bone mineral density* (BMD) was measured by single photon absorptiometer (SPA; Gamma Works, Hungary) in 46 children (6-17 yrs). Later peripheral quantitative computer tomography (pQCT; XCT2000, Stratec Electronics, Germany) was introduced to determine radial volumetric total BMD and trabecular Z-score values of 91 children (6-18 yrs). The results were evaluated comparing with Hungarian reference data [62,63].

2.3.3. *Growth velocity and bone age*

The comparison of age and age for height does not show any difference (age: 6,27 ± 2,65 yrs; age for height: 6,26 ± 2,76 yrs). Bone age was lower than the chronological age (5,73 ± 2,77 yrs; p = 0). The regression's line diverges from the theoretical optimum line in the younger age, but the distribution of the values are almost the same on both sides of the "ideal" line in the older than 10 year of age, or more convincing some values indicate bone age retardation under 10 years (Figure 2).

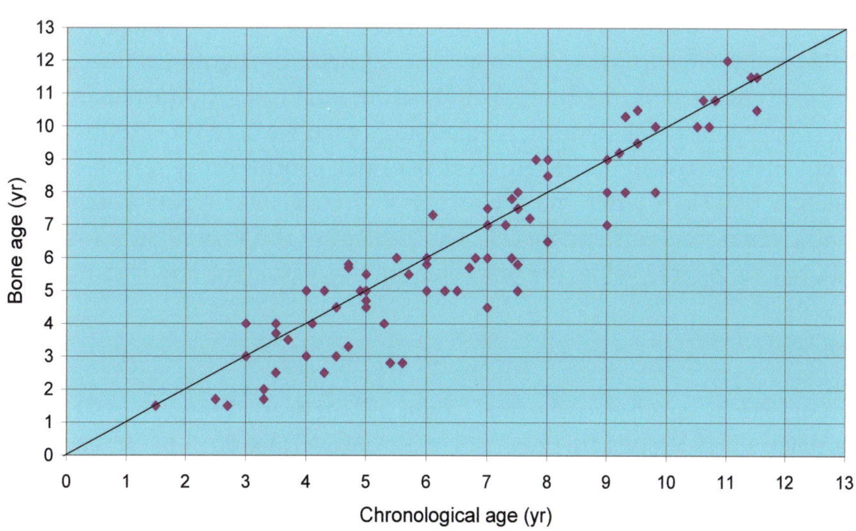

Figure 2. Bone maturation of L-T4 replaced CH patients (n=83)

The publications report usually good results on somatic growth and pubertal development of children with CH detected by neonatal screening and supplemented well with L-T_4 [64-69]. Our results clearly show that the disappearance of bone age retardation is individual. The bone age of children with CH catch up their chronological age in different time at latest about ten years of age.

2.3.4. Bone mineral density

In our first (SPA) study *– 0,24 ± 1,24* mean Z-score values were found; below – 2,0 in 3 cases only. After correction to age for height, one value remained under –2,0 Z-score [62]. However, SPA may measure false results in growing children (areal BMD; its measure is g/cm^2) due to the change of bone size. To avoid this possibility pQCT (volumetric BMD; its measure is g/cm^3) measurements were carried out later. The mean total BMD Z-score of 28 boys was *– 0,19 ± 1,18* and the trabecular BMD Z score: + 0,05 ± 0,9, both in the normal range. Similar values were measured in the group of 63 girls: total Z-score + 0,04 ± 1,15, trabecular Z-scores + 0,1 ± 0,98, but some differences were found in the total density between the younger and older girls (*≤ 11 yr – 0,36 ± 0,9 and > 11 yr + 0,3 ± 1,22*). Pathological (< - 2,0) BMD Z-score did not occur at all among the 28 boys, and only two trabecular density values were in this range among the 63 girls. The total BMD Z-score was found *between – 1,0 and – 1,9 in 5 cases* in both groups, the trabecular Z-score value was in this range very rarely (1 and 2 cases respectively).

One of the most important preventive factors of the adult osteoporosis is the attainment of an optimal peak bone mass. Therefore the importance of the good accretion of bone mineral content during the childhood and adolescence is generally recognized. Thyroid hormones are one of the known influencing factors of the BMD. Hyperthyroxinemia can cause bone resorption resulting in a decreased bone mass. BMD was found decreased in adolescent females treated with high doses of L-T_4 [70].

In the first pediatric studies did not measure decreased bone mineral content in children with congenital hypothyroidism by DXA technique [71,72]. Recently slightly decreased BMD values were published within the normal range [73,74], in one publication by quantitative ultrasound technique [73]. In spite of the different methodology what we used (pQCT: direct volumetric method, not mathematically corrected areal one) our conclusion is similar regarding the development of BMD in children and adolescents with congenital hypothyroidism diagnosed at neonatal screening and replaced by L-T_4. Our results are also very slightly lower compared to controls, but the Z-score values are practically always within the reference range.

2.3.5. Final height

In a cohort of 98 children (65 girls) the final height (FH) or nearly FH (growth ≤ 1 cm in the last year) was determined. Results are presented on the table (Table 8.)

The mean value of FH in boys corresponds to the Hungarian reference data and the 3,1 cm difference in the average of girls does not mean significant deviation. In a detailed presentation interesting data were published on "prepubertal and pubertal growth, timing and duration of

	Boys (33)	Girls (65)
Age (yrs)	17,83 ± 2,56	17,47 ± 2,17
Final height (cm)	177,41 ± 5,77	164,11 ± 6,28

Table 8. Final (and nearly final) height of 98 patients with CH

puberty and attained adult height" of 30 patients, included 17 FH values [66]. The authors emphasize the significant positive correlation between the average L-T_4 daily dose administered during the first 6 months of treatment and attained height. We cannot confirm this observation because of our different protocol (uniform L-T_4 dosage was used during the last two decades).

In a Japan publication a greater peak height velocity and pubertal height gain was presented in their male patients [67]; we also observed some difference between the FH of boys and girls to the advantage of the boys.

2.3.6. *Menarche*

Correct data were gained from 50 girls. Their menarche age is 12,38 ± 1,06 yrs, what is the same as the reference value in Hungary, however the distribution of data is surprising. The manifestation of the first menses happened rather earlier (in 23 girls ≤12 yrs) or later (in 19 girls ≥ 13 yrs) than close to the mean (8 only) indicating the relationship between the thyroid hormone and sexual hormone axes. Italian authors differentiated two groups of girls according to their menarche age (11,5 ± 0,8 yrs versus 12,6 ± 1,2 yrs) like us but both groups attained normal FH similarly to our results [68].

3. Evaluation of psychoneurodevelopment

The somatic development is almost perfect in the children with CH detected by neonatal screening and had optimal thyroid hormone replacement. The same does not apply to their psychoneurodevelopment.

After the first ten years of our neonatal TSH screening program (117 CH/508.590 newborn) the IQ was tested in a cohort of 46 children (39 permanent and 7 transient CH; age 3-8 yrs). Although a normal distribution of IQ values was detected, a strong correlation was observed in 28 children between the IQ and serum thyroglobulin (Tg) level (Tg < 0,3 ng/ml in 3 out of 21 with IQ > 90 and 4 out of 7 with IQ < 90; $p < 0{,}01$ using Yates correction). This early data confirmed the thesis [75,76] that although there is some placental transfer of thyroid hormones during pregnancy, it cannot totally prevent the intrauterine neurological damage in athyroidism [77].

Ten years later we presented more detailed results on the neurodevelopment of CH children [78,79]. The main message is summarized on the next table (Table 9.) The correlation between the date of diagnosis, serum T_4 level before start of replacement, initial L-T_4 dose and the IQ of 58 children (born 1985-95; tested 1993-2000 at age 4,9 ± 2,0 yrs; repeatedly tested 49 of them at age 8,5 ± 2,5 yrs) were analyzed. According to these data the onset of replacement before 2 weeks of life in the newborns with serum T4 level < 3 μg/dl ensure the best IQ; similar data are published [46,47,49].

	Serum T_4 < 3 μg/dl			
	Start of L-T_4 replacement (day)			
	7-13		14-26	
Dose of L-T_4 μg/kg/day	< 10	"/> 10	< 10	"/> 10
Number of patients	3	3	15	8
IQ values	106,3 ± 8,0	108,7 ± 26,5	**101,4 ± 12,2***	101,4 ± 11,4
	Serum T_4 "/> 3 μg/dl			
	Start of L-T_4 replacement (day)			
	7-13		14-26	
Dose of L-T_4 **μ**g/kg/day	< 10	"/> 10	< 10	"/> 10
Number of patients	6	5	14	4
IQ values	115,0 ± 6,7	**113,6 ± 13,6**	103,6 ±8,4	103,8 ± 12,8

* p = 0,05

Table 9. Relationship between some important parameters and the IQ in replaced children with CH

With these experiences we realized the need of regular psychological care. One of us (R.G.) performs this work continuously connecting the endocrine outpatient clinic. Every patient is tested at least once a year.

The recently prepared DQ and IQ results are presented on the next table (Table 10).

Age (year)	Number of patients	DQ/IQ values	Test-methods (norm.: 90-110)
< 3	175	99,65 ± 13,0	Brunet-Lésine
3-8	146	104,44 ± 12,7	Binet
8-10	136	106,3 ± 10,59	Binet
14-16	30	93,25 ± 7,22	WISC-IV*

*Wechsler Intelligence Scale for Children 4th ed. (total quotients). The Processing Speed Q: 95,07 ± 12,74; Verbal Q: 92,81 ± 11,69; Performance Q: 92,55 ± 14,63 and Working memory Q: 89,92 ± 14,95.

Table 10. Developmental and intelligence quotients

The DQ and IQ test-results of the first three age groups are in the normal range. Some neurocognitive abilities might be affected in these children (visuospatial-, visuomotor-, language and speech-, attention and memory).

If the DQ value tested by Brunet-Lésine method suggests a delay in development, we can intervene early enough to help the children. A developmental intervention program is prepared for the children and parents. In these cases the psychoneurological development are regularly controlled. The meetings the family are as often as it is possible or necessary in these cases.

The Binet test is rather verbal test of intelligence (not appropriate to recognize the delay of speech-development, but good for measuring problem-solving, vocabulary employment of experience). Early intervention is necessary in the case of delay in expressive speech and difficulties with coordinative movements (danger of difficulties at school!). Learning disability can be diagnosed in the third class earliest. At the age of 8-10 yrs the Binet test can give acceptable information on the intellectual development. If there are more than one problem of different cognitive abilities, that can mean an increased risk from the point of learning disability. These children have problems with mathematics (not with mechanical reading but with the reading comprehension). The number of children with disability was 9 in this small material: reading disability (3), learning disability in mathematics (3) and ADHD (3).

The WISC-IV test was accredited lately, therefore its use started recently. The results of the first 30 tests (the total IQ and especially the quotients for partial abilities: processing speed-, verbal-, performance- and working memory quotients) tend to be weaker corresponding to the international experiences.

The beneficial effect of early start of replacement and the use of higher initial dose is almost generally accepted. Recently 51 articles were analysed publishing IQ values of children with CH. Normal values were detected in one third of the reports but in the other papers the IQ was found significantly lower comparing to controls [80].

The main conclusions: some of the prenatal effects of hypothyroidism may be irreversible especially in the athyroid babies and may be detected subtle, selective deficits of different abilities in the children with CH in comparison to appropriate reference groups [81,82]. Despite these observations the newborns and children with CH may have better psychoneurological development and long-term outcomes without comparison than before the introduction of the screening system.

Recently a very remarkable material was published by Leger and co-workers [83] on long-term health and socio-economic attainment of French young adult (median age: 23,4 yr) patients with permanent CH detected by neonatal screening between 1978 and 1988 on the basis of self-reported data by questionnaires. Round 1200 answers were evaluated and compared to data of controls. Chronic diseases, hearing impairment, visual problems, overweight were found significantly oftener, moreover socio-economic attainment, health-related quality of life, and full-time employment were lower or less among the CH patients. As limitation of the study is given that "outcome data are based on management procedures used early in the history of the CH screening program" (start of therapy, starting dose etc), however 20,6 % of their patients had abnormal serum TSH values (with median of 12,0 mIU/L) determined within 2 yr of the questionnaire study. Therefore one of the author's conclusions is that the patient's care should modify "to improve compliance with treatment and medical care during the transition from pediatric to adult services" [83].

4. Conclusion

In the era before the neonatal thyroid screening 1:4000 incidence of hypothyroidism was calculated in Hungary on the basis of five years (1966-70) survey by questionnaires from pediatricians. The results of TSH screening (413 permanent CH/1,369.503 newborn = 1:3316) confirmed it during the last quarter of a century (1982-2007). The technique and the incidence did not change significantly in this long period.

Transient form of CH was diagnosed in 8,4 % (26/310). Thyroid scintigraphy in 182 cases showed the following results: dysgenesis occurred in 84 % (agenesis 47 %; ectopic lingual 28 %; hypoplasia 9 %), normal-sized eutopic gland ("thyroid in situ") was found in 10 % and enlarged thyroid (dyshormonogenesis) was seen in 6 %.

Thyroid specific genes involved in CH are summarized in a table. In a cohort of 58 patients PAX8 (exon 2 and exon 3) was analysed without deviation. Congenital malformations were detected in 45 cases, and concomitant disorders in 46/210 CH patients.

Score system for predicting CH is proposed using signs (opened posterior fontanel, umbilical hernia, dry skin, enlarged tongue, constipation, laziness, wide nasal bridge and prolonged jaundice) and TSH value.

According to self-experience 10-15 μg/kg/day initial dose was administered in the last two decades. Recently L-T_4 and L-T_3 combination was applied in some cases resulting in mostly parallel decrease of elevated TSH and FT_4 level.

The children with CH grow generally in a normal tempo but the disappearance of bone age retardation is individual and may be protracted until 10 years of age. Bone mineral density was measured first by single photon absorptiometry, later by peripheral quantitative computer tomography, what may consider as a more precise method for pediatric use. Children with CH detected by neonatal screening have very slightly decreased total BMD values comparing to controls especially in prepubertal girls, but practically always within the reference range.

The final height of boys was found absolutely comparative with the reference values and the decreasing deviation of the girls did not prove to be significant. The mean menarche age corresponds to the Hungarian reference values in average, but not regarding its distribution. This average derives from the values of two different subgroups characterised with an earlier (< 12 yrs) and with a relative delayed (> 13 yrs) sexual development indicating the relationship between the thyroid and sexual hormone axes.

In the 1980s we observed significant correlation between thyroglobulin levels and IQ values detected lower IQ in athyroidism (Tg < 0,3 ng/ml). We presented ten years ago our experience that the onset of L-T_4 replacement during the first two weeks of life, the initial dose > 10 μg/kg/day and the first T_4 level > 3 μg/dl ensure the best IQ in prepubertal (8,5 ± 2,5 yrs) children.

In our recent study, using the Wechsler Intelligence Scale for children, it was found, that the partial abilities – especially the performance and working memory – of the adolescents (14-16 yrs) are commonly decreased and the total Wechsler IQ is also tended to the low normal range (93,25 ± 7,22).

Despite these results the long-term outcomes of the children with CH may consider far better than it was before the neonatal screening.

Finally, a few recent articles are recommended for more up-to-date information [15,53,64,84-88].

Abbreviations

CH - congenital hypothyroidism

TSH - thyroid stimulating hormone

TRH - TSH releasing hormone

TBG- thyroxine binding globulin

DUOX - dual oxidase

T_4 - thyroxine

T_3 - triiodothyronine

FT_4 - free thyroxine

FT_3 - free triiodothyronine

L-T_4 - levothyroxine

L-T_3 - levotriiodothyronine

RIA - RadioImmunoAssay

LIA - Lumino ImmunoAssay

IRMA - ImmunoRadioMetric Assay

DELFIA - Dissociation-Enhanced Lanthanide Fluorescent ImmunoAssay

ELISA - Enzyme-Linked ImmunoSorbent Assay

CPHD - combined pituitary hormone deficiency

GH - growth hormone

PRL - prolactin

RDS - respiratory distress syndrome

TFT - thyroid function test

PAX8 - paired box 8 (gene)

CNS - central nervous system

GORD - gastro-oesophageal reflux disease

T1DM - type 1 diabetes mellitus

Acknowledgements

We should like to thank L Blatniczky MD, PhD, A Kozma MD and B Tobisch, MD their cooperation during the follow up of these children at the outpatient clinic.

Author details

Ferenc Péter, Ágota Muzsnai and Rózsa Gráf

St. John Hospital & United Hospitals of North–Buda, Buda Children's Hospital, Budapest, Hungary

References

[1] (Dussault JH, Laberge C. Dosage de la thyroxine (T4) par methode radioimmunologique dans l'eluat de sang deche: nouvelle méthode de depistage de l'hypothyroidie neonate. Union Med Can 1973;102(10): 2062-2064). 102(10), 2062-2064.

[2] Klein, A. H, Augustin, A. V, & Foley, T. P. Successful laboratory screening for congenital hypothyroidism. Lancet (1974). , 2(7872), 77-79.

[3] Péter, F, Kovács, L, & Blatniczky, L. Erste Ergebnisse des Nationalprogrammes für Hypothyreose-Screening in Ungarn. Experiment Clin Endocrinol (1985). , 86(2), 94-95.

[4] Mäenpää, J. Congenital hypothyroidism. Aetiological and clinical aspects. Arch Dis Child (1972). , 47(12), 914-923.

[5] De Jonge, G. A. Congenital hypothyroidism in the Netherlands. Lancet (1976).

[6] Alm, J, Larsson, A, & Zetterstrom, R. Congenital hypothyroidism in Sweden. Incidence and age at diagnosis. Acta Paediatr Scand (1978).

[7] Péter, F. Medical care of children with thyroid diseases. (Hungarian) Magyar Pediater (1972).

[8] Harris, K. B, & Pass, K. A. Increase in congenital hypothyroidism in New York State and in the United States. Mol Genet Metab (2007). , 91(3), 268-277.

[9]] Deladoëy, J, Bélanger, N, & Van Vliet, G. Random variability in congenital hypothyroidism from thyroid dysgenesis over 16 years in Quebec. J Clin Endocrinol Metab (2007). , 92, 3158-3161.

[10] Olney, R. S, & Grosse, S. D. Vogt Jr RF. Prevalence of congenital hypothyroidism-current trends and future directions: workshop summary. Pediatr (2010). Suppl 2): SS36, 31.

[11] Hinton CFHHarris KB, Borgfeld L, Drummond_Borg M, Eaton R, Lorey F et al. Trends in incidence rates of congenital hypothyroidism related to select demographic factors: data from the United States, California, Massachusetts, New York, and Texas. Pediatr (2010). SS47., 37.

[12] Mengreli, C, Kanaka-gantenbein, C, Girginoudis, P, Magiakou, M. A, Christakopoulou, I, Giannoulia-karantana, A, et al. Screening for congenital hypothyroidism: the significance of threshold limit in false-negative results. J Clin Endocrinol Metab (2010)., 95(9), 4283-4290.

[13] LaFranchi SHIncreasing incidence of congenital hypothyroidism: some answers, more questions. J Clin Endocrinol Metab (2011)., 96(8), 2395-2397.

[14] Deladoëy, J, Ruel, J, Giguére, Y, & Van Vliet, G. Is the incidence of congenital hypothyroidism increasing? A 20-year retrospective population-based study in Quebec. J Clin Endocrinol Metab (2011)., 96(8), 2422-2429.

[15] Mitchell, M. L, Hsu, H-W, & Sahai, I. and the Massachusetts Pediatric Endocrine Work Group. The increased incidence of congenital hypothyroidism: fact or fancy? Clin Endocrinol (2011)., 75(6), 806-810.

[16] Hertzberg, V, Mei, J, & Therrell, B. L. Effect of laboratory practices on the incidence rate of congenital hypothyroidism. Pediatrics (2010). SS53., 48.

[17] Rapaport, R. Congenital hypothyroidism: an evolving common clinical conundrum. J Clin Endocrinol Metab (2010)., 95(9), 4223-4225.

[18] Olivieri, A, Torreasani, T, Donaldson, M, Krude, H, Van Vliet, G, Polak, M, et al. ESPE consensus meeting on congenital hypothyroidism: main recommendations. (Abstr). Horm Res (2012). suppl 1): 38-39.

[19] Maruo, Y, Takahashi, H, Soeda, I, Nishikura, N, Matsui, K, Ota, Y, et al. Transient congenital hypothyroidism caused by biallelic mutations of the dual oxidase 2 gene in Japanese patients detected by a neonatal screening program. J Clin Endocrinol Metab (2008)., 93(11), 4261-4267.

[20] Hoste, C, Rigutto, S, Van Vliet, G, Miot, F, & De Deken, X. Compound heterozygozity for a novel missense mutation and a partial deletion affecting the catalytic core of the H2O2 generating enzyme DUOX2 associated with transient congenital hypothyroidism. Human Mutation (2010). E, 1304-1319.

[21] Péter, F, Blatniczky, L, Kovács, L, & Tar, A. Experience with neonatal screening for congenital hypothyroidism in Hungary. Endocrinol Experiment (1989). , 23(3), 143-151.

[22] Muzsnai, Á. Some aspects for optimalization of hormone substitution in congenital hypothyroidism. (Hungarian) PhD thesis. Budapest, (1991).

[23] Fujiwara, H, Tatsumi, K, Miki, K, Harada, T, & Miyai, K. Takai S-I et al. Congenital hypothyroidism caused by a mutation in the Na+/I− symporter. Nature Genetics (1997)., 16(2), 124-125.

[24] Everett, L. A, Glaser, B, Beck, J. C, Idol, J. R, Buchs, A, Heyman, M, et al. Pendred syndrome is caused by mutations in a putative sulphate transporter gene (PDS) Nature Genetics (1997)., 17(4), 411-422.

[25] Ieiri, T, Cochaux, P, Targovnik, H. M, et al. A 3′ splice site mutation in the thyroglobulin gene responsible for congenital goiter with hypothyroidism. J Clin Invest (1991)., 88(6), 1901-1905.

[26] Abramowicz, M. J, Targovnik, H. M, Varela, V, Cochaux, P, Krawiec, L, Pisarev, M. A, et al. Identification of a mutation in the coding sequence of the human thyroid peroxidase gene causing congenital goiter. J Clin Invest (1992)., 90(4), 1200-1204.

[27] Iwatani, N, Mabe, H, Devriendt, K, Kodama, M, & Miike, T. Deletion of NKX2-1 gene encoding thyroid transcription factor-1 in two siblings with hypothyroidism and respiratory failure. J Pediatr. (2000)., 137(2), 272-276.

[28] Hung, W, & Sarlis, N. J. Molecular genetics of thyroid disorders in the neonate: a review. J Endocr Genetics (2001)., 2(4), 193-213.

[29] Krude, H, Schütz, B, Biebermann, H, Von Moers, A, Schnabel, D, Neitzel, H, et al. Choreoathetosis, hypothyroidism, and pulmonary alterations due to human NKX2-1 haploinsufficiency. J Clin Invest (2002)., 109(4), 475-480.

[30] Moreno, J. C, Bikker, H, Kempers, M. J, Van Trotsenburg, A. S, Baas, F, De Vijlder, J. J, et al. Inactivating mutations in the gene for thyroid oxidase 2 (THOX2) and congenital hypothyroidism. New Engl J Med. (2002)., 347(2), 95-102.

[31] Castanet, M, Park, S. M, Smith, A, Bost, M, Léger, J, Lyonnet, S, et al. A novel loss-of-function mutation in TTF-2 is associated with congenital hypothyroidism, thyroid agenesis, and cleft palate. Human Molec Genetics (2002)., 11(17), 2051-2059.

[32] Bans, I, Ansoy, A. E, Smith, A, Agostini, M, Mitchell, C. S, Park, S. M, et al. A novel missense mutation in human TTF−2 (FKHL15) gene associated with congenital hypothyroidism but not athyreosis. J Clin Endocrinol Metab (2006)., 91(10), 4183-4187.

[33] Tonacchera, M, Banco, M. E, & Montanelli, L. Di Cosmo C, Agretti P, De Marco G et al. Genetic analysis of the PAX8 gene in children with congenital hypothyroidism and dysgenetic or eutopic thyroid glands: identification of a novel sequence variant. Clin Endocrinol (2007)., 67(1), 34-40.

[34] Moreno, J. C, & Visser, T. J. New phenotypes in thyroid dyshormonogenesis: Hypothyroidism due to DUOX2 mutations. In: Van Vliet G, Polak M. (eds). Thyroid gland development and function. Basel: Karger; (2007). , 99-117.

[35] Grüters, A. Thyroid hormone transporter defects. In: Van Vliet G, Polak M. (eds). Thyroid gland development and function. Basel: Karger; (2007). , 118-126.

[36] Zamproni, I, Grasberger, H, Cortinovis, F, Vigone, M. C, Chiumello, G, Mora, S, et al. Biallelic inactivation of the dual oxidase maturation factor 2 (DUOXA2) gene as a novel cause of congenital hypothyroidism. J Clin Endocrinol Metab (2008). , 93(2), 605-610.

[37] Moreno, J. C, Klootwijk, W, Van Toor, H, Pinto, G, Alessandro, D, & Lèger, M. A et al. Mutations in the iodotyrosine deiodinase gene and hypothyroidism. New Engl J Med (2008). , 358(17), 1811-1818.

[38] Afink, G, Kulik, W, Overmars, H, De Randamie, J, Veenboer, T, Van Cruchten, A, et al. Molecular characterization of iodotyrosine dehalogenase deficiency in patients with hypothyroidism. J Clin Endocrinol Metab (2008). , 93(12), 4894-4901.

[39] Hulur, I, Hermanns, P, Nestoris, C, Heger, S, Refetoff, S, Pohlenz, J, et al. A single copy of the recently identified dual oxidase maturation factor (DUOXA) 1 gene produces only mild transient hypothyroidism in a patient with a novel biallelic DUOXA2 mutation and monoallelic DUOXA1 deletion. J Clin Endocrinol Metab (2011). E, 841-845.

[40] Muzsnai, A, Csókay, B, & Péter, F. Thyroid function, associated malformations, gene alterations and its importance in congenital hypothyroidism. In: Péter F. (ed). Progress in paediatric endocrinology. Budapest: Science Press Ltd; (2008). , 88-91.

[41] Park, S. M. Chatterjee VKK. Genetics of congenital hypothyroidism. J Med Genetics (2005). , 42(5), 379-389.

[42] Péter, F, & Muzsnai, A. Congenital disorders of the thyroid: hypo/hyper. Endocrinol Metab Clin N Am (2009). , 38(3), 491-507.

[43] Germak, J. A. Foley Jr TP. Longitudinal assessment of L-thyroxine therapy for congenital hypothyroidism. J Pediatr (1990). , 117(2), 211-219.

[44] Fisher, D. A. Management of congenital hypothyroidism. J Clin Endocrinol Metab (1991). , 72(3), 380-386.

[45] Rovet, J. F, & Ehrlich, R. M. Long-term effects of L-thyroxine therapy for congenital hypothyroidism. J Pediatr (1995). , 126(3), 380-386.

[46] Bargagna, S, Canepa, G, Cossagli, C, et al. Neuropsychological follow-up in early-treated congenital hypothyroidism: a problem-oriented approach. Thyroid (2000). , 10(3), 243-249.

[47] Bongers-schokking, J. J, Koot, H. M, Wiersma, D, & Verkerk, P. H. de Muinck Keizer-Schrama SMPF. Influence of timing and dose of thyroid hormone replcement on de-

velopment in infants with congenital hypotrhyroidism. J Pediatr (2000). , 136(3), 292-297.

[48] Hindmarsh, P. C. Optimisation of thyroxine dose in congenital hypothyroidism. Arch Dis Child (2002). , 86(2), 73-75.

[49] Kempers MJEvan der Sluijs Veer L, Nijhuis-van der Sanden et al. Intellectual and motor development of young adults with congenital hypothyroidism diagnosed by neonatal screening. J Clin Endocrinol Metab (2006). , 91(2), 418-424.

[50] Péter, F, Blatniczky, L, & Breyer, H. About the form and replacement dose of thyroid hormones in the treatment of congenital hypothyroidism (CH). In: Delange F, Fisher DA, Glinoer D (eds). Research in congenital hypothyroidism. New York and London, Plenum Press. (1989). , 338.

[51] Jones, J. H, Gellén, B, Paterson, W. F, Beaton, S, & Donaldson, M. D. Effect of high versus low initial doses of L-thyroxin for congenital hypothyroidism on thyroid function and somatic growth. Arch Dis Child (2008). , 93(11), 940-944.

[52] Balhara, B, Misra, M, & Levitsky, L. L. Clinical monitoring guidelines for congenital hypothyroidism: laboratory outcome data in the first year of life. J Pediatr (2011). , 158(4), 532-537.

[53] LaFranchi SHApproach to the diagnosis and treatment of neonatal hypothyroidism. J Clin Endocrinol Metab (2011). , 96(10), 2959-2967.

[54] Kemper, A. R, Ouyang, L, & Grosse, S. D. Discontinuation of thyroid hormone treatment among children in the United States with congenital hypothyroidism: findings from health insurance claims data. BMC Pediatrics (2010).

[55] Korzeniewski, S. J, Grigorescu, V, Kleyn, M, Young, W. I, Birbeck, G, Todem, D, et al. Transient Hypothyroidism at Year Follow-Up among Cases of Congenital Hypothyroidism Detected by Newborn Screening. J Pediatr. (2012). Aug 7. [Epub ahead of print], 3.

[56] Hennemann, G, Docter, R, Visser, T. J, Postema, P. T, & Krenning, E. P. Thyroxine plus low-dose, slow-release triiodothyronine replacement in hypothyroidism: proof of principle. Thyroid (2004). , 14(4), 271-275.

[57] Gullo, D, Latina, A, & Frasca, F. Le Moli R, Pellegriti G, Vigneri R. Levothyroxine monotherapy cannot guarantee euthyroidism in all athyreotic patients. PloS One. (2011). e22552

[58] Biondi, B, & Wartofsky, L. Combination treatment with T_4 and T_3: toward personalized replacement therapy in hypothyroidism? J Clin Endocrinol Metab (2012). , 97(7), 2256-2271.

[59] Wiersinga, W. M, Duntas, L, Fadeyev, V, & Nygaard, B. Vanderpump MPJ. 2012 ETA guiderlines: the use of L-T4 + L-T3 in the treatment of hypothyroidism. Eur Thyroid J (2012). , 1, 55-71.

[60] Eiben, O, & Pantó, E. The Hungarian National Growth Standards. Antrop Közl (1986). , 30(1), 5-23.

[61] Greulich, W. W, & Pyle, S. I. Radiographic atlas of skeletal development on hand and wrist. 2nd ed. Stanford, University Press, (1959).

[62] Péter, F, Muzsnai, Á, & Kántor, I. Thyroid hormones and bone mineralization in children and adolescents. In: Schönau E, Matkovic V (eds). Paediatric osteology. Prevention of osteoporosis- a paediatric task? Amsterdam etc, Elsevier, (1998). , 183-189.

[63] Péter, F, Muzsnai, Á, & Gyimes, J. Nation-wide survey for normal values of BMD in children measured by mobil pQCT. (Abstr) Horm Res (2002). suppl 2): 80.

[64] Bucher, H, Prader, A, & Illig, R. Head circumference, height, bone age and weigt in 103 children with congenital hypothyroidism before and during thyroid hormone replacement. Helv Paediatr Acta (1985). , 40, 305-316.

[65] Grant, D. B. Growth in early treated congenital hypothyroidism. Arch Dis Child (1994). , 70(6), 464-468.

[66] Dickerman, Z, & De Vries, L. Prepubertal and pubertal growth, timing and duration of puberty and attained adult height in patients with congenital hypothyroidism (CH) detected by the neonatal screening programme for CH- a longitudinal study. Clin Endocrinol (Oxf) (1997). , 47(6), 649-654.

[67] Adachi, M, Asakura, Y, & Tachibana, K. Final height and pubertal growth in Japanese patients with congenital hypothyroidism detected by neonatal screening. Acta Paediatr (2003). , 92(6), 698-703.

[68] Salerno, M, & Micillo, M. Di Maio S, Capalbo D, Ferri P, Lettiero T et al. Longitudinal growth, sexual maturation and final height in patients with congenital hypothyroidism detected by neonatal screening. Europ J Endocrinol (2001). , 145(4), 377-383.

[69] Soliman, A. T, Azzam, S, Elawwa, A, Saleem, W, & Sabt, A. Linear growth and neurodevelopmental outcome of children with congenital hypothyroidism detected by neonatal screening: a controlled study. Indian J Endocrinol Metab (2012). , 16(4), 565-568.

[70] Radetti, G, Castellan, C, Tató, L, Platter, K, Gentili, L, & Adami, S. Bone mineral density in children and adolescent females treated with high doses of L-thyroxine. Horm Res (1993). , 39(1), 127-131.

[71] Saggese, G, Bertelloni, S, Baroncelli, G. I, Costa, S, & Ceccarelli, C. Bone mineral density in adolescent females treated with L-thyroxine: a longitudinal study. Eur J Pediatr (1996). , 155(8), 452-457.

[72] Leger, J, Ruiz, J. C, Guibourdenche, J, Kindermans, C, Garabedian, M, & Czernichow, P. Bone mineral density and metabolism in children with congenital hypothyroidism after prolonged L-thyroxine therapy. Acta Paediatr (1997)., 86(7), 704-10.

[73] Salerno, M, & Lettiero, T. Esposito-del Puente A, Esposito V, Capalbo D, Carpinelli A et al. Effect of long-term l-thyroxine treatment on bone mineral density in young adults with congenital hypothyroidism. Eur J Endocrinol (2004)., 151(6), 689-694.

[74] Kempers, M. J, Vulsma, T, Wiedijk, B. M, De Vijlder, J. J, Van Eck-smit, B. L, & Verberne, H. J. The effect of life-long thyroxine treatment and physical activity on bone mineral density in young adult women with congenital hypothyroidism. J Pediatr Endocrinol Metab (2006)., 19(12), 1405-1412.

[75] Rovet, J, Ehrlich, R, & Sorbara, D. Intellectual outcome in children with fetal hypothyroidism. J Pediatr (1987)., 110(5), 700-704.

[76] Glorieux, I, Desjardins, M, Letarte, J, Morissette, J, & Dussault, J. H. Useful parameters to predict the eventual mental outcome of hypothyroid children. Pediatr Res (1988)., 24, 6-8.

[77] Peter, F, Muzsnai, A, & Szigervari, A. Intellectual assessment of hypothyroid children detected by screening. Acta Med Austr (1992). Sonderheft 1): 60-61.

[78] Gráf-kucsera, R, Péter, F, & Muzsnai, Á. Intellectual development of children with congenital hypothyroidism (CH) detected by newborn screening. In Morreale de Escobar G, de Vijlder JJM, Butz S, Hostalek U (editors) The thyroid and brain. Stuttgart, New York. Schattauer, (2003)., 310-311.

[79] Péter, F, Gráf, R, Blatniczky, L, & Muzsnai, Á. Neuropsychological development of children with congenital hypothyroidism recognized by neonatal screening. (Abstr) Pediatr Res (2001). Suppl 2): 158A.

[80] LaFranchi SHAustin J. How should we be treating children with congenital hypothyroidism? J Pediatr Endocrinol Metab (2007)., 20(5), 559-578.

[81] Oerbeck, B, Sundet, K, Kase, B. F, & Heyerdahl, S. Congenital hypothyroidism: influence of disease severity and L-thyrixine treatment on intellectual, motor, and school-associated outcome in young adults. Pediatrics (2003)., 112(4), 923-930.

[82] Zoeller, R. T, & Rovet, J. Timing of thyroid hormone action in the developing brain: clinical observations and experimental findings. J Neuroendocrinol (2004)., 16(10), 809-818.

[83] Leger, J, Ecosse, E, Roussey, M, Lanoë, J. L, Larroque, B, et al. Subtle health impairment and socioeducational attainment in young adult patients with congenital hypothyroidism diagnosed by neonatal screening: a longitudinal population-based cohort study. J Clin Endocrinol Metab (2011)., 96(6), 1771-1782.

[84] Rastogi, M. V. LaFranchi SH. Congenital hypothyroidism. Orphanet J Rare Dis (2010)., 5(17), 1-22.

[85] Rajput, R, Chatterjee, S, & Rajput, M. Can levothyroxine be taken as evening dose? Comparative evaluation of morning versus evening dose of levothyroxine in trearment of hypothyroidism. J Thyroid Res (2011). Article ID 505239, 5 pages doi: 10.4061/2011/505239., 2011

[86] Péter, F, & Muzsnai, Á. Congenital disorders of the thyroid: hypo/hyper. Pediatr Clin N Am (2011)., 58(5), 1099-1115.

[87] Taylor, P. N, Panicker, V, Sayers, A, Shields, B, Iqbal, A, Bremner, A, et al. A meta-analysis of the associations between common variation in the PDE8B gene and thyroid hormone parameters, including assessment of longitudinal stability of associations over time and effect of thyroid hormone replacement. Eur J Endocrinol (2011)., 164(5), 773-780.

[88] Wheeler, S. M, Willoughby, K. A, Mcandrews, M. P, & Rovet, J. F. Hippocampal size and memory functioning in children and adolescents with congenital hypothyroidism. J Clin Endocrinol Metab (2011). E, 1427-34.

Chapter 4

Congenital Hypothyroidism: Effects on Linear Growth, Catch-Up Growth, GH-IGF-I Axis and Bones

Ashraf T. Soliman, Vincenzo De Sanctis and
El Said M.A. Bedair

Additional information is available at the end of the chapter

http://dx.doi.org/10.5772/53317

1. Introduction

Triiodothyronine (T3) is a primary determinant of normal postnatal somatic growth and skeletal development, and an important regulator of bone and mineral metabolism in human [1, 2]. Before puberty, thyroid hormone appears to be a major prerequisite for normal maturation of bone [3]. Untreated childhood hypothyroidism results in a profound growth retardation and a delayed skeletal maturation. In severe cases, linear growth is almost completely halted. When treatment occurs, growth often resumes at a rate faster and beyond the normal rate for age [3, 4]. This phase of accelerated growth constitutes the "catch-up growth" phenomenon. This may be complete or incomplete depending upon many factors including the age at presentation, the severity of hypothyroidism and its duration, the age at diagnosis, and the genetic target height.

Thyroid hormones are among the important direct biological regulators of growth plate and bone accretion. In addition, thyroid hormones influence and interact with the growth hormone (GH) – Insulin-like growth factor-I (IGF-I) system and other hormones that control stature and bone growth. Hypothyroid patients show low plasma levels of IGF-I and reduced IGF bioactivity, whereas hyperthyroid patients present high plasma IGF-I levels and also low IGF bioactivity. [5] Similar changes have been observed in rats [6]. Besides, a decrease in hepatic IGF-I messenger RNA (mRNA) expression in experimental hypothyroid animals has been reported [7]. In experimental animals the effects of thyroid hormone on the IGFs system can be GH mediated [11] or non-GH mediated [12-14]. The interrelationships between the thyroid function and pituitary GH/serum IGFs axis are complex and not fully understood. GH treatment does not restore serum IGF-I levels in hypothyroid rats [6]. Decreased serum IGF-I levels in hypophysectomized rats increase after treatment with T4 doses in vivo, in a way significantly greater than after GH administration [15], an effect which is not observed in vitro, suggesting the presence of factors, other than GH, involved in the regulation of this axis in vivo.

In human, T4 replacement increases the serum levels of IGF-I and ALS in patients with primary as well as central hypothyroidism [16]. Hypothyroidism in childhood is almost invariably associated with growth failure. After the onset of T4 replacement therapy, growth and skeletal abnormalities usually resolve and a period of catch-up growth ensues. In the past, it has been suggested that catch-up growth in children treated for congenital or juvenile hypothyroidism is complete, and that such children usually reach their expected adult height [17-21], but this is not supported by recent reports showing a failure of catch-up growth in children in whom treatment has been initiated after a long period of untreated hypothyroidism [22-24].

Several mechanisms can contribute to the pathophysiology of growth failure associated with hypothyroidism. These include: abnormalities of GH secretion, IGF-I synthesis and direct action of low thyroxine on growth plate and skeletal growth. [16-19, 24, 25]

2. Postnatal Phases of Growth (Infantile-Childhood-Pubertal (ICP) pattern)

Stature growth is characterized by a pattern of changing height velocity from infancy to adulthood. A high velocity from birth with a rapid deceleration up to about 3 yr of age is seen, followed by a period with a lower and slowly decelerating velocity up to puberty. Puberty starts with an increased velocity and after the age of peak velocity a deceleration is observed until growth ceases. This pattern of growth is known as the infantile-childhood-puberty (ICP) pattern. [26-28]

3. Catch-up growth and patterns of catch-up growth

Catch-up growth is the compensatory total increase in the stature growth, either by increasing the growth velocity and/or by increasing the duration of total growth (delaying growth plate closure), after correction of the limiting factor that inhibited growth. Catch-up growth may be complete or incomplete. Catch-up growth is considered to be complete for an individual child if his final height is within the target range. In groups of patients, complete catch-up growth is expected to result in a mean final height close to the mean target height. Resumption of a normal height velocity once the growth-suppressing problem has been resolved with a return to and then maintenance of normal height growth velocity (GV) does not lead to any catch-up growth as the loss in height standard deviation score (HtSDS) is permanent (not compensated) [26-28].

3.1. Patterns of catch-up growth

Three different types of catch-up growth can be distinguished: Type A is common in infancy and early childhood. When growth restriction ceases, height velocity increases up to 4 times the mean velocity for chronological age in order to compensate rapidly and fully for the height deficit. Once the original curve is re-approached, height velocity returns to normal. A classic example of catch-up growth type A occurs after institution of a gluten-free diet in childhood celiac disease. In catch-up growth type B a small or no increase of height velocity occurs after the growth restriction has ceased as compared with the mean velocity for chronological age. However, growth continues for longer than usual, so that ultimately the growth arrest is compensated. Type C is a mixture of types A and B. When growth restriction ceases, there is an increase in height velocity as well as a delay and prolongation of growth. [26-32]

A catch-up process that brings a child to the 50th percentile or above, for a given population (HtSDS = or > 0) is considered complete. A catch-up that brings a child to > -2 but below 0 is considered incomplete. Complete catch-up growth may be also accepted when the child attains a final height within the genetic potential range (Mid-parental height) (+/- 1 SD) [26].

It has been suggested that acceleration of growth velocity rather than delayed maturation occurs during infancy and early childhood; but during late childhood and adolescence delayed maturation rather than acceleration of growth velocity occurs. This can be explained by the progressive fall of growth plate chondrocyte proliferation, and hence the reduced potential for catch-up with age [26-32].

Canalization means that the individual growth curve parallels the percentile curves of growth charts. In the pre-pubertal period, canalization is clearly seen and therefore a catch-up growth spurt is easily recognizable. However, during pubertal years, catch-up growth may not be clearly separated from pubertal growth spurt [26].

4. Regulation of postnatal longitudinal bone growth

Longitudinal bone growth is achieved by the complex, multistep process known as endochondral ossification, whereby the cartilaginous template of the axial and appendicular skeleton is replaced by bone. This process is initiated when chondrocytes at the epiphyseal growth plate are stimulated to proliferate and then proceed through stages of maturation and hypertrophy. In the region of cellular hypertrophy, the surrounding matrix and vascular tissue undergo calcification. The hypertrophic chondrocytes degenerate and give way to invading osteoblasts, and bone and bone marrow subsequently replace the calcified cartilage at the metaphysis. Endochondral ossification is an important determinant of both the rate and extent of longitudinal bone growth. This growth plate activity is in turn subject to regulation by a number of factors, which might be of genetic, endocrine, paracrine, and autocrine origin. It is the complex interactive effects of these substances on chondrocytes in vivo that determine the final growth response. Endocrine regulators include various hormones such as thyroid hormones, GH, parathyroid hormone/parathyroid hormone related peptide (PTH/PTHrP), as well as several growth factors and cytokines, such as IGF-I and basic fibroblast like growth factor. [32-36]

5. Effect of thyroxine on growth plate and bones

Long bones are formed by endochondral ossification and the skull by intramembranous ossification. During endochondral ossification, mesenchyme-derived chondrocytes form a cartilage model, undergo hypertrophic differentiation and then apoptose. The surrounding collagen X-rich cartilage matrix calcifies and forms a scaffold for bone formation by osteoblasts. Organized columns of proliferating and differentiating chondrocytes persist in the growth plate until adolescence and mediate linear growth and the acquisition of peak bone mass. The epiphyses and metaphyses of long bones originate from separate ossification centers that are separated by a growth plate. By contrast, in intramembranous ossification, osteoblasts differentiate from mesenchyme to form bone directly. Adult bone structure and mechanical strength are preserved by a continuous process of skeletal remodelling during which precise coupling of osteoclastic bone resorption and subsequent osteoblastic bone formation is maintained. [37]

Hypothyroidism slows longitudinal bone growth and endochondral ossification, while hyperthyroidism accelerates both processes. In hypothyroid animals, there is a decrease in the heights of the proliferative and hypertrophic zones, and a decrease in chondrocyte proliferation and chondrocyte hypertrophy and disruption of the normal columnar organization of the growth plate and vascular/bone cell invasion. T3 seems to stimulate the recruitment of cells to the proliferating zone from the germinal zone and facilitate the differentiation of growth plate chondrocytes. [38,39] In thyroid receptor (TRa) knockout mice [40] there is a complete growth arrest, with disorganization of epiphyseal growth plate chondrocytes and delayed cartilage mineralization and bone formation. These abnormalities result from severe hypothyroidism due to impaired thyroid hormone production at weaning, as the skeletal phenotype can be rescued by T4 replacement. [40] In the hypothyroid rat, proliferating chondrocytes fail to form discrete columns and the hypertrophic zone is diminished in width and morphologically indistinct. Expression of collagen X, a specific marker of hypertrophic chondrocyte differentiation is undetectable in the hypothyroid growth plate, indicating that hypertrophic chondrocyte differentiation is severely impaired.

The growth plate is separated from the primary spongiosum by a mineralised interface, essentially sealing off the growth plate from vascular invasion and preventing further bone lengthening, leading to growth retardation. During hypothyroidism, there is disruption of the normal functional continuity between maturing chondrocytes and mineralizing osteoblasts with markedly reduced osteoblast invasion and fewer, thinner bone trabecula. T4 induces the expression of both type II and X collagen, the activity of the differentiation marker alkaline phosphatase, and chondrocyte hypertrophy. [38-40]

In addition, the growth plates of hypothyroid rats also have abnormal cartilage matrix deposition. Normal cartilage matrix is composed of proteoglycans containing chondroitin and heparan sulfates and hyaluronic acid residues. In hypothyroid rats, studies have revealed an abnormal increase in sulfation of heparan sulfate proteoglycans in proliferating chondrocytes. This abnormal matrix is deposited in a patchy irregular fashion suggesting that thyroid hormones influence extra-cellular matrix biology as well as cellular activity of the growth plate. Treatment of these rats with thyroid hormones reverses these changes and studies have shown that this is through the direct actions of T3 on bone, and it is not growth hormone (GH) mediated [38]. T4 but not GH is capable of completely reverting reduced widths of the proliferating and hypertrophic zone, as well as a disturbed growth plate architecture and vascular invasion of the growth plate in hypothyroid rats, establishing a unique role for thyroid hormones in the regulation of bone growth and maturation [39- 44].

In vitro, thyroid hormones also stimulate terminal differentiation of epiphyseal growth plate chondrocytes. [45] Tibial dyschondroplasia (TD), a disorder of broiler chickens, associated with avascular non-mineralised cartilage extending from the epiphyseal growth plate, results from the inability of proliferating chondrocytes to undergo terminal differentiation to hypertrophic chondrocytes. This disorder has been shown to be associated with a markedly reduced expression of iodothyronine deiodinase type 2 (DIO2) in the growth plate [14]. DIO2 acts by catalysing the conversion of T4 to T3. Epiphyseal dysgenesis (Figure 3) in hypothyroidism can be similarly explained by a reduction in T3 which is necessary to stimulate resting zone cells to proliferate and differentiate into chondrocytes, and for vascular invasion of the growth plate [46, 47].

Indian hedgehog (Ihh) is a member of the hedgehog family of secreted ligands and is a master regulator of bone development. Ihh is synthesized by prehypertrophic and hypertrophic chondrocytes [48, 49]. Ihh stimulates production of parathyroid hormone-related peptide (PTHrP) from cells at the periarticular ends of bones. PTHrP acts on the PTH/PTHrP receptor (PPR) to keep proliferating chondrocytes in the proliferative pool. When the source of PTHrP is sufficiently distant, the chondrocytes are no longer stimulated by PTHrP and they stop proliferating and start to synthesize Ihh. In addition, Ihh stimulates chondrocyte proliferation directly and also controls the differentiation of osteoblasts from perichondrial cells during the formation of the bone collar. Thus, interactions between Ihh and PTHrP determine the lengths of proliferating columns of chondrocytes in the growth plate and hence the pace of bone growth. In hypothyroid animals Ihh is mainly located within the upper regions of the proliferative zone and the reserve zone [50]. PTHrP mRNA expression is also altered in the hypothyroid growth plate. Levels of expression are increased and include expression by chondrocytes extending throughout the proliferative and reserve zones. PTH/PTHrP receptor (PPR) is also altered by thyroid status. It is expressed throughout all zones of the growth plate in euthyroid and hypothyroid animals, and restricted to proliferative and prehypertrophic chondrocytes in hypothyroid-T4 treated rats. Thyroid hormone has been shown to stimulate terminal differentiation of growth plate chondrocytes by down regulation of Sox9, a transcription factor present in cells of mesenchymal condensations and proliferating chondrocytes but not in hypertrophic chondrocytes [51]. This terminal differentiation process is associated with expression of cyclin-dependant kinase inhibitors known to regulate the cell cycle checkpoint [52].

These data strongly support a role for thyroid hormones in regulating components of the Ihh/PTHrP feedback loop in the growth plate and thus the pace of chondrocyte differentiation and bone growth.

Fibroblast Growth Factor Receptor-1 (FGFR1) is a T3-target gene in bone. Three FGFRs are known to be essential for skeletal development. Mutations of all three FGFRs can cause variable bony abnormalities, while an activating mutation of FGFR3 is the cause of achondroplasia, the most common genetic form of dwarfism [53, 54]. FGFR1 has been identified as a T3-target gene in osteoblasts [55]. T3 acting via the thyroid hormone receptor (TR) enhances FGF stimulation of FGFR1 activity. Hypothyroid mice display delayed endochondral ossification and have abnormalities of cartilage matrix similar to those described above, namely an increase in heparan sulfate proteoglycans [54]. It is known that heparan sulfate is required for binding of FGF to FGFR and for ligand-induced receptor activity [56, 57]. Therefore, T3-regulated production of heparan sulfate, or modification of its structure, might be the mechanism by which T3 regulates FGFR1 signalling. In addition to the thyroid hormone receptors, receptors for growth hormone (GH), insulin like growth factor-1 (IGF-1), are also expressed by growth plate chondrocytes [58-60]. T3 influences expression of several components of GH/IGF-1 signalling in bone [61, 62].

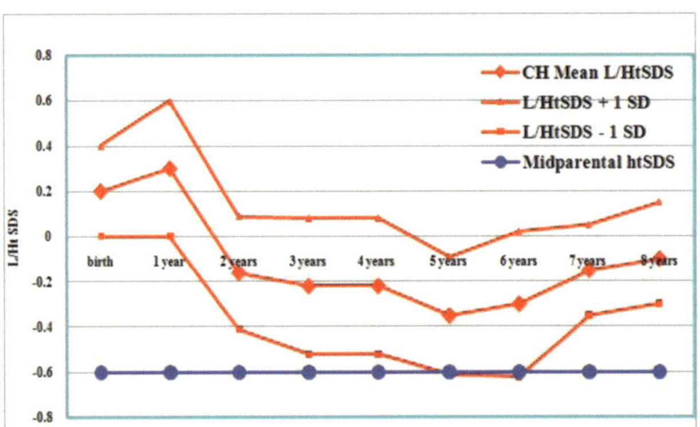

Figure 3. Effect of thyroxine treatment on infants and children with congenital hypothyroidism (CH) (infantile and childhood phases) growth diagnosed through neonatal screening compared to their mid-parental height (MPHtSDS).

In summary, thyroid hormones act through chondrocytes bearing TRs to modulate growth plate proliferation, differentiation, and vascular invasion. These functions are mediated via many possible mechanisms including direct action on the chondrocytes, osteoblasts and mast cells, as well through interaction with other hormones and growth factors acting in endocrine, paracrine and autocrine fashions. Understanding the mechanisms behind the interactions between the T3 signaling pathway and the systemic and paracrine effects of GH/IGF-1 is important in considering the molecular biology of thyroid hormone-dependent skeletal development.

6. Effect of hypothyroidism on bone remodelling and skeleton

Remodelling is crucial for bone health, which is characterized by simultaneous formation and resorption. Thyroid hormones affect bone cells both in vitro and in vivo by stimulating osteoblast and osteoclast cells with more bone resorption and increased skeletal remodelling. Thyroid hormone status within the physiological range affects bone mass and density. In healthy men at age of peak bone mass, between-subject variation in thyroid hormone concentrations affects bone density. Higher levels of FT3, TT3, TT4 and TBG are associated with less favourable bone density and content [63-65].

In experimental adult dogs, thyroxine administration in moderate pharmacologic doses increased the activation frequency, number of bone-forming and -resorbing sites, and the osteoid seam circumference in unaltered bone. Thyroxine, by activating skeletal remodelling, increases bone turnover and both formation and resorption at the tissue level. The increased serum calcium and phosphorus levels and urinary hydroxyproline excretion at several intervals during thyroxine administration are consistent with the morphometric evidence of increased bone turnover and resorption. These findings suggest that thyroxine is a potent activator of skeletal remodelling. [66]

In sheep, thyroidectomy at 105-110 days of gestation results in very low levels of foetal plasma T4 and T3 (no pre-partum rise in fetal plasma T3) and the foetuses have shorter bones and altered metatarsal structure and strength when analysed at or close to term (145 ± 2 days). At and just before term the thyroidectomised sheep data indicated that the structural changes in bone are a result of impaired bone formation whilst resorption was normal. These changes resemble the phenotype reported in adult D2 knockout mice but the precise cellular basis is not known [67]. The reduced bone formation may be a consequence of local effect of T3 on the bones or due to altering signalling pathways such as the GH/IGFI axis which is known to be anabolic to the skeleton.

In human, overt hyperthyroidism is associated with increased bone resorption, low bone mineral density and increased number of fractures in postmenopausal women [68-70]. Both hyperthyroidism and to some extent hypothyroidism are linked to reduction of bone mineral density and, hence, increased risk for fracture. Low thyroid hormone levels, rather than the increased TSH levels, are responsible for the decreased bone resorption during hypothyroidism in thyroid carcinoma patients. The levels of C-cross linking terminal telopeptide of type 1 collagen were lower during hypothyroidism compared to 8 weeks after reinstitution of thyroxine replacement therapy [71,72].

Clinically, the radiological skeletal manifestations of congenital and severe juvenile hypothyroidism include:

a. in the long bones: delay in the appearance of ossification centres (delayed bone age), deformed and irregular shape (epiphyseal dysgenesis) of the already existing centres and metaphyseal widening (splaying);

b. in the skull: the presence of the intrasutural (wormian) bones, widening of the sutures and fontanelles, delayed closure of fontanelle and delayed teeth eruption,

c. in the vertebrae : abnormal flattening, bulleting and inferior lipping and

d. broadening of ribs [73,74].

These radiological changes appeared similar in many aspects to those reported in mucopolysaccharidosis (MPS) and can be explained by the previously mentioned abnormalities in the growth plate chondrocytes, bone cells and matrix [72,75] (Figure 3).

7. Effect of thyroxine on Growth hormone-Insulin-like growth factor-I system

In addition to its local action on the growth plate, thyroid hormones may have indirect effects on the growth plate, mediated by GH and IGF-I. In hypothyroid humans and mice, GH and IGF-I levels are reduced and IGF-I generation is defective. In addition to the local action of thyroxine on growth plate, treatment with thyroxine increases IGF-I secretion and improves IGF-I generation associated with increased growth rate. Moreover, thyroid hormones have been shown to interact with the GH-IGF-I pathway at the level of the growth plate. T3 was shown to promote proliferation of embryonic chicken chondrocytes and cultured rat epiphyseal chondrocytes by enhancing IGF-I mRNA expression. T3/T4 can regulate growth hormone receptor (GHR) expression, in vivo in rat growth plates [75-77].

The effects of T3 and IGF-I on (3H) thymidine incorporation, alkaline phosphatase (ALP) activity and IGF-I receptor mRNA levels are studied in rat epiphyseal chondrocytes cultured in monolayer. ALP activity (a late marker of differentiated epiphyseal chondrocytes) is increased by T3 in a dose-dependent manner with a maximal response at 10 micrograms. IGF-I receptor mRNA levels were increased by 10 micrograms of T3 while no effect of hGH (50 micrograms/l) or IGF-I (25 micrograms/l) was demonstrated. Both T3 and IGF-I are shown to interact with epiphyseal chondrocytes and both substances seem to affect cell proliferation and maturation and therefore longitudinal bone growth. These results indicate that IGF-I is important for proliferation of the cells while T3 initiates the terminal differentiation of epiphyseal chondrocytes [78].

In children with hypothyroidism Soliman et al. [73] have reported a significant decrease of GH response to Clonidine stimulation as well as a decreased IGF-I generation in response to GH stimulation. IGF-I generation shows a small but significant increase in the IGF-I production in response to the exogenous GH. The mean peak is lower than 100 ng/ml, which is the cut off to define GHD stated in the normative data. [73]. This limited, yet significant IGF-I generation after GH administration suggests that the GHD associated with the hypothyroid state was not the sole explanation to the low IGF-I level and supports the possibility of associated GH insensitivity (GHI) state and/or a direct role of thyroxine on hepatic IGF-I production not mediated via GH. In hypothyroid patients, after treatment with thyroxine, marked improvement in the IGF-I generation occurs but this is still lower compared to normal children. Cavaliere H et al. [79] have found significantly decreased basal IGF-I concentrations in primary hypothyroid and endemic cretins with a significant increase after treatment and have described a positive correlation (r = 0.56) between IGF-I and serum T4 and T3 concentrations.

In the mature hypothyroid rats, serum IGF-I levels are partially corrected by GH but are normalised by thyroid hormone replacement [80].

Gaspard T et al. [81] reported that the administration of T4 alone to hypophysectomized or thryoidectomized animals was capable of stimulating the IGF-I activity in the absence of GH. Romos S et al., [82] reported good positive correlation between IGF-I and thyroid hormone concentrations in both neonatal and adult thyroidectomized rats and that the correlation between them was dependent on the dose of T4. Also, Ikeda T et al. [83] stated that the T3, but not T4, directly enhances the release and synthesis of IGF-I in a dose dependent manner in the rat liver. T3 also controls the IGF-I biosynthesis in nerve cells in rats [84]. Collectively, the effects of thyroid hormone on serum IGF levels seem to be mediated only partially via GH but other effects involving either direct thyroid hormone effects, or mediated by some other route, independent of GH, appear to be working.

In children with hypothyroidism, in spite of significant improvement of IGF-I levels after treatment versus before treatment, IGF-I generation is still significantly below age-matched normal children. This defective IGF-I production after treatment suggest that prolonged hypothyroidism may modulate the IGF-I secreting ability of the hepatocytes either through negative effect on their mass (number or size) and/or on the expression of the GHR on their surfaces. In sheep, induction of the hepatic GH receptor and the maturational switch in hepatic IGF-I synthesis are initiated by the pre-partum rise in foetal plasma cortisol [85,86]. Cortisol also stimulates deiodination of thyroxin (T4) to triiodothyronine (T3) and thereby leads to a pre-partum rise in plasma T3 that coincides with the increase in hepatic GH receptor and IGF-I gene expression toward term [86].

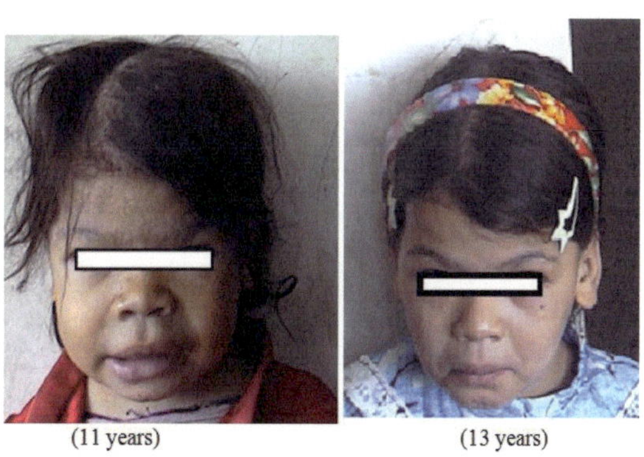

Figure 1. Photograph of patient demonstrating her coarse facial features before treatment [11 years] and improvement after treatment.

Forhead AJ et al., [87] have reported that thyroid hormones regulate hepatic growth hormone receptor (GHR) and IGF-I gene expression in the sheep fetus during late gestation. Thyroid hormone deficiency induced by foetal thyroidectomy abolished the normal pre-partum rise in hepatic GHR mRNA abundance. However, the precise mechanisms by which T3 acts on the GHR gene are unclear [88]. Nuclear thyroid hormone receptors are present in foetal ovine liver during late gestation and have a 10-fold greater affinity for T3 than T4 in utero [89].

The effect of thyroid hormone on the regenerative capacity of hepatocytes may be important. Moro L et al. [89] and Alisi A et al., [90] have proved the role of thyroid hormones on the regenerative capacity of the liver which was reduced during the hypothyroid state and regained to normal after thyroid hormone administration through altering the expression of the proteins involved in the control of cell cycle and apoptosis, decreasing tissue rate of protein synthesis, and retarding growth of the liver and the whole animal [91, 92]. These studies propose an important role of thyroid hormones on the hepatocyte regenerative power and the GHR expression on hepatocytes and suggest that thyroxine deficiency may compromise these functions and dependent loss of IGF-I production capacity.

In adults with GH deficiency, GH administration stimulates peripheral T4 to T3 conversion in a dose-dependent manner. Serum T3 levels are subnormal despite T4 substitution when the patients are off GH but normalised with GH therapy. Energy expenditure increases with GH and correlates with free T3 levels. GH causes a significant blunting of serum TSH. These findings suggest that GH plays a distinct role in the physiological regulation of thyroid function in general, and of peripheral T4 metabolism in particular [93].

Untreated primary hypothyroidism is associated with decreased GH pulsatility, attenuation of GH response to secretagogues and a reduction in IGF-I and IGF Binding Protein-3 (IGFBP-3). Reduced levels of IGF-I that increase with L-thyroxine replacement therapy have also been demonstrated in the setting of subclinical hypothyroidism [94,95]. Conversely, hyperthyroidism is associated with an increase in mean 24 hour GH concentration and secretion rates [96, 97] while serum IGF-I and IGFBP-3 levels have been found to be normal in subclinical hyperthyroidism [84] with a normal or high [94, 98, 99] IGF-I in overt thyrotoxicosis. Administration of T4 to hypophysectomised animals has been shown to stimulate IGF-1 production in the absence of GH, while IGF-BP3 was shown to be GH dependent [100].

In summary, thyroid hormones modulate growth plate growth and part of this effect appears to be mediated by activating GH-IGF-I axis and modulating local GH and/or IGF-I actions.

8. Thyroxine and catch-up growth

Evidence from animal studies suggests that catch-up growth is due, in large part, to a delay in growth plate senescence. Growth plate senescence refers to the normal, programmed changes that occur in the growth plate over time i.e. growth plate chondrocytes may have a finite proliferative capacity that is gradually exhausted, causing growth to slow and eventually to stop. With increasing age, there is a decrease in the linear growth rate, the chondrocyte proliferation rate, the height of the growth plate, and the number of cells in each growth plate zone. Growth plate senescence is not a function of time per se, but of cell proliferation. Hypothyroidism suppresses growth plate chondrocyte proliferation, but it conserves the proliferative capacity of the chondrocytes and therefore it slows their senescence. Consequently, after transient growth inhibition, growth plates retain a greater proliferative capacity, are less senescent, and, hence, show a greater growth rate than expected for age, resulting in catch-up growth [101,102].

Marino R et al. [102] have administered propylthiouracil to newborn rats for 8 wk to induce hypothyroidism and then stopped the propylthiouracil to allow catch-up growth. In untreated controls, the growth plates undergo progressive, senescent changes in multiple functional and structural characteristics. In treated animals, after stopping propylthiouracil, these functional, structural, and molecular senescent changes are delayed, compared with controls. This delayed senescence includes a delayed decline in longitudinal growth rate, resulting in catch-up growth. These findings demonstrate that growth inhibition due to hypothyroidism slows the developmental program of growth plate senescence, including the normal decline in the rate of longitudinal bone growth, thus accounting for catch-up growth.

A proportion of patients with T3 resistance, caused by mutant T3 receptor proteins, suffer from growth retardation and developmental abnormalities of bone [103,104] that reflect tissue hypothyroidism. T4 replacement induces rapid catch-up growth, although this may be incomplete because bone age advances faster than the increase in height [105].

The deficit in final height after treatment appears to correlate with the severity and duration of hypothyroidism. Catch-up growth may be especially compromised if treatment is required at or around the onset of puberty. Boersma B et al, [106] reported that if catch-up growth coincides with the pubertal growth spurt, final height might be compromised, possibly due to very rapid bone maturation. Soliman et al. [73] found that treatment of elder children with neglected hypothyroidism accelerates their bone maturation in the first year of treatment (bone age delay changed from 4.7 +/- 1 years to 3.1 +/- 0.9 years after a year of therapy). In accordance with this, childhood thyrotoxicosis causes accelerated growth and advanced bone age, which may lead to craniosynostosis, premature growth plate closure, and a short stature [107].

9. Growth in Congenital and Juvenile Hypothyroidism Before Versus After Thyroxine Treatment

Poor length growth is apparent as early as the first year of life. Before the neonatal screening was initiated in the 1970s, the percentage of children with congenital hypothyroidism (CH) having a height below the 10th percentile has been shown to range from 19% to 31%. Adult stature without treatment ranges from 1 to 1.6 metres, depending on severity, sex and other genetic factors. Bone maturation and puberty are severely delayed. Ovulation is impeded and infertility is common. Growth arrest, delayed bone age, and epiphyseal dysgenesis occur in congenital hypothyroidism, juvenile hypothyroidism and in some patients with resistance to thyroid hormone, whereas accelerated growth and skeletal maturation are evident in childhood thyrotoxicosis [108-109]. Catch-up growth during thyroid hormone replacement treatment is marked but, unfortunately, may not be complete.

In animals, the dose-response relationship between thyroid hormone and linear growth, has been studied in prepubertal methimazole-induced hypothyroid monkeys. Subsequently, each animal has received 1, 2, 4, or 8 micrograms/kg per day of T4, IM, for 9 weeks. Methimazole administration decreases thyroid hormone and IGF-I levels and decreases leg growth rate. With increasing doses of exogenous T4, serum T4, T3, and IGF-I as well as lower leg growth rate increase significantly. Animals not given T4 has a 65% decrease in lower leg growth rate. Animals given 4 and 8 micrograms/kg per day T4 have 56% and 73% increases, respectively, in lower leg growth rate compared to baseline. Lower leg growth rate correlate better with serum T3, T4 and IGF-I. Serum IGF-I correlate with serum T3. This study proves that increased serum T4 and T3 levels cause progressive increases in growth velocity and IGF-I levels over a range from moderate hypothyroidism to moderate hyperthyroidism. Growth velocity and IGF-I levels correlate more strongly with the serum T3 than with the serum T4 level. [110]

In humans, many case studies and clinical research papers have investigated linear growth and pubertal maturation in neglected hypothyroidism. Their results can be summarised as following:

Case Report: An 11 year- old Egyptian girl has presented with severe short stature and mental retardation. Examination has revealed all features of cretinism with Height SDS (HtSDS) = -7.6 SD, hypotonia, umbilical hernia, myxedematous face, and severe mental retardation with IQ = 30. Low T4 and high TSH (Figure 1, Table 1) with bone age of 4 years are noted with marked epiphyseal dysgenesis, metaphyseal and vertebral changes. L-thyroxine therapy for ten years has been associated with significant and prolonged catch-up growth till the age of 20 years with near-normal adult stature compared to mid-parental height HtSDS = -0.9. Puberty started at the age of 15 y and progressed over 4 years to full maturity. All radiological skeletal abnormalities were corrected after 5 years of thyroxine therapy. Significant increase in IGF-1 level and IGF-I response to GH stimulation was achieved early. In summary, complete catch up of growth with normalization of all radiological changes could occur even in neglected congenital hypothyroidism.

Age [y]	Bone age [y]	HtSDS	GVSDS	T4 ug/dl	TSH mIU/ml	IGF-I ng/dl
Birth	ND	0	ND	ND	ND	ND
11	3	-7.6	3.4	0.5	"/100	25
12	6	-7.2	2	14.7	0.5	75
14	10	-6.5	6	14.00	0.6	98
16	12	-4.6	7	13.8	0.5	
18	14	-2.9	7	12.5	0.5	
20	16	-1.6	ND	13.9	0.8	

Table 1. Growth and hormonal data of a patient with neglected hypothyroidism before and after treatment for 9 years.

http://dx.doi.org/10.5772/53317

Kubicky et al. have described a patient who discontinued treatment few months for 3 years after neonatal diagnosis, and although treated till puberty she had significant growth retardation as an adult. Boersma et al. have described two children with untreated congenital hypothyroidism, and although they have experienced a marked catch-up growth, both of them have reached an adult height below their target height [106, 110].

Soliman et al. [73] have studied 15 children with neglected hypothyroidism aged = 6.4 +/- 4.2 years. Patients had HtSDS = -4.3 +/- 2.5 and delayed bone age (– 4.5 +/- 2), with defective GH response to clonidine and low IGF-I concentration. After two years of treatment with L-thyroxine, their HtSDS has increased from -4.3 +/- 2.5 to -2.7 +/- 2.3. This has been associated with a significant improvement of their GH response to clonidine, increased IGF-I generation in response to GH stimulation. HtSDS increments correlated significantly with free T4 concentrations, and the growth velocity standard deviation score (GVSDS) s correlated significantly with increments in IGF-I concentrations with treatment. Therefore, in neglected hypothyroidism permanent height loss could not be prevented. The capacity to establish a significant, although incomplete, catch-up growth spurt is associated with significant recovery of GH -IGF-I axis and is proved to be possible, even after a long period of thyroid dysfunction. Incomplete catch-up growth after delayed treatment of infants and children with congenital hypothyroidism has been reported in other studies [73,111].

In a retrospective study of 59 children with late diagnosis of hypothyroidism presented at different ages in the Endocrinology clinic of Alexandria University before the establishment of neonatal screening national program, Soliman et al. measured the HtSDS of patients before versus after 2 years of treatment. Results showed significant catch-up growth in those diagnosed during the first two years of life compared to those diagnosed after 6 years of life (Figure 2). Pubertal maturation was delayed in 10/21 patients and accelerated in 3/21. (Unpublished data by authors) (Table 2)

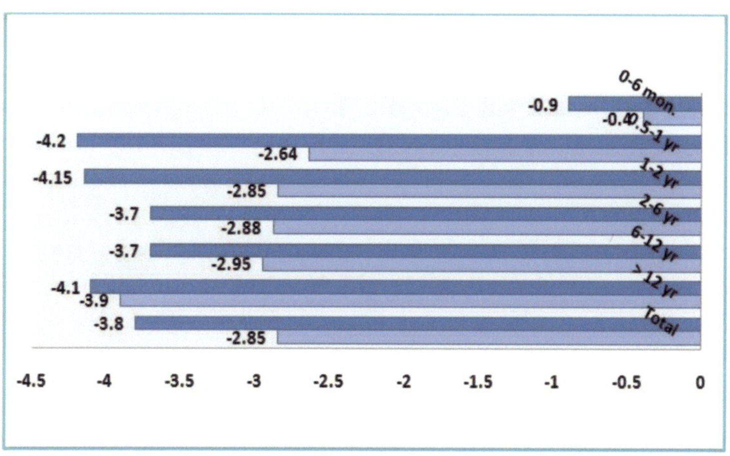

Figure 2. Height Standard Deviation Score [HtSDS] before [dark blue] and after [light blue] one year of treatment of neglected cases of hypothyroidism diagnosed at different ages.

	Delayed Puberty	Normal Puberty	Precocious Puberty
Males [n = 9]	6	2	1
Females [n = 12]	4	6	2
Total [n = 21]	10/21	8/21	3/21

Table 2. Pubertal Data in neglected hypothyroidism

Collectively, these studies demonstrated clearly the deleterious effect of hypothyroidism on all stages of growth [infantile, childhood and pubertal phases] and the incomplete catch-up growth after treatment with thyroxine especially in older children.

10. Growth in Congenital hypothyroidism treated at the neonatal period

Forty years after the worldwide introduction of neonatal screening for congenital hypothyroidism, it is beyond doubt that early diagnosis and thyroxine treatment prevent brain damage. Although benefits of early treatment have never been proven in randomized placebo-controlled trials, studies that described the natural course of congenital hypothyroidism are considered sufficient evidence for its efficacy, at least in severe forms [73, 111-114]. After the introduction of the screening, several studies have reported a normal linear growth in infancy and childhood [115-117], while others have described a slight growth deceleration early in childhood in children with severe CH at diagnosis [118-120]. With respect to the achievement of a normal final height, some studies have suggested that the adequacy of L-thyroxine replacement in the first 6 months of life may influence the adult height of children with CH detected by newborn screening [121]. In contrast, other studies have found no correlation between severity at diagnosis, aetiology, or initial L-thyroxine dosage [122,123]. The only postnatal factor consistently found to be related to adult height has been the age at the start of treatment.

Salerno et al. [122] reported normal linear growth and onset and duration of puberty in both males and females (n= 55) with congenital hypothyroidism (CH) detected by a neonatal screening program and treated with thyroxin. Their data have shown that the onset and the progression of puberty are independent of the aetiology, the severity of CH and the timing of the beginning of treatment. Girls treated with an initial amount of L-thyroxine (L-T4) > 8 microg/kg per day have shown an earlier onset of puberty compared with girls treated with a lower initial dose of L-T4. However, both groups have attained a similar final height, which in both cases was above the target height. No significant relationship has been found between final height and severity of CH at diagnosis, initial L-T4 dosage or aetiology of hypothyroidism.

Soliman et al. [124, 125] have reported that hypothyroid patients (n =45) diagnosed through the neonatal screening program have normal birth length, weight and head circumference compared to normal infants. These data rule out significant effect of foetal hypothyroidism on foetal growth. When treated with an initial T4 dosage (50 ug/day) with adjustment of T4 dose to maintain serum fT4 concentrations within the upper quartile of normal range and

TSH < 4 mIU/ml, these children have adjustment (+/- 0.5 SD) of their mean HtSDS towards their mid-parental height SDS (MPHtSDS) only during the second year of life. In addition, child mean HtSDS is higher than MPHtSDS by an average of 0.4 SD between the 2nd and 8th year of life (Figure 3). Adachi et al. [126] have reported normal adult height of patients with CH detected by neonatal screening which was equivalent to that of the reference population and their target height.

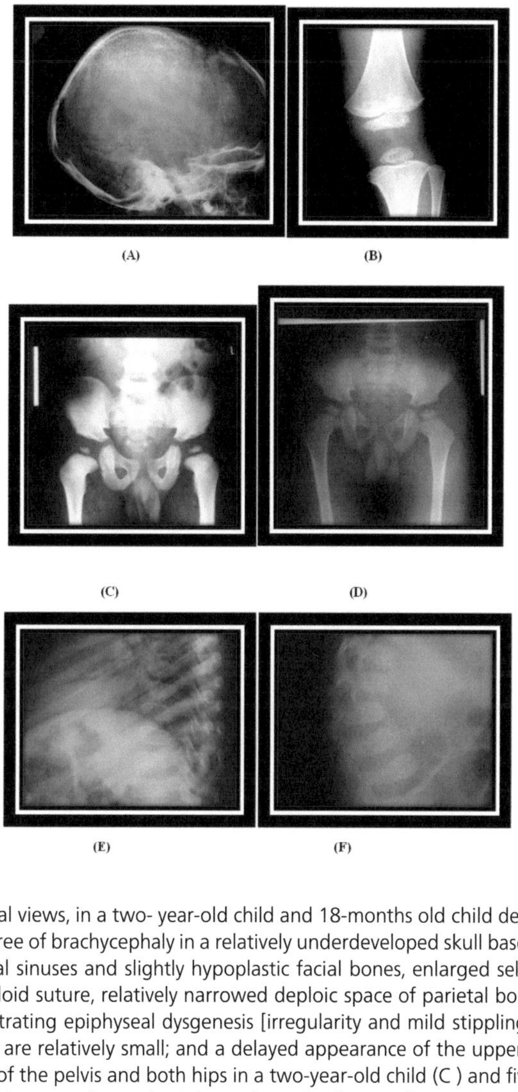

Figure 4. A: Skull X ray, lateral views, in a two- year-old child and 18-months old child demonstrating persistent wide anterior fontanelle, mild degree of brachycephaly in a relatively underdeveloped skull base with increased bone density, underdeveloped paranasal sinuses and slightly hypoplastic facial bones, enlarged sella turcica (Cherry sella), few wormian bones along lambdoid suture, relatively narrowed deploic space of parietal bones and overcrowded teeth. B : AP view of knee demonstrating epiphyseal dysgenesis [irregularity and mild stippling] of the lower femoral and upper tibial epiphyses which are relatively small; and a delayed appearance of the upper fibular epiphysis for age of the patient. C, D. Plain X ray of the pelvis and both hips in a two-year-old child (C) and five-year-old (D) demonstrating epiphyseal dysgenesis of the upper femoral epiphyses (irregular flattened upper femoral epiphysis which are small for age of the patient;underdeveloped) with relatively shallow acetabular roofs and mild coxa vara deformity and relatively small (hypoplastic) iliac bones. E,F : Plain X ray of dorsolumbar region of two different patients demonstrating flattening of the vertebral bodies with relative osteoporosis leading to the appearance of "picture framing" of vertebral bodies (E, and relatively wide disc spaces with typical bullet shape appearance of vertebral bodies (LV1 and LV2) and relatively small body of LV1 with anterior subluaxation of DV12 over LV1 leading to smooth gibbus deformity (F).

Dickerman and de Vries [127] have found normal prepubertal and pubertal growth and achievement of normal adult height in children diagnosed through neonatal screening (n = 30) and have reported a significant correlation with parental height and the mean L-T4 daily dose administered over the first 6 months of treatment. A dose of at least 8.5 micrograms/kg/day is recommended by these authors during this period.

Jones et al. [128] have studied growth of 314 CH children according to initial daily dose of T4: Group 1 (25 ug, n = 152), Group 2 (30-40 ug, n = 63) and Group 3 (50 ug, n = 99). At 3 months weight, length and OFC SDS values have been (-0.39, -0.35, 0.09); (-0.30, -0.47, 0.32) ; and (-0.03, -0.13, 0.18) for Groups 1, 2 and 3, respectively, indicating no difference between the 3 doses on somatic growth between 3 months and 3 years. However, an initial T4 dose of 50 ug daily has normalized thyroid function several months earlier than lower-dose regimes. These data has been confirmed by Salerno et al. [129] who have reported that higher dose has been shown to improve the IQ at 4 years of age, even in patients with severe CH at diagnosis.

These results suggest that conventional management of children with CH detected by neonatal screening with an initial dose > 8 ug/kg/day leads to normal infantile, childhood and pubertal growth with normal adult height and sexual development, and that the major factors determining adult height in these children are the familial genetic growth potential and good compliance to treatment. However, a still unsolved question is whether neonates with mild hypothyroidism benefit from treatment, too [130-134].

11. Growth before and after Juvenile-Acquired hypothyroidism:

In one study, hypothyroidism has been diagnosed and treated in 18 girls and six boys with prolonged juvenile hypothyroidism with a mean age of approximately 10.5 years and bone age = 6.1 years. At diagnosis, the HtSDS scores are -4 +/- 0.5 in boys and -3.12 +/- 0.5 in girls. Treatment up to achieving the final adult has demonstrated incomplete catch-up (HTSDS = -2.1 +/- 0.2) with loss of 6-7 cm of the predicted adult height. Delay in therapy has been a critical factor in the deficit in the final adult height [138]. Another study following 20 girls and 9 boys with juvenile primary hypothyroidism until they reached final height has shown that at presentation the mean age of the boys was 9.5 years (bone age = 6.3 years) and mean age of girls was 8.8 years (bone age= 5.4 years). In the girls, the onset of puberty was 1.2 years later than the normal population but the duration of puberty was reduced. The pattern of growth in girls with treated hypothyroidism is abnormal as growth continues after menarche, at a time when normal girls have almost stopped growing (Figure 5). During the second year after menarche patients still have a mean growth velocity of 4.1 cm/year. These data suggest that juvenile primary hypothyroidism can result in a permanent height deficit and disharmony between growth and sexual maturation in girls, despite adequate treatment [134].

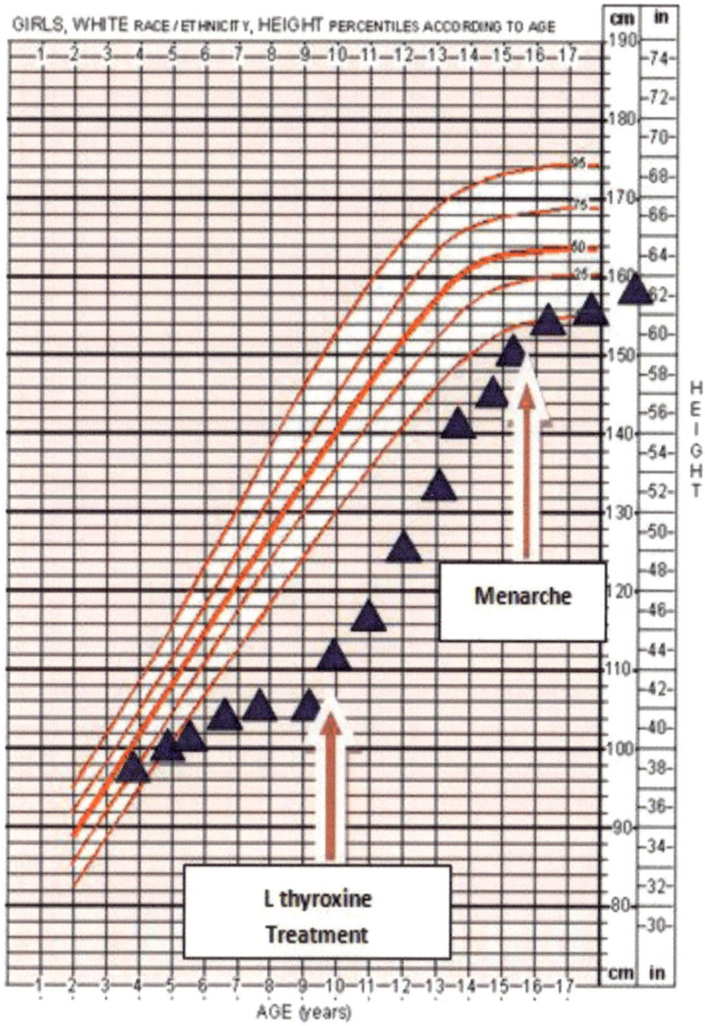

Figure 5. The Pattern of linear growth of a girl with juvenile hypothyroidism after treatment (Note the prolonged growth after menarche and short adult height)

In summary, thyroid hormones act on growth plate, bones and GH-IGF-I axis to modulate growth. These functions are mediated via many possible mechanisms including direct action on the chondrocytes, osteoblasts and mast cells, as well through interaction with other hormones and growth factors acting in endocrine, paracrine and autocrine fashions. Early diagnosis and treatment of infants born with congenital hypothyroidism, through neonatal screening, results in normal linear growth and attaining full growth potential. However, delayed diagnosis and treatment of congenital hypothyroidism and/or acquired hypothyroidism may result in partial catch-up growth and compromise final adult height of patients.

Author details

Ashraf T. Soliman[1*], Vincenzo De Sanctis[2] and El Said M.A. Bedair[3]

*Address all correspondence to: atsoliman@yahoo.com

1 Pediatric Endocrinology, Department of Pediatrics, Hamad General Hospital, Qatar

2 Pediatric and Adolescent Outpatient Clinic, Quisisana Hospital, Italy

3 AlKhor Hospital, Hamad Medical Center, Qatar

References

[1] Allain, T. J., & Mc Gregor, A. M. (1993). Thyroid hormones and bone. *Journal of Endocrinology*, 139-9.

[2] Compston, J. E. (1993). Thyroid hormone therapy and the skeleton. *Clinical Endocrinology*, 39-519.

[3] Underwood, L. E., & Van Wyk, J. J. (1992). Normal and aberrant growth. *In: Williams Textbook of Endocrinology*, 1079-1138, Eds JD Wilson & DW Foster. Philadelphia, PA, USA: WB Saunders Company.

[4] Fisher, D., & Plok, D. (1995). Thyroid disease in the fetus, neonate and child. *In Endocrinology*, 78-798, Ed LJ DeGroot. Philadelphia,PA, USA: WB Saunders.

[5] Miell, J. P., Taylor, A. M., Zini, M., Maheshwari, H. G., Ross, R. J. M., & Valcavi, R. (1993). Effects of hypothyroidism and hyperthyroidism on insulin-like growth factors [IGFs] and growth hormone and IGF binding proteins. *J Clin Endocrinol Metab*, 76, 950-953.

[6] Burstein, P. J., Draznin, B., Johnson, C. J., & Schalch, DS. (1979). The effects of hypothyroidism on growth, serum growth hormone, the growth hormone dependent somatomedin, insulin-like growth factor, and its carrier protein in rats. *Endocrinology*, 104, 1107-1111.

[7] Harakawa, S., Yamashita, S., & Tobinaga, T. (1990). In vivo regulation of hepatic insulin ike growth factor 1 mRNA with thyroid hormone. *Endocrinol Jpn*, 37, 205-211.

[8] Näntö-Salonen, K., Glasscock, G. F., & Rosenfeld, R. G. (1991). The effects of thyroid hormone on insulin-like growth factor [IGF] and IGF-binding protein [IGFBP] expression in the neonatal rat: prolonged high expression of IGFBP-2 in methimazole-induced congenital hypothyroidism. *Endocrinology*, 129, 2563-2571.

[9] Gallo, G., de Marchis, M., Voci, A., & Fugassa, E. (1991). Expression of hepatic mRNAs for insulin-like growth factors-I and-II during the development of hypothyroid rats. *J Endocrinol*, 131, 367-372.

[10] Näntö-Salonem, Rosenfeld. R. G. (1992). Insulin-like growth factor binding protein expression in the hypothyroid rat is age dependent. *Endocrinology*, 131, 1489-1496.

[11] Ramos, S., Goya, L., Alvarez, C., & Pascual-Leone, A. M. (1998). Mechanism of Hypothyroidism Action on Insulin-Like Growth Factor-I and-II from Neonatal to Adult Rats: Insulin Mediates Thyroid Hormone Effects in the Neonatal Period. *Endocrinology, 139*, 12(12), 4782-4792.

[12] Näntö-Salonen, K., Muller, H. L., Hoffman, A. R., Vu, T. H., & Rosenfeld, R. G. (1993). Mechanism of thyroid hormone action on the insulin-like growth factor system: all thyroid hormone effects are not growth hormone mediated. *Endocrinology*, 132, 781-788.

[13] Ikeda, T., Fujiama, K., & Takeuchi, T. (1989). Effect of thyroid hormone on somatomedin C release from perfused rat liver. *Experientia*, 45, 170-180.

[14] Miell, J. P., Taylor, A. M., Zini, M., Maheshwari, H. G., Ross, R. J. M., & Valcavi, R. (1993). Effects of Hypothyroidism and Hyperthyroidism on Insulin-Like Growth Factors [IGFs] and Growth Hormone- and IGF-Binding Proteins. *J Clin Endocrinol Metab*, 76, 950-5.

[15] Gaspard, T., Wondergem, R., Hamamdzic, M., & Klitgaard, H. M. (1978). Serum somatomedin stimulation in thyroxine-treated hypophysectomized rats. *Endocrinology*, 102, 606-611.

[16] Schmid, Christoph., Zwimpfer, Cornelia., Brändle, Michael., Krayenbühl-Alexandre, Pierre., Zapf, Jürgen., & Wiesli, Peter. (2006). Effect of thyroxine replacement on serum IGF-I, IGFBP-3 and the acid-labile subunit in patients with hypothyroidism and hypopituitarism. *Clinical Endocrinology*, 65(6), December, 706-711.

[17] Buchanan, C. R., Stanhope, R., Adlard, P., Jones, J., Grant, D. B., & Preece, MA. (1988). Gonadotropin, growth hormone and prolactin secretion in children with primary hypothyroidism. *Clin Endocrinol [Oxf]*, 29, 427-436.

[18] Chernausek, S. D., Underwood, L. E., Utiger, R. D., & Van Wijk, J. J. (1983). Growth hormone secretion and plasma somatomedin-C in primary hypothyroidism. *Clin Endocrinol [Oxf]*, 19, 337-344.

[19] Burstein, P. J., Draznin, B., Johnson, C. J., & Schalch, DS. (1979). The effect of hypothyroidism on growth, serum growth hormone, the growth hormone-dependent somatomedin, insulin-like growth factor, and its carrier protein in rats. *Endocrinology*, 104, 1107-1111.

[20] Bucher, H., Prader, A., & Illig, R. (1985). Head circumference, height, bone age and weight in 103 children with congenital hypothyroidism before and during thyroid hormone replacement. *Helv Paediatr Acta*, 40, 305-316.

[21] Harnack, G. A., Tanner, J. M., Whitehouse, R. H., & Rodriguez, C. A. (1972). Catch-up in height and skeletal maturity in children on long-term treatment for hypothyroidism. *Z Kinderheilk*, 112, 1-17.

[22] Rivkees, S. A., Bode, H. H., & Crawford, J. D. (1988). Long-term growth in juvenile acquired hypothyroidism: the failure to achieve normal adult stature. *N Engl J Med*, 318, 599-602.

[23] Boersma, B., Otten, B. J., Stoelinga, G. B. A., & Wit, J. M. (1996). Catch-up growth after prolonged hypothyroidism. *Eur J Pediatr*, 155, 362-367.

[24] Pantsiotou, S., Stanhope, R., Uruena, M., Preece, MA, & Grant, D. B. (1991). Growth prognosis and growth after menarche in primary hypothyroidism. *Arch Dis Child*, 66, 838-840.

[25] Weiss, R. E., & Refetoff, S. (1996). Effect of thyroid hormone on growth: lessons from the syndrome of resistance to thyroid hormone. *Endocrinol Metab Clin North Am*, 27, 719-730.

[26] Soliman, A. T., & Awwa, A. (2011). Catch-up growth role of GH-IGF-I and thyroxine. *Victor R. Preedy ed., Handbook of Growth and Growth Monitoring in Health and Disease. Chapter V, New York: Springer*, 935-965.

[27] Boersma, B., Otten, B. J., Stoelinga, G. B. A., & Wit, J. M. (1996). Catch-up growth after prolonged hypothyroidism. *Eur J Pediatr*, 155, 362-367.

[28] Wi, J. M., & Boersma, B. (2002). Catch-up growth: definition, mechanisms, and models. *J Pediatr Endocrinol Metab*, Dec, 15(5), 1229-41.

[29] Williams, J. P. G. (1981). Catch-up growth. *J Embryol Exp Morph*, 65, 89-101.

[30] Holder, N. (1981). Regeneration and compensatory growth. *Br Med Bull*, 37, 227-232.

[31] Lampl, M., Veldhuis, JD, & Johnson, M. L. (1992). Saltation and stasis: a model of human growth. *Science*, 258, 801-803.

[32] De Luca, F. (2006). Impaired growth plate chondrogenesis in children with chronic illnesses. *Pediatr Res.*, May, 59(5), 625-9.

[33] Williams, G. R., Robson, H., & Shalet, S. M. (1998). Thyroid hormone actions on cartilage and bone: interactions with other hormones at the epiphyseal plate and effects on linear growth. *J Endocrinol*, 157, 391-403.

[34] Price, J. S., Oyajobi, B. O., & Russell, R. G. G. (1994). The cell biology of bone growth. *Eur J Clin Nutr*, 48, S131-49.

[35] Lanske, B., Karaplis, A. C., Lee, K., et al. (1996). PTH/PTHrP receptor in early development and Indian hedgehog-regulated bone growth. *Science*, 273, 663-6.

[36] Vortkamp, A., Lee, K., Lanske, B., Segre, G. V., Kronenberg, H. M., & Tabin, C. J. (1996). Regulation of rate of cartilage differentiation by Indian hedgehog and PTH-related protein. *Science*, 273, 613-22.

[37] Bassett, Duncan J. H., & Williams, Graham R. (2009). The skeletal phenotypes of TRα and TRβ mutant mice. *J Mol Endocrinol April*, 1, 42-269.

[38] Lewinson, D., Harel, Z., Shenzer, P., Silbermann, M., & Hochberg, Z. (1989). Effect of thyroid hormone and growth hormone on recovery from hypothyroidism of epiphyseal growth plate cartilage and its adjacent bone. *Endocrinology*, 124, 937-45.

[39] Siebler, T., Robson, H., Bromley, M., Stevens, D. A., Shalet, S. M., & Williams, G. R. (2002). Thyroid status affects number and localization of thyroid hormone receptor expressing mast cells in bone marrow. *Bone*, 30, 259-66.

[40] Fraichard, A., Chassande, O., Plateroti, M., Roux, J. P., Trouillas, J., Dehay, C., Legrand, C., Gauthier, K., Kedinger, M., Malaval, L., Rousset, B., & Samarut, J. (1997). The T3R a gene encoding a thyroid hormone receptor is essential for post-natal development and thyroid hormone production. *EMBO J*, 16, 4412-4420.

[41] Buckler, Jm., Willgerodt, H., & Keller, E. (1986). Growth In Thyrotoxicosis. *Arch Dis Child*, 61, 464-471.

[42] Leger, J., & Czernichow, P. (1989). Congenital Hypothyroidism: Decreased Growth Velocity In The Fi Rst Weeks Of Life. *Biol Neonate*, 55, 218-223.

[43] Stevens, Da., Hasserjian, Rp., Robson, H., Siebler, T., Shalet, Sm., & Williams, Gr. (2000). Thyroid Hormones Regulate Hypertrophic Chondrocyte Differentiation And Expression Of Parathyroid Hormone- Related Peptide And Its Receptor During Endochondral Bone Formation. *J Bone Miner Res*, 15, 2431-2442.

[44] Robson, H., Siebler, T., Stevens, D. A., Shalet, S. M., & Williams, G. R. (2000). Thyroid Hormone Acts Directly On Growth Plate Chondrocytes To Promote Hypertrophic Differentiation And Inhibit Clonal Expansion And Cell Proliferation. *Endocrinology*, 141, 3887-3897.

[45] Ishikawa, Y., Genge, B. R., Wuthier, R. E., & Wu, L. N. (1998). Thyroid hormone inhibits growth and stimulates terminal differentiation of epiphyseal growth plate chondrocytes. *J Bone Miner Res*, Sep, 13(9), 1398-411.

[46] Shen, S., Berry, W., Jaques, S., Pillai, S., & Zhu, J. (2004). Differential expression of iodothyronine deiodinase type 2 in growth plates of chickens divergently selected for incidence of tibial dyschondroplasia. *Anim Genet*, 35, 114-8.

[47] Miura, M., Tanaka, K., Komatsu, Y., Suda, M., Yasoda, A., Sakuma, Y., et al. (2002). Thyroid hormones promote chondrocyte differentiation in mouse ATDC5 cells and stimulate endochondral ossification in fetal mouse tibias through iodothyronine deiodinases in the growth plate. *J Bone Miner Res*, 17, 443-54.

[48] Kronenberg, H. M. (2003). Developmental regulation of the growth plate. *Nature*, 423, 332-6.

[49] Kronenberg, H. M., & Chung, U. (2001). The parathyroid hormone-related protein and Indian hedgehog feedback loop in the growth plate. *Novartis Found Symp*, 232, 144-52.

[50] Stevens, D. A., Hasserjian, R. P., Robson, H., Siebler, T., Shalet, S. M., & Williams, G. R. (2000). Thyroid hormones regulate hypertrophic chondrocyte differentiation and expression of parathyroid hormone-related peptide and its receptor during endochondral bone formation. *J Bone Miner Res*, 15, 2431-42.

[51] Okubo, Y., & Reddi, A. H. (2003). Thyroxine downregulates Sox9 and promotes chondrocyte hypertrophy. *Biochem Biophys Res Commun*, 306, 186-90.

[52] Ballock, R. T., Zhou, X., Mink, L. M., Chen, D. H., Mita, B. C., & Stewart, M. C. (2000). Expression of cyclin-dependent kinase inhibitors in epiphyseal chondrocytes induced to terminally differentiate with thyroid hormone. *Endocrinology*, 141, 4552-7.

[53] De Luca, F., & Baron, J. (1999). Control of Bone Growth by Fibroblast Growth Factors. *Trends Endocrinol Metab*, 10, 61-5.

[54] Ornitz, D. M., & Marie, P. J. (2002). FGF signaling pathways in endochondral and intramembranous bone development and human genetic disease. *Genes Dev*, 16, 1446-65.

[55] Stevens, D. A., Harvey, C. B., Scott, A. J., O'Shea, P. J., Barnard, J. C., Williams, A. J., et al. (2003). Thyroid hormone activates fibroblast growth factor receptor-1 in bone. *Mol Endocrinol*, 17, 1751-66.

[56] Gauthier, K., Plateroti, M., Harvey, C. B., Williams, G. R., Weiss, R. E., Refetoff, S., et al. (2001). Genetic analysis reveals different functions for the products of the thyroid hormone receptor alpha locus. *Mol Cell Biol*, 21, 4748-60.

[57] Schlessinger, J., Plotnikov, A. N., Ibrahimi, O. A., Eliseenkova, A. V., Yeh, B. K., Yayon, A., et al. (2000). Crystal structure of a ternary FGF-FGFR-heparin complex reveals a dual role for heparin in FGFR binding and dimerization. *Mol Cell*, 6, 743-50.

[58] Quarto, R., Campanile, G., Cancedda, R., & Dozin, B. (1992). Thyroid hormone, insulin, and glucocorticoids are sufficient to support chondrocyte differentiation to hypertrophy: a serum-free analysis. *J Cell Biol*, 119, 989-995.

[59] Lewinson, D., Harel, Z., Shenzer, P., Silbermann, M., & Hochberg, Z. (1989). Effect of thyroid hormone and growth hormone on recovery from hypothyroidism of epiphyseal growth plate cartilage and its adjacent bone. *Endocrinology*, 124, 937-45.

[60] Cecillia-Hubner, Camacho. (2010). Normal Physiology of Growth Hormone and Insulin-Like Growth Factors in Childhood. *Endotext.*, February, Chapter 5a, http://www.endotext.org/neuroendo/neuroendo5a/neuroendo5a.htm.

[61] Sriskantharajah, S., O'Shea, P. J., Yao, H., Suzuki, H., Cheng, S. Y., & Williams, G. R. (2004). Regulation of the growth hormone [GH] and insulin-like growth factor-1

[IGF-1] paracrine pathway by thyroid hormone [T3] during bone development. *Endocrine*, Abstracts 7, 142.

[62] Ik, Soo. Kim. Diagnostic Imaging of Musculoskeletal Diseases a Systematic Approach. *In Akbar Bonakdarpour,William R.Reinus, Jasvir S. Khurana, eds. Springer, New York- Dordrecht- Heidelberg-London*, 10.1007/978-1-59745-355-4.

[63] Wexler, J. A., & Sharretts, J. (2007). Thyroid and bone. *Endocrinol Metab Clin North Am*, 36, 673-705.

[64] Bassett, J. H. D., & Williams, G. R. (2003). The molecular actions of thyroid hormones in bone. *Trends Endocrinol Metab*, 14, 356-64.

[65] Greet, Roef., Bruno, Lapauw., Stefan, Goemaere., Hans, Zmierczak., Tom, Fiers., Jean-Marc, Kaufman., & Youri, Taes. (2011). Thyroid hormone status within the physiological range affects bone mass and density in healthy men at the age of peak bone mass. *Eur J Endocrinol*, Jun, 164(6), 1027-34.

[66] High, W. B., Capen, C. C., & Black, H. E. (1981). Effects of thyroxine on cortical bone remodeling in adult dogs: a histomorphometric study. *Am J Pathol*, March, 102(3), 438-446.

[67] Farquharson, C. (2011). Social networking between cells of the foetal skeleton: The importance of thyroid hormones. *J Endocrinol*, Aug, 210(2), 135-6, 2011 Jun 16.

[68] Toivonen, J., Tahtela, R., Laitinen, K., Risteli, J., & Valimaki, MJ. (1998). Markers of bone turnover in patients with differentiated thyroid cancer with and following withdrawal of thyroxine suppressive therapy. *Eur J Endocrinol*, 138(6), 667-673.

[69] Vestergaard, P., & Mosekilde, L. (2003). Hyperthyroidism, Bone Mineral, and Fracture Risk- a meta-analysis. *Thyroid*, 13, 585-593.

[70] Akalin, A., Colakt, O., Alatast, O., & Efe, B. (2002). Bone remodeling markers and serum cytokines in patients with hyperthyroidism. *J Clin Endocrinology*, 57, 125-129.

[71] Dhanwal, D. K., Dennison, E. M., Harvey, N. C., & Cooper, C. (2011). epidemiology of hip fracture: worldwide geographic distribution. *Indian J Orthop*, 45, 15-2.

[72] Botella-Carretero, J. I., varez-Blasco, F., San Millan, J. L., & Escobar-Morreale, H. F. (2007). Thyroid hormone deficiency and postmenopausal status independently increase serum osteoprotegerin concentrations in women. *Eur J Endocrinol*, 156(5), 539-545.

[73] Soliman, A. T., Omar, M., El Awwa, A., Rizk, M. A., El Alaily, R., & Bedair, E. M. A. (2008). Linear Growth, Growth-Hormone Secretion And Igf-I Generation In Children With Neglected Hypothyroidism Before And After Thyroxine Replacement. *J Trop Ped*, 54, 347-349.

[74] Elaine, Murphy. (2004). Thyroid Hormone and Bone Development. *Hot Thyroidology* [1], http://www.hotthyroidology.com, May.

[75] Bassett, J. H. D., Swinhoe, R., Chassande, O., Samarut, J., & Williams, G. R. (2006). Thyroid Hormone Regulates Heparan Sulfate Proteoglycan Expression in the Growth Plate. *Endocrinology*, 147(1), 295-305.

[76] Lewinson, D., Harel, Z., Shenzer, P., Silbermann, M., & Hochberg, Z. (1989). Effect Of Thyroid Hormone And Growth Hormone On Recovery From Hypothyroidism Of Epiphyseal Growth Plate Cartilage And Its Adjacent Bone. *Endocrinology*, 124, 937-945.

[77] Ola, Nilsson., Rose, Marino., & Francesco De, Luca. (2005). Moshe Phillip Endocrine Regulation Of The Growth Plate. *Horm Res*, 64, 157-165.

[78] Ohlsson, C., Nilsson, A., Isaksson, O., Bentham, J., & Lindahl, A. (1992). Effects of tri-iodothyronine and insulin-like growth factor-I [IGF-I] on alkaline phosphatase activity, [3H]thymidine incorporation and IGF-I receptor mRNA in cultured rat epiphyseal chondrocytes. *J Endocrinol*, Oct, 135(1), 115-23.

[79] Cavaliere, H., Knobel, M., & Medeiros-Neto, G. (1987). Effect of Thyroid Hormone Therapy on Plasma Insulin-Like Growth Factor I Levels in Normal Subjects, Hypothyroid Patients and Endemic Cretins. *Hormone Research*, 25(3).

[80] Nato-Salonen, K., Muller, H. L., Hoffman, A. R., Vu, T. H., & Rosenfeld, R. G. (1993). Mechanisms of thyroid hormone action on the insulin-like growth factor system: all thyroid hormone effects are not growth hormone mediated. *Endocrinology*, 132, 781-8.

[81] Gaspard, T., Wondergem, R., Hamamdzic, M., & Klitgaard, H. M. (1978). Serum somatomedin stimulation in thyroxine treated hypophysectomized rat. *Endocrinology*, 102, 606-11.

[82] Ramos, S., Goya, L., Alvarez, C., Martin-Leone, MA, & Pascual, A. M. (2001). Effect of thyroxine administration on the IGF/IGF binding protein system in neonatal and adult thyroidectomized rats. *J Endocrinol*, 169, 111-22.

[83] Ikeda, T., Fujiyama, K., Hoshino, T., Tanaka, Y., Takeuchi, T., Mashiba, H., & Tominaga, M. (1999). Stimulating effect of thyroid hormone on insulin-like growth factor-I release and synthesis by perfused rat liver. *Growth Regul*, 1, 39-41.

[84] Binoux, M., Faivre-Bauman, A., Lassarre, C., Barret, A., & Tixier-Vidal, A. (1985). Triiodothyronine stimulates the production of insulin-like growth factor [IGF] by fetal hypothalamus cell cultured in serum-free medium. *Brain Res*, 353, 319-21.

[85] Li, J., Owens, J. A., Owens, P. C., Saunders, J. C., Fowden, A. L., & Gilmour, R. S. (1996). The ontogeny of hepatic growth hormone receptor and insulin-like growth factor-I gene expression in the sheep fetus during late gestation: developmental regulation by cortisol. *Endocrinology*, 137, 1650-7.

[86] Liggins, G. C. (1994). The role of cortisol in preparing the fetus for birth. *Reprod Fertil Dev*, 6, 141-50.

[87] Forhead, A. J., Li, J., Sunders, J. C., Dauncey, MJ, Gilmour, R. S., & Fowden, A. L. (2000). Control of ovine hepatic growth hormone receptor and insulin-like growth factor-I By thyroid hormones in utero. *Am J Physiol Endocrinol Metab*, 278, 1166-74.

[88] Polk, D., Cheromcha, D., Reviczky, A., & Fisher, D. A. (1989). Nuclear thyroid hormone receptors: ontogeny and thyroid hormone effects on sheep. *Am J Physiol Endocrinol Metab*, 256, 543-9.

[89] Moro, L., Marra, E., Capuano, F., & Greco, M. (2004). Thyroid hormone treatment of hypothyroid rats restores the regenerative capacity and the mitochondrial membrane permeability properties of the liver after partial hepatectomy. *Endocrinology*, 145, 5121-8.

[90] Alisi, A., Demori, I., Spagnuolo, S., Pierantozzi, E., Fugassa, E., & Leoni, S. (2005). Thyroid status affects rat liver regeneration after partial hepatectomy by regulating cell cycle and apoptosis. *Cellular Phsiology and Biochemistry*, 15, 69-76.

[91] Canavan, J. P., Holt, J., Easton, J., Smith, K., & Goldspink, D. F. (1994). Thyroid-induced changes in the growth of the liver, kidney, and diaphragm of neonatal rats. *J cell Physial*, 161, 49-54.

[92] Wolf, M., Ingbar, S. H., & Moses, A. C. (1989). Thyroid hormone and growth hormone interact to regulate insulin-like growth factor-I messenger ribonucleic acid and circulating levels in the rat. *Endocrinology*, 125, 2905-14.

[93] Jorgensen, J. O., Moller, J., Laursen, T., Orskov, H., Christiansen, J. S., & Weeke, J. (1994). Growth hormone administration stimulates energy expenditure and extrathyroidal conversion of thyroxine to triiodothyronine in a dose-dependent manner and suppresses circadian thyrotrophin levels: studies in GH-deficient adults. *Clin Endocrinol [Oxf].*, Nov, 41(5), 609-14.

[94] Akin, F., Yaylali, G. F., Turgut, S., et al. (2009). Growth hormone/insulin like growth factor axis in patients with subclinical thyroid dysfunction. *Growth Horm IGF Res*, 19, 252-255.

[95] Valcavi, R., Valente, F., Dieguez, C., et al. (1993). Evidence against depletion if the growth hormone releasable pool in human primary hypothyroidism: studies with GH-releasing hormone, pyridostigmine and arginine. *J Clin Endocrinol Metab*, 77, 616-20.

[96] Iranmanesh, A., Lizarralde, G., Johnson, M. L., & Veldhuis, JD. (1991). Nature of altered growth hormone secretion in hyperthyroidism. *J Clinical Endocrinol Metab*, 72, 108-115.

[97] Chernausek, S. D., & Turner, R. (1989). Attenuation of spontaneous nocturnal growth hormone secretion in children with hypothyroidism and its correlation with plasma insulin like growth factor 1 concentrations. *J Ped*, 114, 968-972.

[98] Lakatos, P., Foldes, J., Nagy, Z., et al. (2000). Serum insulin-like growth factor-1, insulin-like growth factor binding proteins, and bone mineral content in hyperthyroidism. *Thyroid*, 10, 417-423.

[99] Inukai, T., Takanashi, K., Takabayashi, K., et al. (1999). Thyroid hormone modulates insulin-like growth factor-1 [IFG-1] and IGF-binding protein-3, without mediation by growth hormone, inpatients with autoimmune thyroid diseases. *Horm Metab Res*, 20, 213-216.

[100] Miell, J. P., Taylor, A. M., Zini, M., et al. (1993). Effects of hypothyroidism on insulin-like growth factors [IGFs] and growth hormone and IGF-binding proteins. *Journal of Clinical Endocrinology and Metabolism*, 76, 950-5.

[101] Gafni, R. I., Weise, M., Robrecht, D. T., Meyers, J. L., Barnes, K. M., De -Levi, S., & Baron, J. (2001). Catch-up growth is associated with delayed senescence of the growth plate in rabbits. *Pediatr Res.*, Nov, 50(5), 618-23.

[102] Marino, R., Hegde, A., Barnes, Km., Schrier, L., Emons, Ja., Nilsson, O., & Baron, J. (2008). Catch-Up Growth After Hypothyroidism Is Caused By Delayed Growth Plate Senescence. *Endocrinology.*, Apr, 149(4), 1820-8.

[103] Roy, E., & Weiss, Samuel. Refet. Resistance to Thyroid Hormone [RTH] in the Absence of Abnormal Thyroid Hormone Receptor [TR] [nonTR-RTH]. *Hot Thyroidol. 09/09. Online*, 0207-5220, 2075-220.

[104] Pohlenz, J., Weiss, R. E., Macchia, P. E., Pannain, S., Lau, I. T., Ho, H., & Refetoff, S. (1999). Five new families with resistance to thyroid hormone not caused by mutations in the thyroid hormone receptor beta gene. *J Clin Endocrinol Metab*, 84, 3919-3928.

[105] Rivkees, S. A., Bode, H. H., & Crawford, J. D. (1988). Long-term growth in juvenile acquired hypothyroidism: the failure to achieve normal adult stature. *N Engl J Med*, 318, 599-602, Abstract.

[106] Boersma, B., Otten, B. J., Stoelinga, G. B. A., & Wit, J. M. (1996). Catch-up growth after prolonged hypothyroidism. *Eur J Pediatr*, 155, 362-367.

[107] Segni, M., Leonardi, E., Mazzoncini, B., Pucarelli, I., & Pasquino, A. M. (1999). Special features of Graves' disease in early childhood. *Thyroid*, 9, 871-877.

[108] Hulse, J. A. (1984). Outcome for congenital hypothyroidism,. *Archives of Disease in Childhood*, 59(1), 23-29.

[109] Segni, M., Leonardi, E., Mazzoncini, B., Pucarelli, I., & Pasquino, A. M. (1999). Special features of Graves' disease in early childhood. *Thyroid*, 9, 871-877.

[110] Boersma, B., & Wit, J. M. (1997). Catch-up growth. *Endocr Rev*, 18, 646-61.

[111] Geraldo, A., Medeiros-Neto, L. M., de Assis, William., Nicolau, A., et al. (1965). Congenital and Juvenile Hypothyroidism Due to Thyroid Dysgenesis. *J Nuclear medicine*, 6, 275-286.

[112] Rita, Ann., Kubicky, Evan. Weiner, Carlson, Bronwyn., & De Luca, Francesco. (2012). Effect of Prolonged Discontinuation of L-Thyroxine Replacement in a Child with Congenital Hypothyroidism. *Case Reports in Endocrinology*, Article ID 841947, 5 pages, 10.1155/2012/841947.

[113] Klein, R. Z., & Mitchell, M. L. (2000). Hypothyroidism in infants and children. Neonatal screening. *Braverman LE, Utiger RD, eds. Werner, Ingbar's the thyroid: a fundamental and clinical text. 8th ed. Philadelphia: Lippincott Williams & Wilkins*, 973-988.

[114] Derksen-Lubsen, G., & Verkerk, P. H. (1996). Neuropsychologic development in early treated congenital hypothyroidism: analysis of literature data. *Pediatr Res*, 39, 561-566.

[115] Bucher, H., Prader, A., & Illig, R. (1985). Head circumference, height, bone age and weight in 103 children with congenital hypothyroidism before and during thyroid hormone replacement,. *Helvetica Paediatrica Acta*, 40(4), 305-316, View at Scopus.

[116] Moschini, L., Costa, P., Marinelli, E., et al. (1986). Longitudinal assessment of children with congenital hypothyroidism detected by neonatal screening,. *Helvetica Paediatrica Acta*, 41(5), 415-424.

[117] Moreno, L., Ythier, H., Loeuille, G. A., Lebecq, M. F., Dhondt, J. L., & Farriaux, J. P. (1989). Etude de la croissance et de la maturation osseuse au cours de l'hypotyroidie congenitale depistee en periode neonatale. A propos de 82 observations. *Archives Francaises de Pediatrie*, 46(10), 723-728, View at Scopus.

[118] Grant, D. B. (1994). Growth in early treated congenital hypothyroidism,. *Archives of Disease in Childhood*, 70(6), 464-468, View at Scopus.

[119] Aronson, R., Ehrlich, R. M., Baily, J. D., & Rovet, J. F. (1990). Growth in children with congenital hypothyroidism detected by neonatal screening. *Journal of Pediatrics*, 116(1), 33-37, View at Publisher, View at Google Scholar, View at Scopus.

[120] Heyerdahl, S., Ilicki, A., Karlberg, J., Kase, B. F., & Larsson, A. (1997). Linear growth in early treated children with congenital hypothyroidism,. *Acta Paediatrica*, 86(5), 479-483, View at Scopus.

[121] Dickerman, Z., & De Vries, L. (1997). Prepubertal and pubertal growth, timing and duration of puberty and attained adult height in patients with congenital hypothyroidism [CH] detected by the neonatal screening programme for CH-a longitudinal study,". *Clinical Endocrinology*, 47(6), 649-654, View at Scopus.

[122] Salerno, M., Micillo, M., Di Maio, S., et al. (2001). Longitudinal growth, sexual maturation and final height in patients with congenital hypothyroidism detected by neonatal screening,. *European Journal of Endocrinology*, 145(4), 377-383, View at Scopus.

[123] Bain, P., & Toublanc, J.E. (2002). Adult height in congenital hypothyroidism: prognostic factors and the importance of compliance with treatment. *Hormone Research*, 58(3), 136-142.

[124] Soliman, A., Alsaied, A., Elawwa, A., & Sabt, A. (2012). Linear growth of children with congenital hypothyroidism detected by neonatal screening compared to normal children and their mid-parental height. *Endocrine Abstracts*, 29, 1303.

[125] Ashraf, T. Soliman, Azzam, S., Ahmed., El Awwa, Saleem, Wael., & Aml, Sabt. (2012). Linear growth and neurodevelopmental outcome of children with congenital hypothyroidism detected by neonatal screening: A controlled study. *Indian J Endocrinol Metab.*, Jul-Aug, 16(4), 565-568.

[126] Adachi, M., Asakura, Y., & Tachibana, K. (2003). Final height and pubertal growth in Japanese patients with congenital hypothyroidism detected by neonatal screening. *Acta Paediatr.*, Jun, 92(6), 698-703.

[127] Dickerman, Z., & de Vries, L. (1997). Prepubertal and pubertal growth, timing and duration of puberty and attained adult height in patients with congenital hypothyroidism [CH] detected by the neonatal screening programme for CH--a longitudinal study. *Clinical Endocrinology*, 47(6), 649-54.

[128] Jones, J. H., Gellén, B., Paterson, W. F., Beaton, S., & Donaldson, MD. (2008). Effect of high versus low initial doses of L-thyroxine for congenital hypothyroidism on thyroid function and somatic growth. *Arch Dis Child.*, Nov, 93(11), 940-4, 2008 May 2.

[129] Salerno, M., Militerni, R., Bravaccio, C., Micillo, M., Capalbo, D., & Di Tenore, A. (2002). Effect of different starting doses of levothyroxine on growth and intellectual outcome at four years of age in congenital hypothyroidism. *Thyroid*, Jan, 12(1), 45-52.

[130] Daliva, A. L., Linder, B., Di Martino-Nardi, J., & Saenger, P. (2000). Three-year follow-up of borderline congenital hypothyroidism. *J Pediatr*, 136, 53-56.

[131] Kohler, B., Schnabel, D., Biebermann, H., & Gruters, A. (1996). Transient congenital hypothyroidism and hyperthyrotropinemia: normal thyroid function and physical development at the ages of 6-14 years. *J Clin Endocrinol Metab*, 81, 1563-1567.

[132] Rapaport, R. (2000). Congenital hypothyroidism: expanding the spectrum. *J Pediatr*, 136, 10-12.

[133] Rivkees, S. A., Bode, H. A., & Crawford, J. D. (1988). Long-Term Growth in Juvenile-Acquired Hypothyroidism. *N Engl J Med*, 318, 599-602.

[134] Pantsiouou, S., Stanhope, R., Uruena, M., Preece, M. A., & Grant, D. B. (1991). Growth prognosis and growth after menarche in primary hypothyroidism. *Arch Dis Child.*, July, 66(7), 838-840.

Chapter 5

Growth in Children with Thyroid Dysfunction

Ljiljana Saranac, Hristina Stamenkovic,
Tatjana Stankovic, Ivana Markovic,
Snezana Zivanovic and Zlatko Djuric

Additional information is available at the end of the chapter

http://dx.doi.org/10.5772/55017

1. Introduction

Thyroid hormones (TH) are critical for early brain development, somatic growth, and bone and pubertal maturation. Moreover, they are crucial for survival, both in rodents and humans. In many respects, (TH) may be viewed as tissue growth factors. Effects on growth and development are classified as genomic actions mediated via stimulation of mRNA for pituitary growth hormone (GH) synthesis, secretion and sensitivity. TH potentiate GH stimulation of the synthesis and action of insulin-like growth factor 1 (IGF1) and stimulation of the production of different growth factors (epidermal growth factor, nerve growth factor, and erythropoietin). Cartilage response to IGF1 and osteoblastic/osteoclastic bone remodeling are also regulated by thyroid hormones. Unlike insulin and cortisol levels, which fluctuate widely in response to food ingestion and stress, thyroid hormones are typically maintained at a constant level that keeps the metabolic machinery functioning at a proper rate (Zimmerman-Belsing et al., 2003).

In overt hypothyroidism, the severe impairment of linear growth leads to dwarfism, which is characterised by limbs that are disproportionately short compared with the trunk.

Even in subclinical hypothyroidism, a condition of mild thyroid failure, growth velocity in children is suboptimal.

In this chapter, the impact of TH on growth in different forms of hypothyroidism will be discussed in light of thyroid hormone treatment in pediatric praxis.

2. Causes of acquired primary hypothyroidism in childhood

Acquired primary hypothyroidism (AH) in children and adolescents is predominantly caused by end-stage autoimmune disease arising from a chronic autoimmune thyroiditis (CAT). CAT is the most common cause of AH in nonendemic goitre areas, and it afflicts up to 2% of children and adolescents (Bartalena et al., 2007; Fisher, 1990; Raillison et al., 1975; Tomer & Huber, 2009; Fernandez-Soto et al., 1998). Unlike the overt goitrogenic form of CAT, the atrophic form often remains hidden or misdiagnosed for years. Other causes of acquired hypothyroidism include the following: late-onset thyroid dysgenesis and late-onset dyshormonogenesis; decreased responsiveness to thyroid hormones; TSH deficiency; drug-induced, iatrogenic, or endemic iodine deficiency; and chromosomal disorders and cystinosis (Fisher, 1990).

The importance of the thyroid gland for the human body is largely due to its production of hormones necessary for appropriate energy levels and an active life. These products have pleiotropic effects, which include exerting an immense array of hormonal activities (genomic and non-genomic actions) and playing a critical role in early brain development, somatic growth, bone maturation, and mRNA synthesis for more than 100 proteins that constantly regulate the maintenance of all bodily functions. TH impact every tissue to such an extent that a certain degree of thyroid dysfunction is highly likely to result in multiorgan failure thus often mimicking various diseases (Weetman, 2003; Saranac et al., 2011).

3. Genomic and non–genomic actions of thyroid hormones

T3 binding by the nuclear thyroid receptors (TR) leads to responsive gene transcription, which modulates synthesis of mRNA and proteins—which in turn mediate thyroid hormone effects in various tissues. In the central nervous system, general genomic effects include stimulation of cell migration and neuronal cell maturation and stimulation of dendritic arborisation, synaptic density and increased myelogenesis. Gene products regulated by T3 in the CNS are myelin basic protein, nerve growth factors and their receptors, neurotropin 3, neural cell adhesion molecules, cerebellar PCP-2 and prostaglandin D2 synthase (Fisher & Grueters, 2008).

Genomic effects on growth and development include the following: stimulation of pituitary growth hormone (GH) synthesis and secretion; potentiation of GH stimulation of insulin-like growth factor (IGF) synthesis and action; stimulation of growth factor production (epidermal growth factor, nerve growth factor, erytropoetin); and stimulation of bone metabolism/growth (cartilage response to IGF1 and osteoblastic/osteoclastic bone remodelling).

Thermogenic genomic effects include stimulation of mitochondrial enzyme synthesis; stimulation of UCP-1 and UCP-3 in brown adipose tissue and muscle; and stimulation of membrane Na/K ATPase. Metabolic genomic effects include induction of hepatic lipogenic enzymes; stimulation of hepatic glutamine synthetase and α-aminolevulinic acid synthetase; potentiation of prolactin stimulation of lactalbumin synthesis; and potentiation of GH stimulation of β2 euglobulin synthesis (Fisher & Gruters, 2008; Yen, 2001).

The above effects do not occur immediately but only after hours of TR stimulation. However, some TH effects occur immediately (e.g., stimulation of glucose transport and stimulation of adrenergic receptor binding). Additionally, TH can regulate the number of beta-adrenergic receptors in the heart and may thereby enhance sensitivity to catecholamines. Increased catecholamine effects via increased beta–adrenergic receptor binding and post-receptor responsiveness are prominent manifestations of the hyperthyroid state (tachycardia, tremor and lid lag) and are manifested in the face of normal or lowered circulating concentrations of catecholamines (Fisher, 1990).

4. Thyroid hormones and growth plate

The process of longitudinal bone growth is governed by a complex network of endocrine signals, including growth hormone, IGF1, glucocorticoid, thyroid hormone, oestrogen, androgen, vitamin D and leptin (Nilsson et al., 2005). The growth plate consists of three principal layers: the resting zone, proliferative zone and hypertrophic zone. In hypothyroid animals, the proliferative and hypertrophic zones are decreased in height, and chondrocyte proliferation, chondrocyte hypertrophy and vascular/bone cell invasion are affected. In addition, the normal columnar organisation of the growth plate is disrupted (Stivens et al., 2000). Some of the sceletal effects appear to be due to direct action on the growth plate. Growth plate chondrocytes express thyroid hormone receptor (TR) isoforms TR-α, α-1,and β. Most cases of thyroid hormone resistance in humans are caused by dominant-negative mutations of the TR-β gene, which may also affect TR-α function and show variable sceletal effects (Takeda et al., 1992, Nilsson et al., 2005).

TH are critical for normal bone growth and development. In children, hypothyroidism can cause short stature and delayed closure of the epiphyses. Biochemical studies have shown that TH can affect the expression of various bone markers in the serum, reflecting changes in both bone formation and resorption. TH increase alkaline phosphatase and osteocalcin in osteoblasts. Additionally, osteoclast markers such as urinary hydroxiproline, urinary pyridinium, and deoxypyridinium cross-links are increased in hyperthyroid patients. These observations suggest that both osteoblast and osteoclast activities are stimulated by TH (Yen, 2001).

5. Levels of the thyroid hormone control

There are three levels of the regulation of thyroid hormone concentrations and actions: I constant hormonal serum concentration is maintained by a feedback loop between the hypothalamus, pituitary and thyroid. This centrally regulated system is not sufficient to provide the necessary amount of TH for every tissue and cell in the body. II TH for local needs are provided by the control and regulation of TH entrance by active transmembrane transporters and the tissue-specific action of activating enzymes (D1 and D2 deiodinase) and a deactivating enzyme (D3 deiodinase), whose concentrations are regulated differently in each tissue. III The third level of the regulation of hormonal response depends on the type and activity of TH receptors and is also active at the tissue-specific level. (Bianco et al., 2002; Van der Deure et al., 2010).

Some tissues, such as muscle, have a relatively low deiodinase activity and are dependent, to a great extent, on tri-iodothyronine derived from the thyroid and liver. Other tissues, such as the brain and liver, have a high deiodinase activity, and the availability of tri-iodothyronine is determined within the tissues themselves (Romijn et al., 2003).

Thyroxine-binding globulin (TBG) is the most important carrier protein for T4. In contrast, TBG and albumin seem equally important for T3. The binding reactions are nearly complete, and thus the euthyroid steady-state concentration of free T4 and T3 approximate 0.03% and 0.3% (respectively) of total hormone concentrations. TBG levels are higher in children than in adults and decrease progressively to adult levels during adolescence (Fisher, 1990; Fisher & Grueters, 2008).

6. Different forms of hypothyroidism and their impact on growth

6.1. Central (hypothalamic–pituitary) hypothyroidism

The prevalence of central hypothyroidism approximates 1 in 20,000 births. The most frequent causes of the acquired form are irradiation of the head, chemotherapy for malignant disorders, craniopharyngiomas, granulomatous disease, meningoencephalitis and head trauma. The development of the pituitary gland as well as TSH gene expression is regulated by the multiple pituitary transcription factors. Genetic mutation of these factors has been found to cause familial hypopituitarism with TSH deficiency. The congenital form of central hypothyroidism occurs in anencephaly, holoprosencephaly, septo-optic dysplasia (SOD), medial facial syndromes, TSH β mutations, and HESX1, Pit-1, Prop-1 and LHX3/LHX4 mutations (Kelberman & Dattani, 2008). Congenital central hypothyroidism is also associated with multiple hormonal deficiencies. However, idiopathic forms of hypopituitarism are still often present and hide some forms of autoimmune and congenital disorders (De Graaf et al., 2009).

Growth failure due to GH or TSH deficiency is usually the earliest manifestation of pituitary hypofunction, but other features related to primary disease, neurologic disorder, or hypothalamic dysfunction may be prominent.

Isolated central hypothyroidism is an uncommon disorder associated with short stature in children presenting with low free T4 and normal or low serum TSH concentrations without other evidence of pituitary disease. The diagnosis of central hypothyroidism can be considered in those with a serum free T4 level in the lower half of the normal range and normal TSH concentrations. The TRH test is of diagnostic value in such circumstances.

The prevalence of isolated central hypothyroidism has been reported as 16% in a group of 181 children with idiopathic short stature (Rose, 1995).

In our group of 59 children with growth hormone deficiency, 4 had pituitary dwarfism because of the classic triad (Fig 1): a hypoplastic anterior pituitary, an ectopic posterior pituitary and an invisible or transected pituitary stalk. In 10 children, pituitary structural lesions classified as microadenoma were present on magnetic resonance imaging (MRI) examination (4 micro-prolactinomas and 6 non-functioning pituitary microadenomas). Two children experienced hypopituitarism after head trauma, and an additional 2 experienced hypopituitarism because of suprasellar tumours (germinoma, Fig 2, and teratoma). In one boy, an empty sella syndrome was revealed.

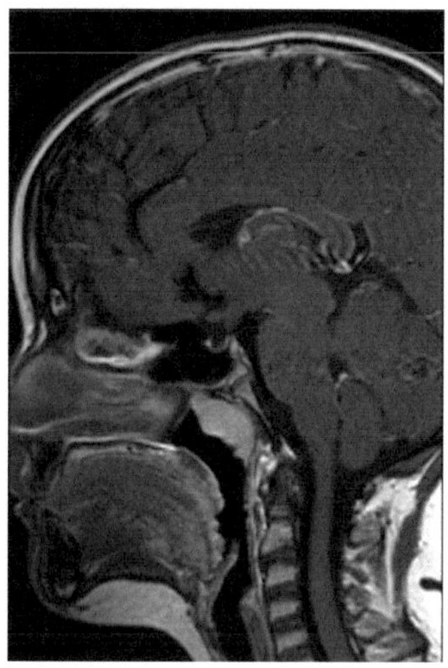

Figure 1. MRI of boy with central hypothyroidism caused by pituitary hypoplasia.

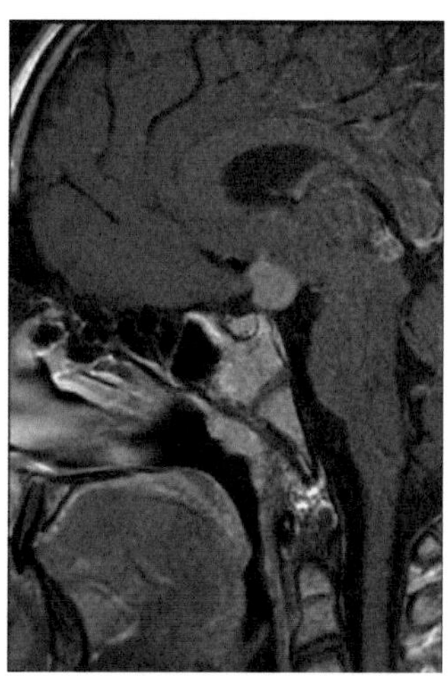

Figure 2. MR sagittal scan of boy with suprasellar germinoma producing central hypothyroidism (TT4 62.41 nmol/L, FT4 8.32 pmol/L, TSH 0.057 mIU/L).

Hypointense pituitary lesions are an important sign of hypothalamic and pituitary dysfunction and a distinguishing marker in children that should be considered for further investigation and endocrinologic surveillance. Thus, MRI investigation is recommended as an effective screening tool. MRI is an important option for use in further evaluation of short children and resistant obesity accompanied by gonadal dysfunction and pubertal disorders.

6.2. Primary, overt hypothyroidism

The clinical manifestations of acquired hypothyroidism in childhood differ from those in adults. The classic manifestations also occur in children but are not as prominent. Instead, the most important sign of acquired hypothyroidism in childhood is a slowing of growth. Weight tends to increase, and, in most instances, weight for age is greater than height for age. The retardation of bone age in hypothyroidism usually equals or exceeds the retardation in linear growth (Fisher, 1990; Hall, 1989; Saranac & Stamenkovic, 2012). Feeling cold, experiencing fatigue, and displaying primary amenorrhoea with no impairment of school performance is also commonly observed in children with acquired hypothyroidism. However, in some children, deterioration in school work and learning difficulties might occur. Clinical signs of severe acquired hypothyroidism unique to childhood are presented in Table 1. Mixedema, generalised or discrete hair loss and firm, often smooth goitre with a palpable Delphian node on the isthmus are clinical signs of autoimmune hypothyroidism. Clinical markers such as segmental vitiligo, hypopigmented rings surrounding dark naevi ("halo naevi"), leukotrichia, premature greying of the hair, and alopecia areata are all, like typical vitiligo, associated with autoimmune disorders (Hall, 1989). An increased frequency of autoimmune thyroid disorders is reported in Turner syndrome (TS) and other non-disjunctional chromosomal disorders, such as Down syndrome, and these disorders seriously affect growth in these children. Hypothyroidism of autoimmune origin is so common in TS that almost every other TS girl will most likely develop hypothyroidism, with the likelihood increasing with age (El-Mansoury et al., 2005; Mortensen et al., 2009; Testa et al., 2006).

Growth retardation
Bone age retardation
Muscle pseudohypertrophy
Sexual disorders
Delayed puberty
Precocious puberty

Table 1. Clinical signs of acquired hypothyroidism unique to childhood (Fisher, 1990)

In primary hypothyroidism, the anterior pituitary shows an increase in thyrotroph cells. Hyperplasia or even adenoma formation may result from long-standing hypothyroidism, particularly hypothyroidism dating from infancy. Enlargement of the pituitary fossa has been demonstrated, and suprasellar extension of the feedback tumour of the cells may occur rarely (Hall, 1989). We recently published a case of a hypothyroid boy with severe growth failure caused by long-standing, neglected hypothyroidism with very high thyrotropin levels and sella enlargement (Saranac & Stamenkovic, 2012).

In cases of long-standing hypothyroidism, the dose of l-thyroxine should be increased gradually to prevent cardiac failure. Most children respond well to a dose of 100 μg/m^2 (Fisher, 1990; Fisher & Grueters, 2008). When clinical features such as loss of body hair occur and increase the possibility of pituitary hypothyroidism, it is dangerous to treat the patient with thyroid hormone without determining the plasma cortisol level and, if necessary, correcting any adrenocortical deficiency (I Iall, 1989).

In clinical practice, the adequacy of TH supplementation is assessed by the measurement of TSH and fT4 concentrations. This approach deserves two comments. First, it is remarkable that the normal values of TSH show a more than ten-fold variation. In clinical practice, because the optimal TSH concentration within this range for individual patients is unknown, titration of the substitution dose of thyroxine within this variation is relatively crude. Secondly, the intrinsic assumption of many doctors using this approach is that a normal TSH concentration reflects adequate TH concentrations not only at the tissue level of the hypothalamus and the pituitary but also in other tissues. However, it is likely that this assumption is erroneous (Romijn et al., 2003).

Some adults require combined l-T3 + l-T4 treatment, although the benefit in humans is controversial. The rationale for this combined treatment is that monotherapy cannot provide euthyroid state in all tissues of the hypothyroid subject. In rodents, it has been clearly demonstrated that there is no single dose of T4 or T3 that normalises TH concentrations simultaneously in all tissues in hypothyroid animals (Escober-Morreale et al., 1996). Therefore, it is highly likely that in patients treated with l-T4, subtle derangements at the tissue level are present with respect to TH availability and, most likely, TH action. Unfortunately, we lack sensitive signs and symptoms needed to evaluate this hypothesis in clinical practice, and we do not have sensitive biochemical markers of TH action at the tissue level other than TSH (Romijn et al., 2003).

Unlike insulin and cortisol levels, which fluctuate widely in response to food ingestion and stress, thyroid hormones are typically maintained at a constant level, resulting in a proper metabolic rate. Thyroid hormones are crucial for survival in both rodents and humans (Zimmerman-Belsing et al., 2003). In many respects, thyroid hormones may be viewed as tissue growth factors. Indeed, normal overall whole body growth does not occur in the absence of thyroid hormones despite adequate levels of growth hormone (GH). TH also influence the function of other endocrine systems. After 3 to 4 years of age, thyroid hormone deficiency is not associated with mental retardation but delayed somatic and linear bone growth. Bone maturation, measured as bone age, is also delayed; diaphyseal bone growth is reduced; and epiphyseal growth and mineralisation largely cease. The effects of thyroid hormones on somatic and skeletal growth are mediated by stimulation of the synthesis and action of growth hormone and growth factors (Griffin & Ojeda, 1998).

Thyroid hormones also potentiate growth hormone stimulation of insulin-growth factor synthesis and action as well as GH and IGFs binding to the receptors and post-receptor events. Additionally, TRH's rise in primary hypothyroidism acts as suppressor of nocturnal growth hormone pulses. In 1989, Chernausek et al. documented the attenuation of spontaneous nocturnal growth hormone secretion in the hypothyroid state and the proportional fall in IGF1 serum concentration.

Catch-up growth is defined as a linear growth rate greater than expected for age after a period of growth inhibition. Growth-inhibiting conditions conserve the limited proliferative capacity of growth plate chondrocytes, thus showing the normal process of growth plate senescence. When the growth-inhibiting condition resolves, the growth plates are less senescent and therefore grow more rapidly than normal for age (Marino et al., 2008,; Shao et al., 2006). If the hypothyroid state is prolonged prior to treatment, catch-up growth may be incomplete. Excessive dosage is marked by disproportionate advancement in skeletal age (Fisher & Grueters, 2008).

In 1991, Pantsiouou found that in spite of appropriate treatment, primary hypothyroidism results in permanent growth failure. In girls, normal harmony between growth and pubertal maturation has been disturbed or lost. Growth continued after menarche, but final height remained far below the age average and predicted height according to mid-parental height. That is why some authors, including Minamitani, recommended the combined treatment with GnRH analogues and GH, besides substitutional l-T4 treatment for optimal growth stimulation.

6.3. Subclinical hypothyroidism

Subclinical hypothyroidism (SCH) is defined by an elevation of serum TSH with circulating free thyroid hormone concentrations that are within the reference range (Evered et al., 1973; Cooper & Biondi 2012). SCH is a common issue in clinical practice that predominantly affects women and has a prevalence of between 2 and 10%, which increases in an age-related fashion. More than three-quarters of individuals with SCH have serum concentrations between 5 and 10 mU/l. Although treatment of the mild thyroid failure of SCH with levothyroxine (l-T4) would seem to be a logical approach to management, only a minority of individuals with SCH have symptoms that are typical of hypothyroidism (Pearce et al., 2012). According to one of the few available follow-up studies on juvenile SCH, this may be a benign and remitting process with a very low risk of evolution toward frank hypothyroidism (Raillison et al., 1975; Moore, 1996).

There is great controversy concerning the clinical significance of SCH and whether or when subjects with SCH should be treated with l-T4. In adults, SCH has been associated with several complications, such as progression into overt hypothyroidism, abnormalities of lipid profile, increased risk of atherosclerosis and cardiovascular morbidity and clinical signs and symptoms of mild disease, including impaired cognitive function (Cerbone et al., 2011). Treatment is currently recommended in SCH subjects with a TSH value above

10 mU/l, whereas treatment for TSH levels between 4.5 and 10 mU/l remains a matter of debate (Wiersinga et al., 2012).

In children, SCH is not yet a well-defined condition due to both the low prevalence of this disorder and the lack of long-term studies.

Some children with CAT experience all types of thyroid dysfunction during the natural course of the disease: mild hyperthyroidism at diagnosis (hashitoxicosis), euthyroid state and gradual progression from subclinical to overt hypothyroidism. An intriguing form of CAT could be subclinical hypothyroidism with mixed signs of hypo- and hyperfunction ("autoimmune dysthyroidism"). Thus, clinical features do not always correspond to hormonal status. The reasons for diagnostic pitfalls, including clinical ambiguity, are challenging for pediatricians and endocrinologists (Saranac & Stamenkovic, 2012).

Even though subclinical hypothyroidism is defined as an asymptomatic disorder in which a euthyroid state is maintained due to TSH elevation, in our experience, this dysfunction type actually has clinical expression despite being labelled as mild, subclinical or compensated. Tunbridge recorded clinical features in adults, which included cold intolerance, dry skin, lack of energy, puffiness around the eyes, acroparaesthesiae and weight gain, and the signs elicited included periorbital swelling, scaling of the skin and a slow pulse rate (minor degrees of hypothyroidism) (Hall, 1989). In children, even the subclinical form of hypothyroidism has an impact on growth, weight regulation, bone maturation and pubertal development.

While the mild clinical picture of hypothyroidism is expected in children, the appearance of the opposite hyperfunction signs in subclinically hypothyroid subjects is intriguing. A possible explanation could be the rise in TRH with neurotransmitter properties that leads to release of TSH, PRL, FSH, and noradrenalin (NA). Tachycardia, nervousness, and emotional lability in subclinically hypothyroid subjects could be attributed to NA released in this way. Moreover, the turnover of NA in the brain of hypothyroid subjects has been found to be elevated (Jovanovic-Micic et al., 1991; Bauer et al., 2008).

The ambiguity in the clinical picture could also be explained by the presence of heterogenic antibodies to the TSH receptor in the same subject. A transient shift from blocking to stimulating antibodies may provoke hyperthyroid signs in the hypothyroid subject (Song et al., 1996; Saranac et al., 2003, 2010).

Reasons not to treat SCH in adults are numerous. Serum TSH is not a perfect marker of thyroid hormone action because of its dependence on hypothalamic TRH, type 2 deiodinase, and the influence of steroids, cytokines, adipokines and neuromediators (e.g., l-dopa). Increased TSH is not a fixed and immutable parameter: it varies according to diurnal, circannual, and physiological and non-thyroidal factors. Normal values of TSH can differ ten-fold within normal reference values. Obesity is a circumstance in which high levels of TSH are frequently discovered, although a lack of thyroid hormone is not generally the culprit. Furthermore, therapy with levothyroxine is not free of inconvenience and risks. Finally, extreme longevity is associated with increased serum thyrotropin levels (Pearce et al., 2012).

In growing child, there are scarce data regarding the evaluation of substitution benefits. Thus, the dilemma of whether to treat subclinical hypothyroidism is still in question. The problem is further complicated by the fact that obese children do present with elevated values of TSH. Several mechanisms leading to hyperthyrotropinaemia have been hypothesised, including increased leptin-mediated production of pro-TRH, impaired feedback due to a decreased number of T3 receptors in the hypothalamus, and variations in peripheral deiodinase activity (Radetti et al., 2008). With respect to growth in SCH, there are ambiguous data. In a prospective evaluation of the natural course of idiopathic subclinical hypothyroidism in childhood and adolescence, Wasniewska et al (2009) did not find any association between TSH changes and FT4 values, clinical status or auxological parameters. The study group consisted of 92 patients (50 boys) with idiopathic SCH. The majority of the patients (88%) normalised or maintained their TSH levels during the 24-month follow-up period. Stature was within normal limits at diagnosis and remained normal at the end of the study. In a cross-sectional controlled study, Cerbone et al (2011) evaluated growth and intellectual outcome in 36 children with persistent SCH who had never been treated with levothyroxine and in the same number of age- and sex-matched controls. The authors concluded that persistent SCH in children is not associated with alterations in growth, bone maturation, BMI, and cognitive function or other complaints that could be ascribed to SCH even after several years. However, the mean duration of follow up was only 3.3 years.

In 17 paediatric patients with SCH, Ergur et al. (2012) documented poor performance on tests measuring attention and neurocognitive capabilities. No significant differences were found between the SCH group and the healthy controls in verbal fluency and encoding tests.

In a small study of 16 children with SCH and diagnosis of CAT, we found suboptimal growth velocity (4.12 cm/year), which significantly improved up to 7.36 cm/year ($p<0.05$) after 12 months of treatment. Mean bone age advancement was 1.6 years/year and did not exceed growth acceleration (1.98 years/year), due to careful dose monitoring. Despite appropriate treatment with l-T4, the mean SD score of height for chronological age remained unachievable in comparison with euthyroid, non-treated CAT patients (Fig 3). During treatment, the T3/T4 ratio in the treated group showed a sharp rise after 1 year of treatment, in accordance with the mean best growth velocity during follow-up period of mean 2.19 years (range 1-4 years) (Fig 4). The mean TSH of the SCH group was 8.98 mU/ml at diagnosis, falling gradually to 4.81 mU/ml after 1 year and 1.98 mU/ml after 2 years of treatment. We concluded that children with SCH had suboptimal growth before treatment, which improved during l-T4 substitution, with simultaneous normalisation of TSH levels. In addition to other favourable effects on thyroid volume and thyroid autoimmunity markers, TH isohormonal therapy provides optimal growth in children with CAT. However, caution is recommended in children who are simply obese, where, despite elevated TSH, l-T4 treatment should be avoided or cautiously considered.

http://dx.doi.org/10.5772/55017

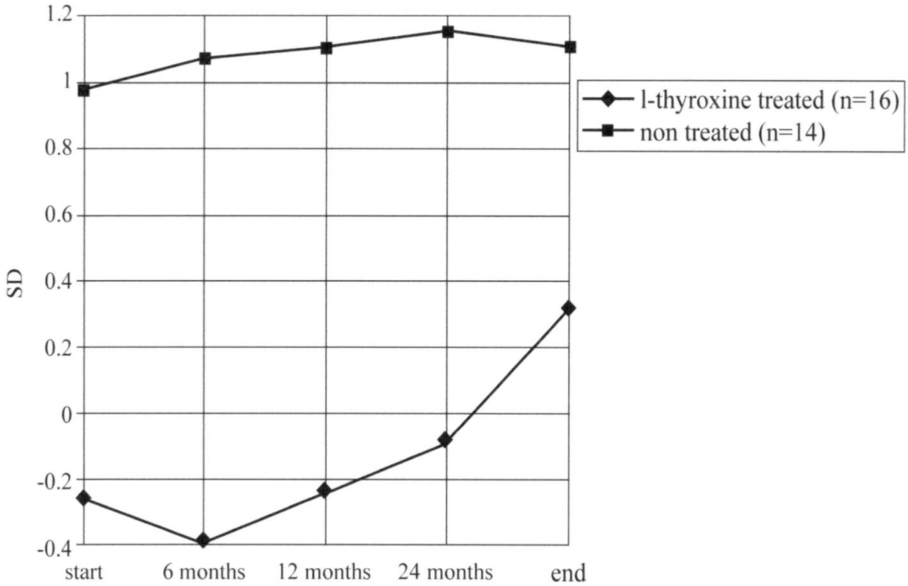

Figure 3. Standard deviation score (SD) changes during follow-up in hypothyroid children (overt+ subclinical hypothyroidism) in comparison with non treated (euthyroid and hyperthyroid). Growth is reflection of thyroid function.

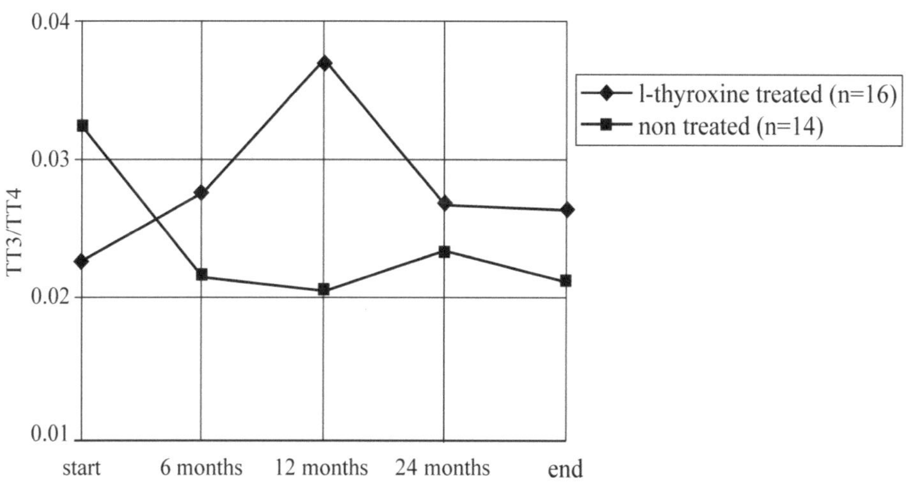

Figure 4. T3/T4 ratio changes in l-thyroxine treated versus non treated children.

7. Conclusion

Screening for congenital hypothyroidism achieved the historical goal of eliminating the most serious endocrine cause of mental retardation, hypothyroid cretinism. However, acquired hypothyroidism remains a frequent cause of interruption of statutoponderal progress, failure to thrive and growth impairment. Dynamic growth is a fundamental characteristic of happy, healthy children who are well nourished and nurtured. Stature represents a phenotypic characteristic that produces significant anxiety in children and their families. A euthyroid state is crucial in this complex, synergistic process in which nutrition, emotions and hormones act simultaneously. Growth is a reflection of thyroid function. Thus, the first step in the hormonal investigation of children with growth failure is the thyroid function assessment. Pediatricians must be educated to select patients suspected of hypothyroidism, to document different forms of hypothyroidism and to treat them properly while simultaneously being attentive to false positive results.

Although hormonal substitution therapy in the treatment of hypothyroidism is extremely successful and has fulfilled its promises, a perfect mimicry of endocrine homeostasis by thyroid hormone replacement is, in general, impossible, especially in growing children.

Acknowledgements

Supported by a grant from the Ministry of Science of Republic of Serbia, No 41018. We are grateful to Mr Mile Randjelovic for excellent technical assistance.

Author details

Ljiljana Saranac[1], Hristina Stamenkovic[1], Tatjana Stankovic[1], Ivana Markovic[2], Snezana Zivanovic[1] and Zlatko Djuric[1]

1 Pediatric Clinic, Faculty of Medicine Nis, University of Nis, Nis, Serbia

2 Institute of Radiology, Faculty of Medicine Nis, University of Nis, Nis, Serbia

References

[1] Bartalena, L, Tanda, M. L, Piantanida, E, Lai, A, Compri, E, & Lombardi, V. (2007). Environnment and thyroid autoimmunity, In: *The Thyroid and Autoimmunity: Merck European Thyroid Symposium Noordwijk*, Wiersinga, WM.; Drexhage, HA.; Weetman, AP, Thieme, 978-3-13134-661-2Stuttgart, 60-73.

[2] Bauer, M, & Goetz, T. Glenn, T; Whybrow, C. ((2008). The thyroid-brain interaction in thyroid disorders and mood disorders. *J Neuroendocrinol*, October 2008), 0953-8194e-ISSN 1365-2826, 20(10), 1101-1114.

[3] Bianco, A. C, Salvatore, D, Gereben, B, Berry, M. J, & Larsen, P. R. (2002). Biochemistry, cellular and molecular biology, and physiological roles of the iodothyronine selenodeiodinases. *Endocrine Rev*, February 2002), 0016-3769X, e-ISSN 1945-7189, 23(1), 38-89.

[4] Cerbone, M, Bravaccio, C, Capalbo, D, Polizzi, M, Wasniewska, M, Cioffi, D, Improda, N, Valenzise, M, Bruzzese, D, De Luca, F, & Salerno, M. (2011). Linear growth and intellectual outcome in children with long-term idiopathic subclinical hypothyroidism. *Eur J Endocrinol*, Epub February 2003), 0804-4643e-ISSN 1479-683X, 164(4), 591-597.

[5] Chernausek, S. D, & Turner, R. (1989). Attenuation of spontaneous nocturnal growth hormone secretion in children with hypothyroidism and its correlation with plasma insulin-like growth factor I concentration. *J Pediatr*, June 1989), 0022-3476e-ISSN 1097-6833, 114(6), 968-972.

[6] Cooper, D. S, & Biondi, B. (2012). Subclinical thyroid disease (Seminar). *Lancet*, March 2012), 0140-6736e-ISSN 1474-547X, 379(9821), 1142-1154.

[7] De Graaf, L, Bellis, A, Bellastella, A, & Hokken-koelega, A. (2009). Antipituitary antibodies in Dutch patients with idiopathic hypopituitarism. *Horm Res*, January 2009), 0301-0163e-ISSN 1423-0046, 71(1), 22-27.

[8] El-Mansoury, M, Bryman, I, Berntorp, K, Hanson, C, Wilhelmsen, L, & Landin-wilhelmsen, K. (2005). Hypothyroidism is common in Turner syndrome: results of a five-year follow up. *J Clin Endocrinol Metab*, April 2005), 0002-1972X, e-ISSN 1945-7197, 90(4), 2131-2135.

[9] Ergur, A. T, Taner, Y, Ata, E, Melek, E, Bakar, E. E, & Sancak, T. (2012). Neurocognitive functions in children and adolescents with subclinical hypothyroidism. *J Clin Res Pediatr Endocrinol*, March 2012), 1308-5727e-ISSN 1308-5735, 4(1), 21-24.

[10] Escobar-Morreale, H. F. del Rey, FE.; Obregon, MJ.; de Escobar, GM. ((1996). Only the combined treatment with thyroxine and triiodothyronine ensures euthyroidism in all tissues of the thyroidectomized rat. *Endocrinology*, June 1996), 0013-7227e-ISSN 1945-7170, 137(6), 2490-2502.

[11] Evered, D. C, Ormaston, B. J, Smith, P. A, Hall, R, & Bird, T. (1973). Grades of hypothyroidism. *Br Med J*, March 1973), 0007-1447, 1(5854), 657-662.

[12] Fernandez-Soto, L, Gonzales, A, Escobar-jimenez, F, Vazquez, R, Ocete, E, Olea, N, & Salmeron, J. (1998). Increased risk of autoimmune thyroid disease in hepatitis C vs hepatitis B before, during, and after discontinuing interferon therapy. *Arch Intern Med*, July 1998), 0003-9926e-ISSN 1538-3679, 158(13), 1445-1448.

[13] Fisher, D. A, & Grueters, A. (2008). Thyroid disorders in childhood and adolescence. In *Pediatric Endocrinology*, ed 3, Kaplan SA, Saunders Elsevier, 978-1-41604-090-3Philadelphia, 237-253.

[14] Fisher, D. A. (1990). The Thyroid, In: *Clinical Pediatric Endocrinology*, ed 2, Kaplan. SA, W. B. Saunders Company, 978-0-72165-283-2Philadelphia, 87-126.

[15] Griffin, J. E, & Ojeda, S. R. (1988). The thyroid. In: *Textbook of Endocrine Physiology*, Griffin JE, Oxford University Press, 0-19505-442-3York, 222-244.

[16] Hall, R. (1989). Thyroid, In: Fundamentals of Clinical Endocrinology, ed 4 Hall, R. & Besser, M, Churchill Livingstone, 978-0-44303-649-1London, 66-152.

[17] Jovanovic-Micic, D, Samardzic, R, & Beleslin, D. (1991). Thyrotropin-releasing hormone: distribution, role and importance (article in Serbian). *Srp Arh Celok Lek*, September-October 1991), 0370-8179, 119(9-10), 263-270.

[18] Kelberman, D, & Dattani, M. T. (2008). Septo-optic dysplasia- novel insights into the aetiology. *Horm Res*, Epub February 2008), 0301-0163e-ISSN 1423-0046, 69(5), 257-265.

[19] Marino, R, Hedge, A, Barnes, K. M, Schrier, L, Emons, J. A, Nilsson, O, & Baron, J. (2008). Catch-up growth after hypothyroidism is caused by delayed growth plate senescence. *Endocrinology*, April 2008), 0013-7227e-ISSN 1945-7170, 149(4), 1820-1828.

[20] Minamitani, K, Murata, A, Ohnishi, H, Wataki, K, Yasuda, T, & Niimi, H. (1994). Attainment of normal height in severe juvenile hypothyroidism. *Arch Dis Child*, May, 1994), 0003-9888e-ISSN 1468-2044, 70(5), 429-430.

[21] Moore, D. C. (1996). Natural course of subclinical hypothyroidism in children and adolescence. *Arch Pediatr Adolesc Med*, March 1996), 1072-4710e-ISSN 1538-3628, 150(3), 293-297.

[22] Mortensen, K. H, Cleemann, L, Hjerrild, B. E, Nexo, E, Locht, H, Jeppesen, E. M, & Gravholt, C. H. (2009). Increased prevalence of autoimmunity in Turner- influence of age. *Clin Exp Immunol*, May 2009), 0009-9104e-ISSN 1365-2249, 156(2), 205-210.

[23] Nilsson, O, Marino, R, De Luca, F, Phillip, M, & Baron, J. (2005). Endocrine regulation of the growth plate. *Horm Res*, Epub October 2005), 0301-0163e-ISSN 1423-0046, 64(4), 157-165.

[24] Pantsiouou, S, Stanhope, R, & Uruena, M. (1991). Growth prognosis and growth after menarche in primary hypothyroidism. *Arch Dis Child*, July 1991), 0003-9888e-ISSN 1468-2044, 66(7), 838-840.

[25] Pearce, S, Vaisman, M, & Wemeau, J. L. (2012). Management of subclinical hypothyroidism: The thyroidologists view. *Eur Thyroid J*, Epub February 2012), 2235-0640e-ISSN 2235-0802, 1(1), 45-50.

[26] Radetti, G, Kleon, W, Buzi, F, Crivellaro, C, & Pappalardo, L. di Iorgi, N.; Maghnie, M. ((2008). Thyroid function and structure are affected in childhood obesity. *J Clin Endocrinol Metab*, December 2008), 0002-1972X, e-ISSN 1945-7197, 93(12), 4749-4754.

[27] Rallison, M. L, Dobyns, B. M, Keating, F. R, Rall, J. E, & Tyler, F. H. (1975). Occurence and natural history of chronic autoimmune thyroiditis in childhood. *J Pediatr*, May 1975), 0022-3476e-ISSN 1097-6833, 86(5), 675-682.

[28] Romijn, J. A, Smit, J. W, & Lamberts, W. J. (2003). Intrinsic imperfection of endocrine replacement therapy. *Eur J Endocrinol*, August 2003) 0804-4643e-ISSN 1479-683X, 149(2), 91-97.

[29] Rose, S. R. (1995). Isolated central hypothyroidism in short stature. *Pediatr Res*, December 1995), 0031-3998e-ISSN 1530-0447, 38(6), 967-973.

[30] Saranac, L, & Stamenkovic, H. (2012). Different Faces of Chronic Autoimmune Thyroiditis in Childhood and Adolescence. In: *A New Look at Hypothyroidism*, Drahomira Springer (Ed), InTech, Rijeka, 978-9-53510-020-1, 125-132.

[31] Saranac, L, Miljkovic, M, Stamenkovic, H, Mileusnic-milenovic, R, Petrovic, G, & Kamenov, B. (2003). Late onset transient thyroid dysfunction in children born to mothers with autoimmune thyroid disease. *Facta Universitatis Series Medicine and Biology*, March 2003), 0000-0354, 10(1), 52-56.

[32] Saranac, L, Zivanovic, S, & Novak, M. High fT3 (free triiodothyronine), new syndrome or innocent bystander. *Endocrine Abstracts 2010: 22 771Abstr European Congress of Endocrinology*, Prague, April 24-28, (2010).

[33] Saranac, L, Zivanovic, S, Bjelakovic, B, Stamenkovic, H, Novak, M, & Kamenov, B. (2011). Why is the thyroid so prone to autoimmune disease. *Horm Res Paediatr*, February 2011), 1663-2818e-ISSN 1663-2826, 75(3), 157-165.

[34] Shao, Y. Y, Wang, L, & Ballock, R. T. (2006). Thyroid hormone and the growth plate. *Rev Endocrin Metab Disord*, December 2006), 1389-9155e-ISSN 1573-2606, 7(4), 265-271.

[35] Song, Y. H, Li, Y, & Maclaren, N. K. (1996). The nature of autoantigens targeted in autoimmune endocrine diseases. *Immunol Today*, May 1996), 0167-5699, 17(5), 232-238.

[36] Stevens, D. A, Hasserjian, R. P, Robson, H, Siebler, T, Shalet, S. M, & Williams, G. R. (2000). Thyroid hormones regulate hypertrofic chondrocyte differentiation and expression of parathyroid hormone-related peptide and its receptor during endochondral bone formation. *J Bone Miner Res*, December 2000), 0884-0431e-ISSN 1523-4681, 15(12), 2431-2442.

[37] Takeda, K, Sakurai, A, Degroot, L. J, & Refetoff, S. (1992). Recessive inheritance of thyroid hormone resistance caused by complete deletion of the protein-coding region of the thyroid receptor-beta gene. *J Clin Endocrinol Metab*, January 1992), 0002-1972X, e-ISSN 0021-972X, 74(1), 49-55.

[38] Testa, A, Castaldi, P, Fanti, V, Fiore, G. F, Grieco, V, & De Rosa, G. (2006). Prevalence ov HCV antibodies in autoimmune thyroid disease. *Eur Rev Med Pharmacol Sci*, July-August 2006), 1128-3602, 10(4), 183-186.

[39] Tomer, Y, & Huber, A. (2009). The etiology of autoimmune thyroid disease: a story of genes and environment. *J Autoimmun*, May-June 2009), ISNN 0896-8411, 32(3-4), 231-239.

[40] Van Der Deure, W. M, Peeters, R. P, & Visser, T. J. (2010). Molecular aspects of thyroid hormone transporters, including MCT8, MCT10, and OATPS, and the effects of genetic variation in these transporters. *J Mol Endocrinol*, January 2010), 0952-5041e-ISSN 1479-6813., 44(1), 1-11.

[41] Wasniewska, M, Salerno, M, Cassio, A, Corrias, A, Aversa, T, Zirilli, G, Capalbo, D, Bal, M, Mussa, A, & De Luca, F. (2009). Prospective evaluation of the natural course of idiopathic subclinical hypothyroidism in childhood and adolescence. *Eur J Endocrinol*, March 2009), 0804-4643e-ISSN 1479-683X, 160(3), 417-421.

[42] Weetman, A. P. (2003). Autoimmune thyroid disease: propagation and progression. *Eur J Endocrinol*, January 2003), 0804-4643e-ISSN 1479-683X, 14(1), 1-9.

[43] Wiersinga, W. M, Duntas, L, Fadeyev, V, & Nygaard, B. Vaderpump, MPJ. ((2012). ETA Gidelines: the use L-T4+ L-T3 in the treatment of hypothyroidism. *Eur Thyroid J*, Epub June 2012), 2235-0640e-ISSN 2235-0802, 1(2), 55-71.

[44] Yen, P. M. (2001). Physiological and molecular basis of thyroid hormone action. *Physiol Rev*, July 2001), 0031-9333e-ISSN 1522-1210, 81(3), 1097-1142.

[45] Zimmerman-Belsing, T, Brabant, G, Holst, J. J, & Feldt-rasmusen, U. (2003). Circulating leptin and thyroid dysfunction. *Eur J Endocrinol*, October 2003), 0804-4643e-ISSN 1479-683X, 149(4), 257-271.

Chapter 6

Approach to Subclinical Hypothyroidism in Children

Yardena Tenenbaum-Rakover

Additional information is available at the end of the chapter

http://dx.doi.org/10.5772/55134

1. Introduction

1.1. Definition of SCH

SCH is defined when serum TSH concentration is above the statistically upper limit of the reference range while serum free T_4 (FT_4) concentration is within its reference range (Biondi & Cooper, 2008; Surks et al., 2005). Other names for SCH include compensated, early, latent, mild, minimally symptomatic, preclinical hypothyroidism and euthyroid hyperthyrotropinemia (Chu & Crapo, 2001). It suggests a compensated early state of primary thyroid failure wherby an increased level of TSH is required to maintain notmal levels of thyroid hormones. The reference TSH levels in a normal population aged 12 and older (excluding individuals with medications or diseases that might influence thyroid function) were assessed at 0.45 to 4.12 mIU/l (2.5^{th}–97.5^{th} percentile) (Hollowell et al., 2002). Although there were age, gender, and ethnic group differences, they were small and it was therefore not considered necessary to adjust the reference for these parameters. Additional studies assessing the normal TSH reference in children have shown broad differences between adult and children that were dependent on the patient's age (Elmlinger et al., 2001; Hübner et al., 2002; Kapelari et al., 2008 ; Soldin et al., 2009; Strich et al., 2012; Zurakowski et al., 1999), indicating that the definition of SCH is age-dependent. A panel of experts divided patients with SCH into two groups: patients with mildly increased serum TSH levels (4.5–10 mIU/l) and patients with more severely increased serum TSH levels (>10 mIU/l) (Surks et al., 2004).

2. Prevalence of SCH

The prevalence of SCH is about 4% to 10% in the adult population (Biondi & Cooper, 2008; Hollowell et al., 2002; Surks et al., 2004), with a higher prevalence in women and the elderly.

The prevalence of congenital hypothyroidism (CH) has increased in the last two decades from 1 in 4000 births (Grüters et al., 1993) to as high as 1 in 2000 births in the Hispanic population in the United States (Harris & Pass, 2007). Explanations for the increase in prevalence of CH in the United States include lower TSH cut-off levels, increasing numbers of preterm or very low weight babies who can be affected by a transient rise in TSH levels and reflect more benign or transient cases (Grüters & Krude, 2011) and higher numbers of neonates with Hispanic background in the tested population. The precise incidence of SCH in children is not well defined; however, a prevalence of about 1 in 8260 births was found in Europe for transient CH and SCH (Klett & Schönberg, 1981).

3. Etiology of SCH

The different causes of SCH in children are summarized in Table 1. The most common cause in children, as well as in adults, is AITD. In the newborn, hyperthyrotropinemia can reflect a physiological condition, as well as maternal AITD and perinatal exposure to iodine. Loss-of-function mutations of genes that are involved in thyroid development and thyroid hormone synthesis may also present as euthyroid hyperthyrotropinemias at birth or later on in life. Additional etiologies are acquired thyroid infiltration diseases, thyroid injury, and secondary effects of medication that influences thyroid hormone synthesis or clearance of thyroid hormones. Mild hyperthyrotropinemia may be a consequence of obesity. Laboratory interference in the assay process is not a rare cause for elevated TSH. Many of these causes result in overt hypothyroidism with time, or even at presentation.

AITD	Risk factors: family history of AITD-associated autoimmune disorders (diabetes mellitus type 1, celiac disease, pernicious anemia, viteligo, atrophic gastritis, etc.) as part of autoimmune polyglandular syndrome type 1 & 2. In Down syndrome and Turner's syndrome
Congenital hyperthyrotropinemia	Iodine exposure or endemic iodine deficiency, maternal AITD, maternal drug treatment like propylthiouraciland metimazole
Persistent TSH after subacute thyroiditis or painless thyroiditis	
Thyroid injury	Partial thyroidectomy, radioactive iodine therapy, external radiotherapy of head and neck, chemotherapy
Drugs	Iodine and iodine-containing medications (amiodorone, radiographic contrast agents), lithium, interferon α, sulfonamides
Inadequate replacement therapy of hypothyroidism	Inadequate dosage, noncompliance, drug interactions (iron, calcium carbonate, dietary soy), increased T_4

	clearance (phenytoin, carbamazepine, phenobarbital), malabsorption
β-thalassemia major	Due to hemosiderosis
After bone marrow transplantation	
Thyroid infiltration	Amyloidosis, sarcoidosis, hemochromatosis, cystinosis, primary thyroid lymphoma
Obesity	
Genetic	Loss-of-function mutations in *TSHR*, *GNAS*, *PAX8*, *TTF-1*, *DUOX2*
Laboratory interferences	Macro-TSH, hetrophylic antibodies, thyroid autoantibodies, RF

Table 1. Causes of SCH in children

3.1. Transient hyperthyrotropinemia in newborns

Hyperthyrotropinemia in newborns is mainly a physiological condition reflecting the TSH surge which occurs immediately after birth. Additional etiologies for this condition include iodine deficiency that is common in areas of endemic goiter or secondary to iatrogenic iodine overload during fetal and postnatal life. Significant exposure to iodine may be caused by transplacental crossing of iodine to the fetus or secretion of iodine into the breast milk consumed by the newborn. In addition, the newborn, and especially premature newborns, can be exposed to iodine overload through contrast medium in imaging studies or to iodine in topical agents. Rare causes of neonatal hyperthyrotropinemia are transplacental passage of thyroid-blocking antibodies and antithyroid drugs from mother to fetus in maternal autoimmune diseases. Genetic etiologies include TSH resistance (RTSH), mainly due to mutations in *TSHR*. Additional inherited defects include mutations in *DUOX2*, *PAX8*, *TTF-1* and *GNAS1*. Long-term follow-up and laboratory and imaging evaluation are needed to define the specific etiology and to select the appropriate clinical approach in each case. Sakka et al. (2009) reported significant elevations in TSH levels in children born after in-vitro fertilization. The authors hypothesized that this might represent an epigenetic developmental abnormality related to preimplantation manipulation of the embryo.

3.2. Maturation of thyroid hormone metabolism

Fetal thyroid develops under the influence of increasing TSH levels during the last half of gestation. Serum TSH increases from low levels at 18 weeks to a peak of 7–10 mU/l at term. Fetal hypothalamic–pituitary feedback matures during the second trimester (Fiser & Klein, 1981; Fisher & Polk, 1989; Rakover et al., 1999). More recent studies sampling fetal cord blood have shown measurable TSH levels at as early as 15 weeks gestation which peak in the second trimester and then plateau at that level until term (Hume et al., 2004; Thorpe-Beeston et al., 1991). At birth, in response to extrauterine exposure, there is acute release of TSH (TSH surge) that peaks at a concentration of about 70 mU/l at 30 min and remains elevated for 3 to 5 days after birth. The increase in FT_4 levels at birth is TSH-dependent. Increased FT_4 secretion continues for 1 to 2 months after birth. Normal pediatric age-dependent references for thyroid hormones have shown TSH concentrations as high as 9.64 mIU/l in the first months after birth, suggesting that hyperthyrotropinemia in the first year of life reflects normal phenomena and does not necessarily require further evaluation or therapy (Hübner et al., 2002).

3.3. Maternal Autoimmune Thyroid Diseases (AITDs)

Transplacental transfer of thyroid-stimulating antibodies (TSAbs) and TSH binding inhibitor antibodies (TBIAbs) from mother to fetus has been described in the presence of maternal AITDs. In maternal Graves' disease, the infant is at risk for congenital hyperthyroidism (Ogilvy-Stuart et al., 2002), CH and euthyroid hyperthyrotropinemia (Fu et al., 2005). Fu et al. (2005) reported on 78 mothers with AITDs; about half of their babies had transient hyperthyrotropinemia, seven had overt hypothyroidism and one had hyperthyroidism (Fu et al., 2005). The severity of the clinical presentation correlated with the levels of maternal autoantibodies. Congenital hyperthyroidism resulted from maternal transfer of TSAbs. Transient CH or hyperthyrotropinemia resulted from the mother consuming anti-thyroid drugs such as metimazole and propylthiouracil, which have a short half life of a few days (Cheron et al., 1981), and from transplacental transfer of TBIAbs, which are eliminated from the infant's serum after a few months in parallel to the elimination of maternal immunoglublulins. Papendieck et al. (2009) described 28 newborns of mothers with Graves' disease diagnosed with neonatal hyperthyroidism (9 newborns), primary hypothyroidism (14) and central hypothyroidism (5). Spontaneous remission was shown in all of the affected babies between 16 days and 8 months apart from 2 babies who had permanent hypothyroidism. The authors concluded that infants born to mothers with Graves' disease should be assessed by a pediatric endocrinologist to better identify thyroid diseases in the offspring. In maternal Hashimoto's thyroiditis, the infant is at risk for transient CH or hyperthyrotropinemia due to transplacental transfer of TBIAbs. To determine the incidence of transient CH due to TRAbs, all dried neonatal blood specimens from the neonatal screening in North America were screened for TRAbs (Brown et al., 1996) and only 2% of babies diagnosed with CH were positive for TRAbs, suggesting that maternal AITD is a rare etiology of CH. The occurrence of transient hypothyroidism due to maternal Hashimoto's thyroiditis was reported mainly as a case report (Matsuura et al.,1980; Zakarija et al., 1990; Wada et al., 2000). We described transient CH in three siblings born to a mother with well-controlled Hashimoto's thyroiditis with extremely high levels of TBIAbs (Rakover et al., 1990). The baby had high TBIAbs concentrations and as reflected by sequential serum measurements, these antibodies disappeared after 4 months. In one sibling, the thyroid gland was absent in a ^{99m}TC scan performed on the first days of life but repeated scan after the age of 2 years, revealed a gland of normal size and position. Absence of distal femoral epiphysis at birth was shown. Interestingly, the three siblings had minor abnormal neurological signs in late childhood such as dyslexia, attention deficit disorder and coordination disorders. These neurological findings, along with the lack of distal femoral epiphysis at birth, suggested *in-utero* fetal hypothyroidism. A less favorable intellectual outcome was reported in babies with transient CH born to mothers positive for TBIAbs compared to babies with permanent hypothyroidism of other etiologies, especially if unrecognized maternal hypothyroidism was present *in utero* (Matsuura et al., 1990; Wada et al., 2000). Our findings as well as other reports raised the dilemma of whether prenatal follow-up, after umbilical cord blood sampling and intra-amnionic L-T_4 injections, if indicated, is required to prevent late neurological sequels in these cases (Abalovich et al., 2007; De Groot et al., 2012; Wada et al., 2000). It is recommended that all babies born to mothers with AITDs be reviewed in the first 3 days of life and a thyroid function test be taken to identify those babies with transient CH that require L-T_4 therapy, or babies with congenital hyperthyroidism requiring anti-thyroid drugs (Ogilvy-Stuart et al., 2002). The approach for *in-utero* treatment of fetal thyroid disease is still a matter of debate (De Groot et al., 2012).

3.4. Exposure to iodine

Abnormal thyroid function due to either iodine deficiency or iodine overload has been described in prenatal and postnatal periods. In cases of iodine overload, the Wolff-Chaikoff mechanism blocks the uptake of iodine by the thyroid gland resulting in reduced T_4 production and in turn increased TSH secretion via a negative feedback mechanism. Sava et al. (1984) showed that newborns from areas of iodine deficiency in Sicily were at higher risk for hyperthyrotropinemia; the increase in risk was related to the degree of iodine deficiency as reflected by iodine cord blood measurements. On recall, only two patients were diagnosed with CH which required L-T_4 therapy for as long as 1 year. The authors suggested the need for maternal iodine prophylaxis therapy in areas of endemic iodine deficiency. Transient thyroid function abnormalities have also been observed in neonates born to mothers with excessive iodine intake. Maternal iodine exposure was reported accompanying excess iodine in the diet (Nishiyama et al., 2004), use of iodine compounds such as povidone iodine in topical applications, exposure to contrast medium during pregnancy and the use of antiseptic agents in obstetric departments (Grüters et al., 1983). Prenatally, maternal iodine crosses the placenta and concentrates in the fetal thyroid gland, whereas postnatally, the newborn is exposed to iodine through the breast milk (Chanoine et al., 1988; Koga et al., 1995). Premature babies are particularly susceptible to iodine-induced hypothyroidism due to immaturity of the thyroid–pituitary negative feedback mechanism and to higher exposure to iodine-containing agents in intensive care (Delange et al., 1984). Uses of iodine in Cesarean sections and in neonatal intensive care units are additional causes for newborn iodine overload and therefore it is recommended to avoid iodine compounds in deliveries and in the neonate intensive care units. In newborns, exposure to iodine may be attributed to umbilical iodine application as well. Iodine overload may cause either transient hyperthyroidism with symptoms of tachycardia and failure to gain weight (Rakover & Adar, 1989) or may present as CH or persistent hyperthyrotropinemia. Nishiyama et al. (2004) described 15 babies with transient CH or persistent hyperthyrotropinemia born to mothers in Japan who consumed a high iodine diet during their pregnancies; among them, 12 babies were treated with L-T_4. The authors recommended that food be labeled with their precise amount of iodine to avoid high intake of iodine by pregnant women. CH and hyperthyrotropinemia in cases of iodine overload or deficiency are transitory; however, whether transient hypothyroidism or hyperthyrotropinemia can result in permanent neurological sequels in these cases is not clear, and it is therefore recommended that sort-term L-T_4 therapy be considered on an individual basis.

4. Genetic etiology of SCH

4.1. TSH Resistance syndrome (RTSH)

RTSH is a condition in which thyroid cells show reduced sensitivity to TSH. This condition is characterized by elevated serum TSH concentration, a normal or hypoplastic thyroid gland and normal to very low levels of thyroid hormones (Refetoff, 2003). The diagnosis of RTSH defect is based on the absence of thyroid antibodies, a lack of goiter, measurable serum thyroglobulin, and familial occurrence of hyperthyrotropinemia or hypothyroidism. Most of the cases of RTSH are attributed to mutations in the *TSHR* but in many cases, no such mutations were found, suggesting that additional genes are associated with RTSH syndrome (Xie et al., 1997). The diagnostic work-up of RTSH should exclude *PAX8* mutations, which are characterized by thyroid dysgenesis associated with kidney abnormalities (Grüters et al., 2003; Park & Chatterjee, 2005) and mutations in *GNAS1*, which encodes Gsα subunit, causing pseudohypoparathyroidism (PHP). Another form of RTSH is an autosomal dominantly inherited disease characterized by euthyroid hyperthyrotropinemia, for which the specific gene has not yet been identified. This condition has been linked to a locus on chromosome 15q25.3-26.1 (Grasberger et al., 2005). Loss-of-function mutations of *DUOX* genes are an additional cause for transient hyperthyrotropinemia.

4.2. TSH Receptor (*TSHR*)

Loss-of-function mutations in *TSHR* manifest with a variable clinical spectrum of phenotypes ranging from severe uncompensated RTSH presenting with CH, or partially compensated RTSH presenting with SCH or even with normal thyroid function (for review see Tenenbaum-Rakover, 2012). CH is commonly detected by TSH-based neonatal screening but may missed by total T_4 (TT_4)-based screening since, in many cases, TT_4 levels are within the normal range at birth. The degree of CH is variable and depends on the genotype. Severe forms manifest as overt CH; moderate forms manifest as hypothyroidism identified by neonatal screening without clinical symptoms of hypothyroidism and mild forms present with hyperthyrotropinemia and normal thyroid hormone levels. Most of the described cases of CH are detected by neonatal screening with elevated TSH and normal TT_4 levels, but without any clinical symptoms or signs of hypothyroidism (de Roux et al., 1996; Tenenbaum-Rakover et al., 2009). Nevertheless, L-T_4 therapy is initiated in most cases to prevent future consequences of untreated CH. At the age of 2 to 3 years, when L-T_4 is withdrawn, thyroid hormones remain low in the severe mutations; however in milder mutations, despite extremely elevated TSH levels, thyroid hormone levels are normal, indicating compensated hypothyroidism (Tenenbaum-Rakover et al., 2009). ^{99m}TC scan commonly reveals a normal or hypoplastic gland but in some cases, an absence of thyroid gland has been demonstrated, suggesting thyroid agenesis. On the other hand, the presence of detectable thyroglobulin as well as the demonstration of a thyroid gland in the normal position in ultrasonographic imaging exclude thyroid agenesis and indicate a diagnosis of RTSH. The affected patients who are not identified by neonatal screening are commonly identified by routine laboratory tests in childhood or even as adults and are commonly asymptomatic. Most of the described cases are heterozygous for

TSHR mutations, but biallelic mutations have been reported as well. To date, about 50 different *TSHR* mutations have been reported, presenting with a spectrum of phenotypes ranging from overt CH to mild euthyroid hyperthyrotropinemia. Subjects with euthyroid hyperthyrotropinemia commonly have stable TSH levels and do not develop overt hypothyroidism with time. The phenotype correlates with the genotype as the latter is reflected in the severity of hyperthyrotropinemia and the decrease in FT_4 levels. Screening for *TSHR* mutations should be considered in individuals with apparent nonautoimmune SCH. In view of the variability in phenotypes and outcomes among individuals with this condition, careful long-term follow-up is recommended and replacement therapy should be considered on an individual basis according to thyroid hormone levels in the clinical context. In cases with loss-of-function mutations in *TSHR* presenting with CH, early initiation of L-T_4 therapy is recommended to prevent late-effect consequences of hypothyroidism as in other etiologies of CH. However, withdrawal of L-T_4 at the age of 2 to 3 years revealed transient hypothyroidism in some cases, putting the need for lifelong replacement therapy into question (Alberti et al., 2002; Tenenbaum-Rakover et al., 2009). SCH caused by *TSHR* mutations with mild to moderate loss of function maintains stable compensated RTSH and may not necessitate thyroid hormone replacement. Moreover, most patients with RTSH do not present with symptoms of hypothyroidism or with biochemical parameters of uncompensated hypothyroidism, such as elevated creatinine phosphokinase (CPK) and liver enzymes and hyperlipidemia (Tenenbaum-Rakover et al., 2009). The presence of normal FT_4 levels argues against the need for replacement treatment, especially when inadvertent overtreatment, producing subclinical hyperthyroidism, can have undesirable effects (Samuels et al., 2008). Contrasting with this approach, it has been shown that some subjects with RTSH have a slight decrease in FT_4 levels compared to controls, although remaining within the normal range, which may point to a condition of compensated hypothyroidism in these affected patients. In addition, the possibility of secondary pituitary enlargement in patients with extreme hyperthyrotropinemia may support L-T_4 replacement therapy. In view of the variability in phenotypes for the different types of mutations, as well as between individuals with the same genotypes, it is recommended that careful follow-up and cautious administration of L-T_4 be considered based on individual thyroid hormone levels in the clinical context.

4.3. Pseudohypoparathyroidism (PHP)

Loss-of-function mutations in *GNAS1*, which encodes Gsα subunit, cause PHP and lead to a syndrome of resistance to multiple G-coupled receptor hormones. Resistance to parathyroid hormone (PTH) is the main feature of PHP (Mantovani, 2011; Mantovani et al., 2002). RTSH is commonly clinically manifested during childhood or adulthood but may present at birth as CH identified by neonatal screening. In most cases, hypothyroidism is mild and may present with hyperthyrotropinemia for long durations without any clinical symptoms of hypothyroidism. ^{99m}TC scan generally demonstrates a hypoplastic gland in a normal position but absence of a thyroid gland, demonstrated by ultrasonographic imaging, has been reported as well. SCH is the presenting laboratory finding of PHP in many cases. RTSH is commonly found in PHP-Ia but is also reported in PHP-Ib. The phenotype of patients with PHP-Ia includes Albright osteodystrophy presenting with brachydactyly, round face, short stature, central obesity, subcutaneous ossifications and variable degree of mental retardation. Clinicians should be aware of this rare syndrome; in those cases of SCH occurring in obese subjects or with Albright osteodystrophy phenotype, PHP should be suspected and further hormonal and molecular evaluations should be considered.

4.4. Dual Oxidase maturation factor (*DUOX*)

Loss-of-function mutations in *DUOX* have been reported in children with CH and in transient hyperthyrotropinemia of the newborn (De Marco et al., 2011; Hoste et al., 2010; Maruo et al., 2008; Moreno et al., 2002). Hydrogen peroxide (H_2O_2) is an essential co-substrate for oxidation of iodine and iodination of thyroglobulin by the thyroid peroxidase (TPO) enzyme. DOUX1 and DOUX2 proteins have a crucial role in H_2O_2 generation and therefore in thyroid hormone synthesis. The structure of these proteins includes seven putative transmembrane domains. Moreno et al. (2002) showed that biallelic mutations of *DUOX2* result in organification defect presenting with permanent CH, whereas monoallelic mutations result in transient CH or hyperthyrotropinemia (OMIM#606758) (Moreno et al., 2002). In contrast, sequencing of *DUOX2* in Japanese children diagnosed with transient congenital hyperthyrotropinemia revealed eight novel mutations of the *DUOX2* gene, all with biallelic mutations (Maruo et al., 2008). The authors concluded that even complete inactivation of *DUOX2* causes transient, but not permanent CH, due to the presence of DUOX1, which maintains the supply of H_2O_2 required for oxidation after the neonatal period. However, late onset of hypothyroidism or SCH may appear in adulthood during periods of increased requirement for thyroid hormones, such as in pregnancy (Ohye et al., 2008). The organification defect is characterized by normal position and location of the thyroid gland in a ^{99m}TC scan, high iodine uptake with partial positive perchlorate discharge test. Goiter may be present or develop over time (Moreno et al., 2002; Ohye et al., 2008).

4.5. Thyroid dysgenesis

Three transcription factors have been identified as involved in thyroid development: *TTF-1*, *TTF-2* and *PAX8*. The discovery of these transcription factors in a knockout mouse model was followed by descriptions of the phenotypes in humans. Human mutations in *TTF-2* are very rare and present with CH, cleft palate and spiky hair (OMIM#602617). Patients with *TTF-1* and *PAX8* mutations present with either CH or persistent congenital hyperthyrotropinemia; the former are associated with lung and neurological involvement while the latter are associated with kidney abnormalities.

4.5.1. TTF-1 mutations

TTF-1, also known as NKX2.1, is a transcription factor involved in thyroid development. Ttf1-null mice were born dead, lacking a thyroid gland, lung parenchyma and pituitary gland, and with severe defects in the ventral forebrain. Heterozygous mice presented a euthyroid phenotype with reduced motor-coordination skills (Park & Chatterjee, 2005). In humans, *TTF-1* mutations have been reported in children presenting with SCH, lung involvement presenting with neonatal respiratory distress and neurological involvement presenting with hypotonia, persistent ataxia, dysarthria, microcephaly, choreathetosis and developmental delay (OMIM #600635). *TTF-1* mutations are inherited in an autosomal dominant manner. Patients present with variable thyroid phenotypes ranging from permanent severe CH to persistent congenital hyperthyrotropinemia resembling RTSH (Devriendt et al., 1998; Krude et al., 2002; Pohlenz et al., 2002) with hypoplasticity or agenesis of the thyroid gland or the gland in a normal position (Krude et al., 2002). *TTF-1* mutations may also present with isolated benign hereditary chorea without thyroid phenotype (Breedveld et al., 2002).

4.5.2. PAX8 mutations

PAX8 is thyroid transcription factor which is a key gene in mammalian embryonic development. Homozygous Pax8-null mice die shortly after weaning and their survival is dependent on thyroxin replacement therapy. Mutations in the *PAX8* gene in humans are characterized by thyroid dysgenesis associated with kidney abnormalities (Damante 1998; Grüters et al., 2003; Narumi et al., 2011; Park & Chatterjee, 2005; Vilain et al., 2001) inherited in an autosomal dominant manner (OMIM#167415). The thyroid gland is hypoplastic (Vilain et al., 2001) or in an ectopic location. Partial organification defect and partial iodide transport defect have been reported (Jo et al., 2010). To date, 31 mutations have been described in the *PAX8* gene, presenting as permanent CH or as mild SCH (Narumi et al., 2011; Narumi et al., 2012). Screening for *PAX8* gene mutations in 300 Chinese patients with CH revealed only two subjects with heterozygous *PAX8* mutations, suggesting that *PAX8* mutation is a very rare etiology for CH (Liu et al., 2012).

5. Outcome of neonatal hyperthyrotropinemia

Neonatal hyperthyrotropinemia may be transitory or permanent. Transient congenital hyperthyrotropinemia has been shown in iodine deficiency or due to iodine overload and in both of these cases, full recovery is expected within days to a month after the cause has been removed. In maternal AITD, TRAbs disappear within 4 to 8 months. A less favorable intellectual outcome was reported in these cases, probably due to *in-utero* fetal hypothyroidism (Matsuura et al., 1990; Wada et al., 2000). In cases of persistent congenital hyperthyrotropinemia, minor thyroid abnormalities (Calaciura et al., 2002; Daliva et al., 2000; Leonardi et al., 2008; Miki et al., 1989; Zung et al., 2010) have been reported in late childhood. Longitudinal studies assessing the outcome of subjects with neonatal hyperthyrotropinemia have shown a prevalence of 50% SCH with morphological alterations of the thyroid in early childhood (3 years) (Calaciura et al., 2002), which decreases in follow-up to 30% in late childhood (8 years), suggesting that persistent hyperthyrotropinemia represents minor congenital thyroid abnormalities (Leonardi et al., 2008). In about 50% of the subjects morphological, immunological or genetic abnormalities were found. A high rate of thyroid autoantibodies was identified at the age of 2 to 3 years in about 25% of the subjects (Calaciura et al., 2002); morphological changes such as enlarged or hypoplastic thyroid gland or its hemiagenesis were shown in 10% of the cases. Zung et al. (2010) showed that subjects with persistent vs. transient hyperthyrotropinemia had a higher rate of abnormal thyroid imaging and therefore thyroid imaging was recommended to distinguish between the persistent and transient forms. Moreover, genetic analysis revealed heterozygous mutations of *TPO* and *TSHR* (Calaciura et al., 2002) in about 5% of the children with SCH following transient neonatal hyperthyrotropinemia. These findings indicate that hyperthyrotropinemia at birth may represent an inherited thyroid disease that interferes with thyroid hormone synthesis or thyroid genesis. In contrast to these studies, Köhler et al. (1996) showed no increase in the risk of thyroid abnormalities and normal neurological development as well as normal growth in children with hyperthyrotropinemia at birth; they therefore recommended avoiding longitudinal surveys of these children to prevent parents' anxiety (Köhler et al., 1996). In summary, neonatal hyperthyrotropinemia may be persistently associated with either autoimmune disease, inherited thyroid hormone synthesis defects or morphological changes, and therefore long-term follow-up throughout childhood is recommended in cases where TSH levels are persistently above the normal range during the first year of life.

6. Pediatric-age-dependent thyroid hormone reference

The commonly available normal reference range provided by commercial companies for thyroid hormone levels in routine laboratories is for adults. Using this may result in an erroneous interpretation of the results of thyroid function in children. Moreover, great variability exists between the pediatric references published in the literature (Elmlinger et al., 2001; Hübner et al., 2002; Kapelari et al., 2008; Soldin et al., 2009; Strich et al., 2012; Zurakowski et al., 1999). The variability in the normal reference range is attributed to different types of assays, different ethnic and age groups and different sample sizes. Even in the same assay, different laboratories can provide different normal ranges (Hübner et al., 2002; Kapelari et al., 2008; Strich et al., 2012). The variability between assays results from the different standards, antibodies and methods used [two-site immunoassay commonly gives lower results than radioimmunoassays (RIAs)]. Furthermore, the references established for children in different age groups make use of different populations; for example, hospitalized children (Hübner et al., 2002; Kapelari et al., 2008) have lower FT_3 concentration due to non-thyroidal illness, whereas references using routine laboratory samples (Strich et al., 2012) may include samples from children bearing unidentified thyroid diseases, which may cause an upward bias in the TSH levels. Despite these limitations, it is still clear that childhood references are very different from adult references. Strich et al. (2012) showed that in 11,000 samples of children aged 0 to 18 years taken from a routine laboratory database, the upper limit of TSH was 1 mIU/ml above the provided reference and the lower normal range of FT_3 was 0.5 to 2 pmol/l higher than the reference. Hübner et al. (2002) analyzed thyroid hormone levels in children with the ADVIA® Centaur ™ analyzer. They showed elevated TSH levels in the first year of life with an upper limit of 9.64 mIU/l, which decreased gradually to 4.9 mIU/l at the age of 18 years. The same trend was shown with FT_4, decreasing from 17.2 to 14.7 pmol/l from 1 to 18 years of age. The upper limit of FT_3 levels showed the same, albeit less pronounced trend, from 8.2 to 6.63 pmol/l. The authors suggested using continuous-age-dependent reference ranges in children who show better agreement with biological reality, as these are more reliable than discontinuous reference ranges. No significant sex-specific effects on age-adjusted hormone levels were shown (Hübner et al., 2002; Kapelari et al., 2008). In recent years, there has been some controversy regarding the normal TSH range for adult populations following the laboratory guidelines from the National Academy of Clinical Biochemistry, indicating that 85% of normal adult individuals have TSH levels below 2.5 mIU/l. These findings raised a debate over whether subjects with TSH levels above 2.5 mIU/l have SCH and should be further followed-up by repeated TSH measurements (Surks et al., 2004; Wartofsky & Dickey, 2005). In summary, age-dependent references should be used to interpretate thyroid functions in childhood. Hyperthyrotropinemia as high as 6.0 mIU/l (Hübner et al., 2002) with normal thyroid hormone levels and without clinical symptoms, during the first months of life can be considered within the upper normal limit for age and therefore not requiring L-T_4 therapy. Follow-up with repeated thyroid function tests is recommended in cases of persistent hyperthyrotropinemia to identify those infants which may develop late onset overt hypothyroidism.

7. Laboratory pitfalls

In about 0.5 to 5% of patient samples, hyperthyrotropinemia with normal thyroid hormone levels results from laboratory interference (Ismail et al., 2002). Such interference includes the presence of heterophilic antibodies, rheumatic factor (RF), autoimmune antithyroid hormone antibodies and the presence of macro-TSH.

7.1. Heterophilic antibodies

Heterophilic antibodies are antibodies produced against poorly defined antigens of various animal immunoglobulins. The best known heterophilic antibodies are human antimouse antibodies (HAMAs). Since immunometric assays use animal antihuman antibodies, the presence of human antimouse immunoglobulins in an individual's serum could interfere with the antigen–antibody binding reaction, resulting in falsely high or low hormonal levels. This interference is very rare in competitive RIAs but well recognized in the two-site sandwich immunometric assays (Després & Grant, 1988; Halsall et al., 2009; Kaplan & Levinson, 1999). High false-positive results are commonly reported in the latter, whereas false low levels are reported in competitive RIAs. High levels of α-fetoprotein, human chorionogonadotropin, follicle-stimulating hormone, luteinizing hormone, ferritin and tumor markers were described in TSH measurements secondary to the presence of heterophilic antibodies. Since TSH is commonly measured in routine evaluations for various medical complaints, elevated TSH level due to the presence of heterophilic antibodies is not a rare finding. Transient neonatal hyperthyrotropinemia identified by neonatal screening was reported by Czernichow et al. (1981), attributed to maternal heterophilic antibodies. The antibodies disappeared from the circulation within 2 months in the infants and within 4 to 6 months in the mothers (Czernichow et al., 1981). When heterophilic interference is suspected, further evaluation is indicated. The first step is to assess the sample using other immunoassays with different antibodies. The sample should be remeasured after dilution (Ross et al., 2008). Nonlinearity in sample dilution indicates the presence of laboratory interference. Preincubation of a patient's sample with antiheterophilic tube or mouse serum confirms the diagnosis of heterophilic antibodies. The clinician should be aware that hyperthyrotropinemia with normal thyroid hormone levels and without clinical symptoms of hypothyroidism in the newborn or in childhood may be the result of interference by heterophilic antibodies. The diagnosis of hyperthyrotropinemia due to heterophilic antibodies cancels the need for further expensive laboratory and imaging investigations and avoids unnecessary L-T_4 therapy.

7.2. Thyroid hormone autoantibodies

Thyroid hormone autoantibodies are present in about 1 to 7% of patients with autoimmune thyroid diseases, mainly Graves' disease. Antibodies against thyroglobulin and thyroid peroxidase are very common in Hashimoto's thyroiditis and Graves' disease; however, antibodies against thyroid hormones T_3 and T_4 are less common and anti-TSH autoantibodies are even rarer. The presence of thyroid hormone autoantibodies interferes with the assay procedure, giving higher hormonal levels (Després & Grant, 1998). We had one case of a 16-year-old girl with Graves' disease (unpublished data) who presented with severe symptoms of hypothyroidism, 4 months after 8 mCi of I-131 therapy, with bradycardia and excessive weight gain. Thyroid function was confusing, with extremely high TSH 136 mIU/dl (0.35–5.5 mIU/dl), extremely high FT_4 > 6 (0.88–12.76 ng/ml); low FT_3 30 ng/dl (60–180 ng/dl) and extremely high thyroid stimulating immunoglobulin (TSI) 164 IU/l, anti-TPO > 1000 U/ml and antithyroglobulin > 3000 U/ml. Measuring FT_4 in another assay using different antibodies revealed low FT_4, confirming the clinical diagnosis of hypothyroidism post-radioactive iodine therapy. The increase in FT_4 and TSI concentrations was associated with the autoimmune overreaction post-I-131 therapy with production of anti-FT_4 autoantibodies. This case demonstrates the importance of being aware of the existence laboratory interferences for making correct clinical decisions.

7.3. Macro-TSH

Macro-TSH is a macromolecule that is formed when anti-TSH IgG combines with a TSH molecule. Due to their large size, these macromolecules are less efficiently cleared from the circulation by the kidneys, and therefore accumulate in the serum. Since they are nonfunctioning, they have no clinical significance and therefore may lead to unnecessary therapy. This condition is commonly described in patients with asymptomatic hyperprolactinemia caused by macroprolactinemia (Batista et al., 2012). Macro-TSH is rarer than macroprolactinemia with only about 13 cases described to date (Halsall et al., 2006; Loh et al., 2012; Mendoza, 2009; Newman et al., 2006; Rix et al., 2011; Sakai et al., 2009). The presence of macro-TSH should be suspected when the patient is asymptomatic and has elevated TSH level which does not correlate with additional thyroid function. Nonlinearity when the subject's serum is diluted indicates the presence of interfering antibodies. The presence of macro-TSH is proven by adding polyethylene glycol (PEG) to the patient's serum. Recovery results less than 50 to 30% of the pre-PEG results indicate the presence of macro-TSH. The diagnosis of macro-TSH is confirmed by gel-filtration chromatography but this technique is not routinely available. The presence of macro-TSH is not part of AITD or autoimmunity. Misdiagnosis of CH identified by TSH-based neonatal screening was described in newborns which were later found to have macro-TSH of maternal origin (Halsall et al., 2006; Newman et al., 2006; Rix et al., 2011). It is suggested that maternal TSH levels be measured in cases of euthyroid neonates with elevated serum TSH and normal thyroid hormone. When maternal TSH is persistently elevated, the presence of macro-TSH should be considered. Further analysis, including recovery with PEG, is indicated to avoid unnecessary L-T_4 treatment. Macro-TSH spontaneously disappears from the infant's serum at the age of 6 to 8 months in parallel with the elimination of maternal immunoglobulins.

In summary, clinicians should be aware of false laboratory results attributed to interference in the immunoassay methods, mainly in evaluating euthyroid hyperthyrotropinemia. In cases in which there are discrepancies between the clinical presentation and the laboratory results, antibody interference should be suspected. This may be followed up by further laboratory evaluation. Accurate diagnosis leads to a better clinical approach and may allow avoiding unnecessary treatment.

8. Obesity and hyperthyrotropinemia

Obesity in children has become a great medical concern in the last two decades. Thyroid function tests are part of the diagnostic work-up in children who are overweight or obese. Moderate elevation in TSH levels in up to 20% of obese children has been demonstrated in many studies (Eliakim et al., 2006; Grandone et al., 2010; Reinehr, 2011; Reinehr et al., 2006; Shalitin et al., 2009). Among them, only 7 to 20% showed positive thyroid autoantibodies (Eliakim et al., 2006; Grandone et al., 2010). It has been speculated that hyperthyrotropinemia in obesity is a result of elevated leptin which stimulates the hypothalamic–pituitary–thyroid axis (Reinehr, 2011). The question is whether the elevation in TSH is the cause for or a consequence of obesity and whether it merits treatment with L-T_4. Reiter et al. (2006) did not find any association between hyperthyrotropinemia and lipid profile, whereas Shalitin et al. (2009) showed a positive correlation between hyperthyrotropinemia and waist circumference and triglyceride levels, supporting the need to treat those children. The fact that hyperthyrotropinemia was accompanied by normal FT_4 and elevated FT_3 levels (Reinehr et al., 2006) disagrees with the hypothesis of SCH as the cause for obesity in these children. Moreover, weight loss led to a significant reduction in TSH levels (Eliakim et al., 2006; Grandone et al., 2010; Reinehr et al., 2006) and L-T_4 therapy had no significant influence on body weight or lipid profile (Eliakim et al., 2006). Most of the studies agree that hyperthyrotropinemia in obesity is a consequence rather than a cause, and therefore L-T_4 therapy is unnecessary in obese children (Eliakim et al., 2006; Grandone et al., 2010; Reinehr, 2011; Reinehr et al., 2006).

9. Autoimmune Thyroid Disease (AITD) — Hashimoto's thyroiditis

Hashimoto's thyroiditis is characterized by the presence of thyroid autoantibodies [anti-thyroid peroxidase (TPO) and anti-thyroglobulin (TG)], with or without goiter. This condition is characterized by hypoechogenicity of the thyroid gland in ultasonographic imaging and lymphocytic infiltration of the gland in fine-needle aspiration. The disease commonly appears in adolescence, with predominantly females affected. Among children with acquired hypothyroidism, 66% had AITD (Hunter et al., 2000), and about 30% to 50% had a family history of thyroid diseases (de Vries et al., 2009). The risk of overt hypothyroidism in adults with thyroid autoantibodies is estimated at 4.3% per year (Vanderpump & Tunbridge, 2002); however, there are only a few pieces of data on the natural history of Hashimoto's thyroiditis in children (Gopalakrishnan et al., 2008; Jaruratanasirikul et al., 2001; Moore, 1996; Radetti et al., 2006; Rallison et al., 1991). Hypoechogenicity of the thyroid gland in ultrasound imaging is a useful tool for the diagnosis of AITD (Marcocci et al., 1991; Pedersen et al., 2000; Wolgang et al., 2002), showing higher sensitivity than the thyroid autoantibody tests (100 vs. 63.3%) (Rago et al., 2001). Marwaha et al. (2008) showed that among children with hypoechogenic appearance of the gland, 41.4% were positive for FNA, 30.6% were positive for TPO antibodies and 46.8% showed abnormal thyroid function. They concluded that ultrasound echogenicity is useful tool for the diagnosis of AITD in children but less sensitive compared to adults (Marwaha et al., 2008). Moreover, the occurrence of hypoechogenicity has been found to predict evolution toward hypothyroidism over time in euthyroid subjects (Marcocci et al., 1991; Rago et al., 2001). Disagreement also exists with regard to the criteria for L-T_4 therapy in childhood SCH (de Vries et al., 2009; Padberg et al., 2001; Radetti et al., 2006; Svensson et al., 2006). Thyroid function in Hashimoto's thyroiditis in children at presentation is variable. Özen et al. (2011) found that 36.7% of children were euthyroid, 32.7% had SCH, 16.6% were hypothyroid, 7.9% had subclinical hyperthyroidism and 5.9% presented with hyperthyroidism (Hashitoxicosis) (Özen et al., 2011). The main complaint was goiter presenting in 57.85% of patients, most of which were female (5.7:1, F:M). Similar findings were found by others showing that about 70% of children are either euthyroid or have SCH (Demirbilek et al., 2007; de Vries et al., 2009; Skarpa et al., 2011). Moore (1996) showed a benign course of SCH in children and adolescents with AITD and therefore suggested careful follow–up rather than treating them empirically. Gopalakrishnan et al. (2008) found that only 12.5% of children with either goiterous euthyroid or SCH develop overt hypothyroidism within 2 years. In contrast, Jaruratanasirikul et al. (2001) showed that 50% of subjects with SCH develop overt hypothyroidism within 5 years, supporting the need for long-term monitoring of thyroid function in patients with thyroid autoantibodies. de Vries et al. (2009) suggested that L-T_4 therapy of euthyroid children with AITD, if appropriately monitored, is not harmful and may even be beneficial. Further benefit consisted of reducing thyroid volume in those patients with goiter with or without overt hypothyroidism (Svensson et al., 2006). Padberg et al. (2001) demonstrated that prophylactic L-T_4 therapy of patients with euthyroid AITD reduces both serological and cellular markers of autoimmune thyroiditis, indicating that L-T_4 therapy might be useful for stopping progression of the disease. In contrast, the findings in an adult population that unnecessary long-term thyroxine therapy or overdose is associated with increase risk for osteopenia, cardiac disease and other harmful effects (Samuels et al., 2008) argues against regular therapy in children with AITD-associated SCH.

10. Natural history

The annual rate of progression of SCH to overt hypothyroidism (elevated TSH with low thyroid hormones) in an adult population was 4.3% in women with positive thyroid autoantibodies and only 2% when antibodies were negative (Biondi & Cooper, 2008). Huber et al. (2002), in a prospective study, found that 28% of women with SCH developed overt hypothyroidism after 10 years of follow-up. In children, the risk for progression to overt hypothyroidism is less common and recovery is more frequent. About 25% of subjects with goiterous thyroiditis had spontaneous remission and 33% developed hypothyroidism over 20 years of follow-up (Rallison et al., 1991). Radetti et al. (2006) showed, retrospectively, in 160 children with AITD in an over 5-year follow-up that abnormal thyroid functions occur in 34.3% at presentation whereas 47.55% had abnormal thyroid function at last visit. However, 10% of patients with SCH became euthyroid. TSH concentrations showed large fluctuations over time. The presence of goiter and elevated thyroid autoantibodies at presentation together with an increase in thyroid autoantibodies and TSH levels in the course of the follow-up were predictive factors for development of overt hypothyroidism. After 5 years, more that 50% became or remained euthyroid, and therefore a poor predictive outcome could be shown in individual patients. The authors suggested that medical therapy should be considered only when significant deterioration of thyroid function appears (Radetti et al., 2006).

11. Treatment

The dilemma of whether to treat children with SCH is a matter of debate. The risk of developing overt hypothyroidism in an adult population with SCH was estimated at between 2 to 4.3% per year, with higher occurrence in patients with positive thyroid autoantibodies and increased TSH at presentation (Vanderpump & Tunbridge, 2002). In adults, despite extensive studies and discussion, two different approaches still exist; one expert panel reviewed the available evidence and concluded that patients with TSH above 10 mIU/l with normal FT_4 levels may be treated, whereas subjects with TSH between 4.5 and 10 mIU/l should be followed-up without treatment considering the adverse effects of L-T_4 on mineral health and heart and the lack of evidence to support the benefits of the treatment (Surks et al., 2004). On the other hand, a joint statement of experts from three endocrine societies (American Association of Clinical Endocrinologists, American Thyroid Association, Endocrine Society) recommended treatment of subjects with TSH between 4.5 and 10 mIU/l, arguing that lack of evidence does not necessarily mean lack of benefit (Gharib et al., 2004). Moreover, in view of the recent suggestion to revise the reference range for adult TSH from 0.3 to 3 mIU/l by the National Health and Nutrition Examination Survey in United States, indicating that values above this range can be considered early thyroid failure, additional subjects will be included in the range of TSH within which thyroxine therapy is justified (Hollowell et al., 2002). In children, most of the subjects with SCH remain euthyroid over time, and therefore careful follow-up rather than treating them empirically was suggested (Moore, 1996; Radetti et al., 2006). It is commonly accepted that children with TSH above 10 mIU/l should be treated even if the FT_4 is within a normal range while those with TSH between 4.5 and 10 mIU/l with thyroid autoantibodies should be followed up with repeated thyroid function tests but without treatment (Gopalakrishnan & Marwaha, 2007). Still, the benefit of L-T_4 therapy has been questioned and some studies have shown no difference in metabolic parameters or neurocognitive function between treated and untreated subjects (Aijaz et al., 2006; Biondi & Cooper, 2008). On the other hand, it has been shown that L-T_4 therapy of patients with euthyroid AITD reduces both serological and cellular markers of autoimmune thyroiditis, indicating that L-T_4 therapy might be useful in stopping disease progression (Padberg et al., 2001) and reducing thyroid volume in those patients with goiter (Svensson et al., 2006). Stable euthyroid hyperthyrotropinemia is a common condition that usually does not present with clinical symptoms or signs. Furthermore, biochemical parameters such as increased liver enzyme, hypercholesterolemia or elevated CPK are negative, indicating a euthyroid state. It is therefore recommended not to treat children without evidence of clinical hypothyroidism. However, those children with TSH above 10 mIU/l or with a trend toward increasing TSH and decreasing FT_4 over time might benefit from L-T_4 therapy. Side effects of L-T_4 therapy on the heart with such as resting tachycardia and on individuals' behavior, such as restlessness and sleep disturbances, should be considered in the clinical decisions for initiation of therapy. In euthyroid hyperthyrotropinemia caused by heterozygous loss-of-function mutation of *TSHR*, TSH levels tend to be stable over the years and therefore no therapy is indicated (Tenenbaum-Rakover, 2012). In newborns, a different approach should be taken since delay in therapy may result in permanent intellectual damage. In the case of TSH levels above 10 mIU/l, early initiation of therapy should be considered, even if thyroid hormones are within the normal range. In view of the controversy that still exists around L-T_4 therapy in SCH, it is recommended that the decision to initiate therapy be considered on an individual basis taking into account the benefits and possible side effects. In pregnant women and in newborns, initiation of therapy should be more urgent, whereas in other cases, sequential thyroid function tests along with clinical follow-up and further investigation, including laboratory, imaging and molecular analyses, might be a more reasonable approach prior to initiation of therapy.

12. Conclusion

The variable causes of SCH in children of different age groups were reviewed. The outcome of SCH in infancy and during childhood was shown to be dependent on etiology. Long-term follow-up is recommended since SCH may develop into overt hypothyroidism. Initiation of L-T_4 therapy in children, similar to adults, is still a matter of debate. In newborns, early initiation of therapy should be considered even if thyroid hormones are within the normal range to prevent possible late neurological sequels; in older children, on the other hand, it is recommended that the decision to initiate therapy be considered on an individual basis, taking into account its benefits and possible side effects.

http://dx.doi.org/10.5772/55134

Acknowledgements

Thanks to Camille Vainstein for professional language editing.

Author details

Yardena Tenenbaum-Rakover*

Address all correspondence to: rakover_y@clalit.org.il

Ha'Emek Medical Center, Afula and The Ruth & Rappoport Faculty of Medicine, Technion, Haifa, Israel

References

[1] Abalovich, M, Amino, N, Barbour, L. A, Cobin, R. H, De Groot, L. J, Glinoer, D, Mandel, S. J, & Stagnaro-green, A. (2007). Management of thyroid dysfunction during pregnancy and postpartum: an Endocrine Society Clinical Practice Guideline. *Journal of Clinical Endocrinology and Metabolism,* Suppl.8, (August 2007), 0002-1972X, 92, S1-S47.

[2] Alberti, L, Proverbio, M. C, Costagliola, S, Romoli, R, Boldrighini, B, Vigone, M. C, Weber, G, Chiumello, G, Beck-peccoz, P, & Persani, L. (2002). Germline mutations of TSH receptor gene as cause of nonautoimmune subclinical hypothyroidism. *Journal of Clinical Endocrinology and Metabolism,* June 2002), 0002-1972X, 87(6), 2549-2555.

[3] Aijaz, N. J, Flaherty, E. M, Preston, T, Bracken, S. S, Lane, A. H, & Wilson, T. A. Neurocognitive function in children with compensated hypothyroidism: lack of short term effects on or off thyroxin. *BMJ Endociene disordes,* March (2006). 1472-6823, 6(20), 2.

[4] Batista, R. L, Toscanini, A. C, Glezer, A, Siqueira, M. G, Benabou, S, Fonoff, E. T, Tavares, W. M, & Teixeira, M. J. Cunha Neto, M.B. ((2012). Approach to the patient with persistent hyperprolactinemia and negative sellar imaging. *Journal of Clinical Endocrinology and Metabolism,* July 2012), 0002-1972X, 97(7), 2211-2216.

[5] Biondi, B, & Cooper, D. S. (2008). The clinical significance of subclinical thyroid dysfunction. *Endocrine Reviews,* February 2008), 0016-3769X, 29(1), 76-131.

[6] Breedveld, G. J, Van Dongen, J. W. F, Danesino, C, Guala, A, Percy, A. K, Dure, L. S, Harper, P, Lazarou, L. P, Van Der Linde, H, Joosse, M, & Gruters, A. MacDonald, M.E.; de Vries, B.B.A.; Arts, W.F.M.; Oostra, B.A.; Krude, H. & Heutink, P. ((2002).

Mutations in TITF-1 are associated with benign hereditary chorea. *Human Molecular Genetics*, April 2002), 0964-6906, 11(8), 971-979.

[7] Brown, R. S, Bellisario, R. L, Botero, D, Fournier, L, Abrams, C. A, Cowger, M. L, David, R, Fort, P, & Richman, R. A. (1996). Incidence of transient congenital hypothyroidism due to maternal thyrotropin receptor-blocking antibodies in over one million babies. *Journal of Clinical Endocrinology and Metabolism*, March 1996), 0002-1972X, 81(3), 1147-1151.

[8] Calaciura, F, Motta, R. M, Miscio, G, Fichera, G, Leonardi, D, Carta, A, Trischitta, V, Tassi, V, Sava, L, & Vigneri, R. (2002). Subclinical hypothyroidism in early childhood: a frequent outcome of transient neonatal hyperthyrotropinemia. *Journal of Clinical Endocrinology and Metabolism*, July 2002), 0002-1972X, 87(7), 3209-3214.

[9] Chanoine, J. P, Boulvain, M, Bourdoux, P, Pardou, A, Van Thi, H. V, Ermans, A. M, & Delange, F. (1988). Increased recall rate at screening for congenital hypothyroidism in breast fed infants born to iodine overloaded mothers. *Archives of Disease in Childhood*, October 1988), 0003-9888, 63(10), 1207-1210.

[10] Cheron, R. G, Kaplan, M. M, Larsen, P. R, Selenkow, H. A, & Crigler, J. F. Jr. ((1981). Neonatal thyroid function after propylthiouracil therapy for maternal Graves' disease. *New England Journal of Medicine*, February 1981), 0028-4793, 304(9), 525-528.

[11] Chu, J. W, & Crapo, L. M. (2001). The treatment of subclinical hypothyroidism is seldom necessary. *Journal of Clinical Endocrinology and Metabolism*, October 2001), 0002-1972X, 86(10), 4591-4599.

[12] Czernichow, P, Vandalem, J. L, & Hennen, G. Transient neonatal hyperthyrotropinemia: a factitious syndrome due to the presence of heterophilic antibodies in the plasma of infants and their mothers. *Journal of Clinical Endocrinology and Metabolism*, August (1981). 0002-1972X, 53(2), 387-393.

[13] Daliva, A. L, & Linder, B. DiMartino-Nardi, J. & Saenger, P. ((2000). Three-year follow-up of borderline congenital hypothyroidism. *Journal of Pediatrics*, January 2000), 0022-3476, 136(1), 53-56.

[14] Damante, G. (1998). Thyroid defects due to Pax8 gene mutations. *European Journal of Endocrinology*, December 1998), 0804-4643, 139(6), 563-566.

[15] De Groot, L, Abalovich, M, Alexander, E. K, Amino, N, Barbour, L, Cobin, R. H, Eastman, C. J, Lazarus, J. H, Luton, D, Mandel, S. J, Mestman, J, Rovet, J, & Sullivan, S. (2012). Management of Thyroid Dysfunction during Pregnancy and Postpartum: An Endocrine Society Clinical Practice Guideline. *Journal of Clinical Endocrinology and Metabolism*, August 2012), 0002-1972X, 97(8), 2543-2565.

[16] Delange, F, Dalhem, A, Bourdoux, P, Lagasse, R, Glinoer, D, Fisher, D. A, Walfish, P. G, & Ermans, A. M. (1984). Increased risk of primary hypothyroidism in preterm infants. *Journal of Pediatrics*, September 1984), 0022-3476, 105(3), 462-469.

[17] De Marco, G, Agretti, P, & Montanelli, L. Di Cosmo, C.; Bagattini, B; De Servi, M.; Ferrarini, E.; Dimida, A.; Freitas Ferreira, A.C.; Molinaro, A.; Ceccarelli, C.; Brozzi, F.; Pinchera, A.; Vitti, P. & Tonacchera, M. ((2011). Identification and functional analysis of novel dual oxidase 2 (DUOX2) mutations in children with congenital or subclinical hypothyroidism. *Journal of Clinical Endocrinology and Metabolism,* August 2011), 0002-1972X, 96(8), E1335-E1339.

[18] Demirbilek, H, Kandemir, N, Gonc, E. N, Ozon, A, Alikasifoglu, A, & Yordam, N. (2007). Hashimoto's thyroiditis in children and adolescents: a retrospective study on clinical, epidemiological and laboratory properties of the disease. *Journal of Pediatric Endocrinology and Metabolism,* November 2007), 0033-4018X, 20(11), 1199-1205.

[19] De Roux, N, Misrahi, M, Brouner, R, Houang, M, Carel, J. C, & Granier, M. Le Bouc, Y.; Ghinea, N.; Boumedienne, A.; Toublanc, J.E. & Milgrom, E. ((1996). Four families with loss of function mutations of the thyrotropin receptor. Journal of Clinical Endocrinology and Metabolism, December 1996), 0002-1972X, 81(12), 4229-4235.

[20] Després, N, & Grant, A. M. (1998). Antibody interference in thyroid assays: a potential for clinical misinformation. *Clinical Chemistry,* March 1998), 0009-9147, 44(3), 440-454.

[21] Devriendt, K, Vanhole, C, Matthijs, G, & De Zegher, F. (1998). Deletion of thyroid transcription factor-1 gene in an infant with neonatal thyroid dysfunction and respiratory failure. (Letter) *New England Journal of Medicine,* April 1998), 0028-4793, 338(18), 1317-1318.

[22] De Vries, L, Bulvik, S, & Phillip, M. (2009). Chronic autoimmune thyroiditis in children and adolescents: at presentation and during long-term follow-up. *Archives of Disease in Childhood,* January 2009), 0003-9888, 94(1), 33-37.

[23] Eliakim, A, Barzilai, M, Wolach, B, & Nemet, D. (2006). Should we treat elevated thyroid stimulating hormone levels in obese children and adolescents? *International Journal of Pediatric Obesity,* April 2006), 1747-7166, 1(4), 217-221.

[24] Elmlinger, M. W, Kühnel, W, Lambrecht, H. G, & Ranke, M. B. (2001). Reference intervals from birth to adulthood for serum thyroxine (T4), triiodothyronine (T3), free T3, free T4, thyroxine binding globulin (TBG) and thyrotropin (TSH). *Clinical Chemistry and Laboratory Medicine,* October 2001), 1437-4331, 39(10), 973-979.

[25] Fisher, D. A, & Klein, A. H. (1981). Thyroid development and disorders of thyroid function in the newborn. *New England Journal of Medicine,* March 1981), 0028-4793, 304(12), 702-712.

[26] Fisher, D. A, & Polk, D. H. (1989). Development of the thyroid. *Baillieres Clinical Endocrinology and Metabolism,* November 1989), 0095-0351X, 3(3), 627-657.

[27] Fu, J, Jiang, Y, Liang, L, & Zhu, H. (2005). Risk factors of primary thyroid dysfunction in early infants born to mothers with autoimmune thyroid disease. *Acta Paediatrica*, August 2005), 1651-2227, 94(8), 1043-1048.

[28] Gharib, H, Tuttle, R. M, Baskin, H. J, Fish, L. H, Singer, P. A, & Mcdermott, M. T. (2004). Subclinical thyroid dysfunction: a joint statement on management from the American Association of Clinical Endocrinologists, the American Thyroid Association, and the Endocrine Society. Endocrine Practice, November-December 2004), 0153-0891X, 10(6), 497-501.

[29] Gopalakrishnan, S, & Marwaha, R. K. (2007). Juvenile autoimmune thyroiditis. *Journal of Pediatric Endocrinology and Metabolism,* September 2007), 0033-4018X, 20(9), 961-970.

[30] Gopalakrishnan, S, Chugh, P. K, Chhillar, M, Ambardar, V. K, Sahoo, M, & Sankar, R. (2008). Goitrous autoimmune thyroiditis in a pediatric population: a longitudinal study. *Pediatrics,* September 2008), 0031-4005, 122(3), e670-e674.

[31] Grandone, A, Santoro, N, Coppola, F, Calabrò, P, & Perrone, L. Del Giudice, E.M. ((2010). Thyroid function derangement and childhood obesity: an Italian experience. *BMC Endocrine Disorders,* May 2010), 1472-6823, 10, 8.

[32] Grasberger, H, Vaxillaire, M, Pannain, S, Beck, J. C, Mimouni-bloch, A, Vatin, V, Vassart, G, Froguel, P, & Refetoff, S. (2005). Identification of a locus for nongoitrous congenital hypothyroidism on chromosome 15q25.3-26.1. *Human Genetics*, December 2005), 0340-6717, 118(3-4), 348-355.

[33] Grüters, A, & Krude, H. (2011). Detection and treatment of congenital hypothyroidism. *Nature Reviews Endocrinology*, October 2011), 1759-5029, 8(2), 104-113.

[34] Grüters, A, Allemand, l, Heidemann, D, & Schürnbrand, P. H. P. ((1983). Incidence of iodine contamination in neonatal transient hyperthyrotropinemia. *European Journal of Pediatrics,* September 1983), 0340-6199, 140(4), 299-300.

[35] Grüters, A, Delange, F, Giovannelli, G, Klett, M, Rochiccioli, P, Torresani, T, Grant, D, Hnikova, O, Maenpää, J, Rondanini, G. F, et al. (1993). Guidelines for neonatal screening programmes for congenital hypothyroidism. Working group on congenital hypothyroidism of the European Society for Paediatric Endocrinology. *European Journal of Pediatrics,* December 1993), 0340-6199, 152(12), 974-975.

[36] Grüters, A, Biebermann, H, & Krude, H. (2003). Neonatal thyroid disorders. *Hormone Research,* Suppl.1, (January 2003), 0301-0163, 59, 24-29.

[37] Halsall, D. J, Fahie-wilson, M. N, Hall, S. K, Barker, P, Anderson, J, Gama, R, & Chatterjee, V. K. (2006). Macro thyrotropin-IgG complex causes factitious increases in thyroid-stimulating hormone screening tests in a neonate and mother. *Clinical Chemistry,* 2006 October 2006), 0009-9147, 52(10), 1968-1969.

[38] Halsall, D. J, English, E, & Chatterjee, V. K. (2009). Interference from heterophilic antibodies in TSH assays. *Annals of Clinical Biochemistry,*July 2009), 0004-5632, 46(4), 345-346.

[39] Harris, K. B, & Pass, K. A. (2007). Increase in congenital hypothyroidism in New York State and in the United States. *Molecular Genetics and Metabolism,* July 2007), Erratum in: *Molecular Genetics and Metabolism,* Vol.94, No.1, (May 2008), p. 140, 1096-7192, 91(3), 268-277.

[40] Hoste, C, Rigutto, S, Van Vliet, G, Miot, F, & De Deken, X. (2010). Compound heterozygosity for a novel hemizygous missense mutation and a partial deletion affecting the catalytic core of the H_2O_2-generating enzyme DUOX2 associated with transient congenital hypothyroidism. *Human Mutation,*April 2010), 1098-1004, 31(4), E1304-E1319.

[41] Hollowell, J. G, Staehling, N. W, Flanders, W. D, Hannon, W. H, Gunter, E. W, Spencer, C. A, & Braverman, L. E. (2002). Serum TSH, T(4), and thyroid antibodies in the United States population (1988 to 1994): National Health and Nutrition Examination Survey (NHANES III). *Journal of Clinical Endocrinology and Metabolism,* February 2002), 0002-1972X, 87(2), 489-499.

[42] Huber, G, Staub, J. J, Meier, C, Mitrache, C, Guglielmetti, M, Huber, P, & Braverman, L. E. (2002). Prospective study of the spontaneous course of subclinical hypothyroidism: prognostic value of thyrotropin, thyroid reserve, and thyroid antibodies. *Journal of Clinical Endocrinology and Metabolism,* July 2002), 0002-1972X, 87(7), 3221-3226.

[43] Hübner, U, Englisch, C, Werkmann, H, Butz, H, Georgs, T, Zabransky, S, & Herrmann, W. (2002). Continuous age-dependent reference ranges for thyroid hormones in neonates, infants, children and adolescents established using the ADVIA Centaur Analyzer. *Clinical Chemistry and Laboratory Medicine,* October 2002), 1437-4331, 40(10), 1040-1047.

[44] Hume, R, Simpson, J, Delahunty, C, Van Toor, H, Wu, S. Y, Williams, F. L, & Visser, T. J. (2004). Scottish Preterm Thyroid Group. Human fetal and cord serum thyroid hormones: developmental trends and interrelationships. *Journal of Clinical Endocrinology and Metabolism,* August 2004), 0002-1972X, 89(8), 4097-4103.

[45] Hunter, I, & Greene, S. A. MacDonald, T.M. & Morris, A.D. (2000). Prevalence and aetiology of hypothyroidism in the young. Archives of Disease in Childhood, September 2000), 0003-9888, 83(3), 207-210.

[46] Ismail, A. A, Walker, P. L, Barth, J. H, Lewandowski, K. C, Jones, R, & Burr, W. A. (2002). Wrong biochemistry results: two case reports and observational study in 5310 patients on potentially misleading thyroid-stimulating hormone and gonadotropin immunoassay results. *Clinical Chemistry,* November 2002), 0009-9147, 48(11), 2023-2029.

[47] Jaruratanasirikul, S, Leethanaporn, K, Khuntigij, P, & Sriplung, H. (2001). The clinical course of Hashimoto's thryoiditis in children and adolescents: 6 years longitudinal

follow-up. *Journal of Pediatric Endocrinology and Metabolism,* February 2001), 0033-4018X, 14(2), 177-184.

[48] Jo, W, Ishizu, K, Fujieda, K, & Tajima, T. (2010). Congenital hypothyroidism caused by a PAX8 gene mutation manifested as sodium/iodide symporter gene defect. *Journal of Thyroid Research,* Article ID 619013, 2042-0072, 2010(2010)

[49] Kapelari, K, Kirchlechner, C, Högler, W, Schweitzer, K, Virgolini, I, & Moncayo, R. (2008). Pediatric reference intervals for thyroid hormone levels from birth to adulthood: a retrospective study. *BMC Endocrine Disorders,* November 2008), 1472-6823, 8, 15.

[50] Kaplan, I. V, & Levinson, S. S. (1999). When is a heterophile antibody not a heterophile antibody? When it is an antibody against a specific immunogen *Clinical Chemistry,* May 1999), 0009-9147, 45(5), 616-618.

[51] Klett, M, & Schönberg, D. (1981). Neonatal screening for hypothyroidism in the Federal Republic of Germany (author's transl)]. Deutsche Medizinische Wochenschrift, January 1981), 0012-0472, 106(1), 6-12.

[52] Koga, Y, Sano, H, Kikukawa, Y, Ishigouoka, T, & Kawamura, M. (1995). Effect on neonatal thyroid function of povidone-iodine used on mothers during perinatal period. Journal of Obstetrics and Gynaecology, December 1995), 1701-2163, 21(6), 581-585.

[53] Köhler, B, Schnabel, D, Biebermann, H, & Gruters, A. (1996). Transient congenital hypothyroidism and hyperthyrotropinemia: normal thyroid function and physical development at the ages of 6-14 years. *Journal of Clinical Endocrinology and Metabolism,* April 1996), 0002-1972X, 81(4), 1563-1567.

[54] Krude, H, Schutz, B, Biebermann, H, Von Moers, A, Schnabel, D, Neitzel, H, Tonnies, H, Weise, D, Lafferty, A, Schwarz, S, Defelice, M, Von Deimling, A, & Van Landeghem, F. DiLauro, R., Gruters, A. ((2002). Choreoathetosis, hypothyroidism, and pulmonary alterations due to human NKX2-1 haploinsufficiency. *Journal of Clinical Investigation,* February 2002), 0021-9738, 109(4), 475-480.

[55] Leonardi, D, Polizzotti, N, Carta, A, Gelsomino, R, Sava, L, Vigneri, R, & Calaciura, F. (2008). Longitudinal study of thyroid function in children with mild hyperthyrotropinemia at neonatal screening for congenital hypothyroidism. *Journal of Clinical Endocrinology and Metabolism,* July 2008), 0002-1972X, 93(7), 2679-2685.

[56] Liu, S. G, Zhang, S. S, Zhang, L. Q, Li, W. J, Zhang, A. Q, Lu, K. N, Wang, M. J, Yan, S. L, & Ma, X. (2012). Screening of PAX8 mutations in Chinese patients with congenital hypothyroidism. *Journal of Endocrinological Investigation,* (January 2012), [Epub ahead of print], 0391-4097, 0391-4097.

[57] Loh, T. P, Kao, S. L, Halsall, D. J, Toh, S. A, Chan, E, Ho, S. C, Tai, E. S, & Khoo, C. M. Macro-thyrotropin: a case report and review of literature. *Journal of Clinical Endocrinology and Metabolism,* June (2012). 0002-1972X, 97(6), 1823-1828.

[58] Mantovani, G. (2011). Clinical review: Pseudohypoparathyroidism: diagnosis and treatment. *Journal of Clinical Endocrinology and Metabolism,* October 2011), 0002-1972X, 96(10), 3020-3030.

[59] Mantovani, G, Ballare, E, Giammona, E, Beck-peccoz, P, & Spada, A. (2002). The gsalpha gene: predominant maternal origin of transcription in human thyroid gland and gonads. Journal of Clinical Endocrinology and Metabolism, October 2002), 0002-1972X, 87(10), 4736-4740.

[60] Marcocci, C, Vitti, P, Cetani, F, Catalano, F, Concetti, R, & Pinchera, A. (1991). Thyroid ultrasonography helps to identify patients with diffuse lymphocytic thyroiditis who are prone to develop hypothyroidism. *Journal of Clinical Endocrinolology & Metabolism,* January 1991), 0002-1972X, 72(1), 209-213.

[61] Maruo, Y, Takahashi, H, Soeda, I, Nishikura, N, Matsui, K, Ota, Y, Mimura, Y, Mori, A, Sato, H, & Takeuchi, Y. (2008). Transient congenital hypothyroidism caused by biallelic mutations of the dual oxidase 2 gene in Japanese patients detected by a neonatal screening program. *Journal of Clinical Endocrinology and Metabolism,* November 2008), 0002-1972X, 93(11), 4261-4267.

[62] Marwaha, R. K, Tandon, N, Kanwar, R, Ganie, M. A, Bhattacharya, V, Reddy, D. H, Gopalakrishnan, S, Aggarwal, R, Grewal, K, Ganguly, S. K, & Mani, K. (2008). Evaluation of the role of ultrasonography in diagnosis of autoimmune thyroiditis in goitrous children. *Indian Pediatrics,* April 2008), 0019-6061, 45(4), 279-284.

[63] Matsuura, N, & Konishi, J. (1990). Transient hypothyroidism in infants born to mothers with chronic thyroiditis-a nationwide study of twenty-three cases. The Transient Hypothyroidism Study Group. *Endocrinology Japan,* June 1990), Erratum in: *Endocrinology Japan,* Vol.37, No.5, (October 1990) p. 767, 0013-7219, 37(3), 369-379.

[64] Matsuura, N, Yamada, Y, Nohara, Y, Konishi, J, Kasagi, K, Endo, K, Kojima, H, & Wataya, K. (1980). Familial neonatal transient hypothyroidism due to maternal TSH-binding inhibitor immunoglobulins. *New England Journal of Medicine,* September 1980), 0028-4793, 303(13), 738-741.

[65] Mendoza, H, Connacher, A, & Srivastava, R. (2009). Unexplained high thyroid stimulating hormone: a "BIG" problem. *BMJ Case Reports,* pii: bcr01.2009.1474, Epub Apr 14 2009, 0175-7790X, 1757-790.

[66] Miki, K, Nose, O, Miyai, K, Yabuuchi, H, & Harada, T. (1989). Transient infantile hyperthyrotrophinaemia. *Archives of Disease in Childhood,* August 1989), 0003-9888, 64(8), 1177-1182.

[67] Moore, D. C. (1996). Natural course of'subclinical' hypothyroidism in childhood and adolescence. Archives of Pediatrics and Adolescent Medicine, March 1996), 1072-4710, 150(3), 293-297.

[68] Moreno, J. C, Bikker, H, Kempers, M. J, Van Trotsenburg, A. S, Baas, F, De Vijlder, J. J, Vulsma, T, & Ris-stalpers, C. (2002). Inactivating mutations in the gene for thyroid

oxidase 2 (THOX2) and congenital hypothyroidism. *New England Journal of Medicine,* July 2002), 0028-4793, 347(2), 95-102.

[69] Narumi, S, Yoshida, A, Muroya, K, Asakura, Y, Adachi, M, Fukuzawa, R, Kameyama, K, & Hasegawa, T. (2011). PAX8 mutation disturbing thyroid follicular growth: a case report. *Journal of Clinical Endocrinology and Metabolism,* December 2011), 0002-1972X, 96(12), E2039-E2044.

[70] Narumi, S, Araki, S, Hori, N, Muroya, K, Yamamoto, Y, Asakura, Y, Adachi, M, & Hasegawa, T. (2012). Functional characterization of four novel PAX8 mutations causing congenital hypothyroidism: new evidence for haploinsufficiency as a disease mechanism. *European Journal of Endocrinology,* (Aug 2012), [Epub ahead of print], 0804-4643, 0804-4643.

[71] Newman, J. D, Bergman, P. B, Doery, J. C, & Balazs, N. D. (2006). Factitious increase in thyrotropin in a neonate caused by a maternally transmitted interfering substance. *Clinical Chemistry,* March 2006), 0009-9147, 52(3), 541-542.

[72] Nishiyama, S, Mikeda, T, Okada, T, Nakamura, K, Kotani, T, & Hishinuma, A. (2004). Transient hypothyroidism or persistent hyperthyrotropinemia in neonates born to mothers with excessive iodine intake. *Thyroid,* December 2004), 1050-7256, 14(12), 1077-1083.

[73] Ogilvy-stuart, A. L. (2002). Neonatal thyroid disorders. *Archives of Disease in Childhood- Fetal and Neonatal Edition,* November 2002), 1359-2998, 87(3), F165-F171.

[74] Ohye, H, Fukata, S, Hishinuma, A, Kudo, T, Nishihara, E, Ito, M, Kubota, S, Amino, N, Ieiri, T, Kuma, K, & Miyauchi, A. (2008). A novel homozygous missense mutation of the dual oxidase 2 (DUOX2) gene in an adult patient with large goiter. *Thyroid,* May 2008), 1050-7256, 18(5), 561-566.

[75] Özen, S, Berk, Ö, Simsek, D. G, & Darcan, S. (2011). Clinical course of Hashimoto's thyroiditis and effects of levothyroxine therapy on the clinical course of the disease in children and adolescents. *Journal of Clinical Research in Pediatric Endocrinology,* April 2011), 1308-5727, 3(4), 192-197.

[76] Padberg, S, Heller, K, Usadel, K. H, & Schumm-draeger, P. M. (2001). One-year prophylactic treatment of euthyroid Hashimoto's thyroiditis patients with levothyroxine: is there a benefit? Thyroid, March 2001), *1050-7256,* 11(3), 249-255.

[77] Papendieck, P, Chiesa, A, Prieto, L, & Gruñeiro-papendieck, L. (2009). Thyroid disorders of neonates born to mothers with Graves' disease. *Journal of Pediatric Endocrinology and Metabolism,* June 2009), 0033-4018X, 22(6), 547-553.

[78] Park, S. M, & Chatterjee, V. K. (2005). Genetics of congenital hypothyroidism. *Journal of Medical Genetics,* May 2005), 0022-2593, 42(5), 379-389.

[79] Pedersen, O. M, Aardal, N. P, Larssen, T. B, Varhaug, J. E, Myking, O, & Vik-mo, H. (2000). The value of ultrasonography in predicting autoimmune thyroid disease. *Thyroid*, March 2000), 1050-7256, 10(3), 251-259.

[80] Pohlenz, J, Dumitrescu, A, Zundel, D, Martine, U, Schonberger, W, Koo, E, Weiss, R. E, Cohen, R. N, Kimura, S, & Refetoff, S. (2002). Partial deficiency of thyroid transcription factor 1 produces predominantly neurological defects in humans and mice. *Journal of Clinical Investigation*, No., (MONTH 2002), 0021-9738, 109, 469-473.

[81] Raber, W, Gessl, A, Nowotny, P, & Vierhapper, H. (2002). Thyroid ultrasound versus antithyroid peroxidase antibody determination: a cohort study of four hundred fifty-one subjects. *Thyroid*, August 2002), 1050-7256, 12(8), 725-731.

[82] Radetti, G, Gottardi, E, Bona, G, Corrias, A, Salardi, S, & Loche, S. Study Group for Thyroid Diseases of the Italian Society for Pediatric Endocrinology and Diabetes (SIEDP/ISPED)((2006). The natural history of euthyroid Hashimoto's thyroiditis in children. *Journal of Pediatrics*, December 2006), 0022-3476, 149(6), 827-832.

[83] Rago, T, Chiovato, L, Grasso, L, Pinchera, A, & Vitti, P. (2001). Thyroid ultrasonography as a tool for detecting thyroid autoimmune diseases and predicting thyroid dysfunction in apparently healthy subjects. Journal of Endocrinology Investigation, November 2001), 0391-4097, 24(10), 763-769.

[84] Rakover, Y, & Adar, H. (1989). Thyroid function disturbances in an infant following maternal topical use of polydine]. *Harefuah* May 1989), 0017-7768, 116(10), 527-529.

[85] Rakover, Y, Sadeh, O, Sobel, E, Shneyour, A, & Kraiem, Z. (1990). A case of transient hypothyroidism: sequential serum measurements of autoantibodies inhibiting thyrotropin-stimulated thyroid cAMP production in a neonate. *Acta Endocrinologica (Copenh)*, July 1990), 0001-5598, 123(1), 118-122.

[86] Rakover, Y, Weiner, E, Mosh, N, & Shalev, E. (1999). Fetal pituitary negative feedback at early gestational age. *Clinical Endocrinology*, June 1999), 0300-0664, 50(6), 809-814.

[87] Rallison, M. L, Dobyns, B. M, Meikle, A. W, Bishop, M, Lyon, J. L, & Stevens, W. (1991). Natural history of thyroid abnormalities: prevalence, incidence, and regression of thyroid diseases in adolescents and young adults. *The American Journal of Medicine*, October 1991), 0002-9343, 91(4), 363-370.

[88] Refetoff, S. (2003). Resistance to thyrotropin. *Journal of Endocrinological Investigation*, August 2003), 0391-4097, 26(8), 770-779.

[89] Reinehr, T. (2011). Thyroid function in the nutritionally obese child and adolescent. *Current Opinion in Pediatrics*, August 2011), 1040-8703, 23(4), 415-420.

[90] Reinehr, T, De Sousa, G, & Andler, W. (2006). Hyperthyrotropinemia in obese children is reversible after weight loss and is not related to lipids. *Journal of Clinical Endocrinology and Metabolism*, August 2006), 0002-1972X, 91(8), 3088-3091.

[91] Rix, M, Laurberg, P, Porzig, C, & Kristensen, S. R. (2011). Elevated thyroid-stimulating hormone level in a euthyroid neonate caused by macro thyrotropin-IgG complex. *Acta Paediatrica*, September 2011), 1651-2227, 100(9), e135-e137.

[92] Ross, H. A, Menheere, P. P. C. A, Thomas, C. M. G, Mudde, A. H, Kouwenberg, M, & Wolffenbuttel, B. H. R. (2008). Interference from heterophilic antibodies in seven current TSH assays. *Annals of Clinical Biochemistry*, November 2008), 0004-5632, 45(6), 616.

[93] Sakai, H, Fukuda, G, Suzuki, N, Watanabe, C, & Odawara, M. (2009). Falsely elevated thyroid-stimulating hormone (TSH) level due to macro-TSH. *Endocrine Journal*, April 2009), 0918-8959, 56(3), 435-440.

[94] Sakka, S. D, Malamitsi-puchner, A, Loutradis, D, Chrousos, G. P, & Kanaka-gantenbein, C. (2009). Euthyroid hyperthyrotropinemia in children born after in vitro fertilization. *Journal of Clinical Endocrinology and Metabolism,* April 2009), 0002-1972X, 94(4), 1338-1341.

[95] Samuels, M. H, Schuff, K. G, Carlson, N. E, Carello, P, & Janowsky, J. S. (2008). Health status, mood, and cognition in experimentally induced subclinical thyrotoxicosis. Journal of Clinical Endocrinology and Metabolism, May 2008), 0002-1972X, 93(5), 1730-1736.

[96] Sava, L, Delange, F, Belfiore, A, Purrello, F, & Vigneri, R. (1984). Transient impairment of thyroid function in newborn from an area of endemic goiter. *Journal of Clinical Endocrinology and Metabolism,* July 1984), 0002-1972X, 59(1), 90-95.

[97] Shalitin, S, Yackobovitch-gavan, M, & Phillip, M. (2009). Prevalence of thyroid dysfunction in obese children and adolescents before and after weight reduction and its relation to other metabolic parameters. Hormone Research, March 2009), 0301-0163, 71(3), 155-161.

[98] Skarpa, V, Kappaousta, E, Tertipi, A, Anyfandakis, K, Vakaki, M, Dolianiti, M, Fotinou, A, & Papathanasiou, A. (2011). Epidemiological characteristics of children with autoimmune thyroid disease. *Hormones (Athens),* July-September 2011), 1109-3099, 10(3), 207-214.

[99] Soldin, O. P, Jang, M, Guo, T, & Soldin, S. J. (2009). Pediatric reference intervals for free thyroxine and free triiodothyronine. *Thyroid,* July 2009), 1050-7256, 19(7), 699-702.

[100] Strich, D, Edri, S, & Gillis, D. (2012). Current normal values for TSH and FT3 in children are too low: evidence from over 11,000 samples. *Journal of Pediatric Endocrinology and Metabolism,* March 2012), 0033-4018X, 25(3-4), 245-248.

[101] Surks, M. I, Ortiz, E, Daniels, G. H, Sawin, C. T, Col, N. F, Cobin, R. H, Franklyn, J. A, Hershman, J. M, Burman, K. D, Denke, M. A, Gorman, C, Cooper, R. S, & Weissman, N. J. (2004). Subclinical thyroid disease: scientific review and guidelines for diagnosis

and management. Journal of the American Medical Association, January 2004), 0098-7484, 291(2), 228-238.

[102] Surks, M. I, Goswami, G, & Daniels, G. H. (2005). The thyrotropin reference range should remain unchanged. *Journal of Clinical Endocrinology and Metabolism,* September 2005), 0002-1972X, 90(9), 5489-5496.

[103] Svensson, J, Ericsson, U. B, Nilsson, P, Olsson, C, Jonsson, B, Lindberg, B, & Ivarsson, S. A. (2006). Levothyroxine treatment reduces thyroid size in children and adolescents with chronic autoimmune thyroiditis. *Journal of Clinical Endocrinology and Metabolism,* May 2006), 0002-1972X, 91(5), 1729-1734.

[104] Tenenbaum-rakover, Y. (2012). The clinical spectrum of thyrotropin receptor gene (tshr) mutations. In: *Hypothyroidism- Influences and Treatments,* D. Springer, (Ed.), InTech, 978-9-53510-021-8Available from: http://www.intechopen.com/articles/show/title/the-clinical-spectrum-of-tsh-receptor-tshr-mutations

[105] Tenenbaum-rakover, Y, Grasberger, H, Mamanasiri, S, Ringkananont, U, Montanelli, L, Barkoff, M. S, Dahood, A. M, & Refetoff, S. (2009). Loss-of-function mutations in the thyrotropin receptor gene as a major determinant of hyperthyrotropinemia in a consanguineous community. *Journal of Clinical Endocrinology and Metabolism,* May 2009), 0002-1972X, 94(5), 1706-1712.

[106] Thorpe-beeston, J. G, Nicolaides, K. H, Felton, C. V, Butler, J, & Mcgregor, A. M. (1991). Maturation of the secretion of thyroid hormone and thyroid-stimulating hormone in the fetus. *New England Journal of Medicine*, February 1991), 0028-4793, 324(8), 532-536.

[107] Vanderpump, M. P, & Tunbridge, W. M. (2002). Epidemiology and prevention of clinical and subclinical hypothyroidism. Thyroid, October 2002), 1050-7256, 12(10), 839-847.

[108] Vilain, C, Rydlewski, C, Duprez, L, Heinrichs, C, Abramowicz, M, Malvaux, P, Renneboog, B, Parma, J, Costagliola, S, & Vassart, G. (2001). Autosomal dominant transmission of congenital thyroid hypoplasia due to loss-of-function mutation of PAX8. *Journal of Clinical Endocrinology and Metabolism,* January 2001), 0002-1972X, 86(1), 234-238.

[109] Wada, K, Kazukawa, I, Someya, T, Watanabe, T, Minamitani, K, Minagawa, M, Wataki, K, Nishioka, T, & Yasuda, T. (2000). Maternal hypothyroidism in autoimmune thyroiditis and the prognosis of infants. *Endocrine Journal*, Suppl., (March 2000), 0918-8959, 47, S133-S135.

[110] Wartofsky, L, & Dickey, R. A. (2005). The evidence for a narrower thyrotropin reference range is compelling. *Journal of Clinical Endocrinology and Metabolism,* September 2005), 0002-1972X, 90(9), 5483-5488.

[111] Raber, W, Gessl, A, Nowotny, P, & Vierhapper, H. (2002). Thyroid ultrasound versus antithyroid peroxidase antibody determination: a cohort study of four hundred fifty-one subjects. *Thyroid,* Augost 2002), 1050-7256, 12(8), 725-531.

[112] Xie, J, Pannain, S, Pohlenz, J, Weiss, R. E, Moltz, K, Morlot, M, Asteria, C, Persani, L, Beck-peccoz, P, Parma, J, Vassart, G, & Refetoff, S. (1997). Resistance to thyrotropin (TSH) in three families is not associated with mutations in the TSH receptor or TSH. Journal of Clinical Endocrinology and Metabolism, December 1997), 0002-1972X, 82(12), 3933-3940.

[113] Zakarija, M, Mckenzie, J. M, & Eidson, M. S. (1990). Transient neonatal hypothyroidism: characterization of maternal antibodies to the thyrotropin receptor. *Journal of Clinical Endocrinology and Metabolism,* May 1990), 0002-1972X, 70(5), 1239-1246.

[114] Zung, A, Tenenbaum-rakover, Y, Barkan, S, Hanukoglu, A, Hershkovitz, E, Pinhas-hamiel, O, Bistritzer, T, & Zadik, Z. (2010). Neonatal hyperthyrotropinemia: population characteristics, diagnosis, management and outcome after cessation of therapy. Clinical Endocrinology, February 2010), 0300-0664, 72(2), 264-271.

[115] Zurakowski, D. Di Canzio, J. & Majzoub, JA. ((1999). Pediatric reference intervals for serum thyroxine, triiodothyronine, thyrotropin, and free thyroxine. *Clinical Chemistry,* July 1999), 0009-9147, 45(7), 1087-1091.

Section 3

Challenging Laboratory Findings

Chapter 7

Subclinical Hypothyroidism; Natural History, Long-Term Clinical Effects and Treatment

Jandee Lee and Woong Youn Chung

Additional information is available at the end of the chapter

http://dx.doi.org/10.5772/53688

1. Introduction

Subclinical hypothyroidism, defined as a mild degree of thyroid dysfunction biochemically, is a common clinical disease. It is marked by elevated serum concentrations of thyroid stimulating hormone (TSH) and normal serum concentrations of free thyroxine (fT4) and triiodothyronine (T3). Subclinical hypothyroidism can be divided into two categories, depending on the magnitude of the increase in serum TSH, with concentrations of 4.5-10 mU/L considered mild disease and TSH >10 mU/L considered severe disease. However, the definition and clinical significance of subclinical hypothyroidism are confounded by controversies over the exact upper limit of the reference range for se um TSH.

Subclinical hypothyroidism occurs in 4-20% of the adult population, a wide range that results from differences in age, gender, body-mass index, race, dietary iodine intake, and the cut-off concentrations of serum TSH used to define this condition. For example, most epidemiological surveys have reported that the prevalence of mild thyroid dysfunction was higher in older than in younger populations. In addition, overt or subclinical hypothyroidism occurs more frequently in areas of abundant iodine intake than in iodine-deficient areas, suggesting that iodine supplementation may increase the incidence of this disease. Subclinical hypothyroidism may be persistent or transient. In some of these patients, the transient expression of TSH-receptor blocking antibodies may indicate the recovery of thyroid function. Thus, it may be reasonable to reassess antibodies to thyroid hormones, including TSH-receptor blocking antibodies, in patients previously diagnosed with hypothyroidism to determine whether the latter is transient or permanent.

On average, 2-28% of patients with subclinical hypothyroidism progress to overt hypothyroidism, depending on age, gender, and the presence of anti-thyroid antibodies. However, baseline TSH concentration has been shown to be the most significant factor associated with progression to overt hypothyroidism. For example, a recent prospective study reported that the rate of overt hypothyroidism was about 10% in the entire study population, but was 2%, 20%, and 73% in patients with initial TSH concentrations of 5.0-9.9 mU/L, 10.0-14.9 mU/L, and 15.0-19.9 mU/L, respectively.

Subclinical hypothyroidism may be associated with depressed systolic function at rest and left ventricular diastolic dysfunction at rest and during exercise. Persistent subclinical hypothyroidism may also affect the vascular smooth muscle cells, increasing systemic vascular resistance and arterial stiffness. Studies on the risks of cardiovascular disease and mortality due to coronary heart disease in these patients, however, have yielded conflicting results. To date, the clinical significance of cardiovascular effects after long-term subclinical hypothyroidism has not been definitively clarified.

The relationship between subclinical hypothyroidism and lipid metabolism is also unclear. Subclinical hypothyroidism has been associated with variable increases in total cholesterol and LDL-cholesterol, higher plasma concentrations of oxidized LDL-cholesterol, and inconsistent changes in serum concentrations of HDL-cholesterol. These lipid patterns, however, may also be affected by age, gender, smoking status, the cause and duration of thyroid dysfunction, and serum TSH concentration. All of these findings have suggested that there are no definitive TSH cutoffs for association with lipids.

Subclinical hypothyroidism may also be associated with mood disorders such as major depression. Moreover, the life-time prevalence of major depressive disorder may be greater in individuals with than without subclinical hypothyroidism. These findings, however, do not suggest a direct causal link between subclinical hypothyroidism and mood disturbance. Studies of the relationships between cognitive function and thyroid hormone levels within the normal reference range have produced somewhat conflicting results. Some studies have reported that higher TSH is associated with poorer cognitive function, whereas others found that higher TSH is correlated with better cognitive performance. These studies indicate that variations in serum TSH concentrations in individuals having normal thyroid hormone concentrations (fT4, T3) may be related to cognitive impairment, especially in older individuals. Further investigations of the relationships between serum TSH concentrations and mood disturbance or cognitive function may be required.

In this chapter, we summarize the definition, causes, diagnosis, and treatment of subclinical hypothyroidism. We also discuss the clinical effects of this illness, including the effects of long-term subclinical hypothyroidism on the cardiovascular system, lipid metabolism, mood disorders and cognitive function.

2. Subclinical hypothyroidism

2.1. Definition

The term subclinical indicates the presence of a disease without obvious symptoms, suggesting that the disease may be at an early stage. Subclinical thyroid disease is based on the delicate sensitivity of the hypothalamic-pituitary-thyroid (HPT) axis. Subclinical hyperthyroid and hypothyroid conditions are laboratory-based diagnoses. By definition, subclinical hypothyroidism is characterized by abnormal serum TSH and normal fT4 and T3 concentrations.

In 2002, a scientific review and consensus committee, which included representatives from the American Thyroid Association (ATA), the American Association of Clinical Endocrinologists (AACE), and the US Endocrine Society, convened a panel of experts to define subclinical thyroid disease, review the literature concerning the risks and benefits of treatment, and make recommendations about evaluation and population-based screening (Surks et al, 2004). This committee defined subclinical hypothyroidism as "a serum TSH concentration above the statistically defined upper limit of the reference range when serum free T4 concentration is within its reference range". However, the definition and the clinical significance of subclinical hypothyroidism are confounded by controversies over the correct upper limit of the reference range for serum TSH. Meticulous studies from the United States and elsewhere have addressed this reference range, taking into account the influence of the inclusion or exclusion of subjects with a personal or family history of thyroid disease and patients positive for antithyroid antibodies. Because subclinical hypothyroidism is only detected as an abnormal TSH concentration, defining the TSH reference range is critical. Circulating TSH is heterogeneous in glycosylation and biological activity. Assays vary widely because current TSH immunometric assays involve the use of monoclonal antibodies that differ in specificity and may therefore bind to different TSH isoforms. Therefore, variations in the reference intervals obtained with different methods reflect differences in epitope recognition of different TSH isoforms. Since these differences make it difficult to establish a universal upper TSH reference limit, the use of thyroid antibody tests has resulted in a progressive decrease in the upper limit of the normal range over the last decades, from 10.0-7.0 mU/L to 4.0-5.0 mU/L (Biondi & Cooper, 2008).

Lymphocytic infiltration of the thyroid gland is present in up to 40% of healthy women. Moreover, competitive immunoassays have shown that 10% of the general population is positive for antithyroglobulin antibody (Tg Ab) and 12% are positive for detectable antithyroid peroxidase (TPO) antibody levels (Biondi et al, 2005). Furthermore, ultrasound characteristics can reveal the typical pattern of hypoechogenicity, heterogeneity, and increased blood flow seen in autoimmune thyroiditis. A hypoechoic or irregular echo ultrasound pattern may precede positivity for TPO Abs in patients with autoimmune thyroid disease, and TPO Abs may not be detected in more than 20% of individuals with ultrasound evidence of thyroid autoimmunity (Vejbjerg et al, 2006). A high thyroid autoantibody titer (usually against TPO Ab and/or Tg Ab, or more rarely, TSH receptor Ab) is frequently associated with a persistently elevated serum TSH concentration. Although the thyroid gland is usually goitrous, it may also be normal or atrophic, its hypoechogenicity at ultrasound evaluation could allow clinicians to identify individuals with subclinical hypothyroidism due to autoimmune disease (Biondi, 2012).

Therefore, it has been recommended that the reference serum TSH concentration be determined using blood sampled in the morning from fasting euthyroid subjects with no family history of thyroid disease, who are not taking any medication, have no visible or palpable goiter or pathological thyroid ultrasonography findings, and are not positive for TPO Ab or Tg Ab (Kratzsch et al, 2005). Evidence from the National Health and Nutritional Examination Survey (NHANES III) of a large 'reference' population without evidence of thyroid disease indicated that 95% of adults have serum TSH concentrations of 0.45-4.12 mU/L, indicating that the widely applied upper limit of normal for serum TSH of around 4.5 mU/L remains appropriate (Hollowell et al, 2001). A panel of experts has classified subjects with subclinical hypothyroidism into two categories, based on the degree of serum TSH elevation and pathophysiological consequences; these include patients with mild (4.5-10 mU/L) and more severely elevated (TSH>10 mU/L) serum TSH (Surks et al, 2004).

Subclinical hypothyroidism should be diagnosed only after a detailed personal and family history, pharmacological evaluation and an accurate clinical assessment. Some familial disorders, including a family history of autoimmune thyroid disease and/or endocrine or systemic autoimmune disorders, and genetic disorders such as Down, Turner and Klinefelter syndromes, should be investigated to identify subjects with an increased predisposition to developing autoimmune thyroiditis. In addition, a high thyroid autoantibody titer is frequently associated with a persistently elevated serum TSH concentration. The ultrasonographic hypoechogenicity of the thyroid gland can be used to identify individuals with subclinical hypothyroidism due to autoimmune disease (Wilson & Curry, 2005).

Prior to treatment, patients should be evaluated for transient and false causes of mild increases in TSH. Reference TSH ranges by age, race and body mass index can help avoid misclassifying patients with increased serum TSH (Biondi, 2012). Interestingly, serum TSH concentrations are higher in white than in black populations, suggesting that TSH is influenced by genetics and ethnicity/race. Moreover, increased serum TSH might not always reflect mild thyroid hormone deficiency in elderly subjects from iodine sufficient areas because the distribution of serum TSH shifts to higher concentrations with age. An increased serum TSH concentration in older individuals may reflect recovery from acute illness or the use of drugs that can interfere with thyroid function (Surks et al, 2004). Since serum TSH concentrations are higher in overweight and obese individuals than in lean subjects, subclinical hypothyroidism may be falsely diagnosed in overweight and obese patients, especially in those negative for thyroid autoantibodies. However, this altered thyroid hormone pattern can be reversed by losing weight (Biondi, 2010).

2.2. Causes

The most frequent causes of subclinical hypothyroidism are autoimmune thyroiditis and previous treatment for hyperthyroidism. In about 60-80% of patients, subclinical hypothyroidism has been associated with TPO Abs, a marker of chronic lymphocytic (Hashimoto's) thyroiditis. Hashimoto's thyroiditis is more common in females than in males, with the overall incidence increasing with age in both sexes. Transient or persistent increases in serum TSH may occur after subacute, post-partum or painless thyroiditis and after an infiltrative disease (Riedel's thyroiditis, amyloidosis, hemochromatosis and cystinosis) or infectious disorder of the thyroid gland. Patients treated for overt thyroid failure often have subclinical hypothyroidism because of inadequate thyroid hormone supplementation, poor adherence, drug interactions, or inadequate monitoring of treatment (Cooper & Biondi, 2012). Between 17.6% and 30% of patients with overt hypothyroidism were reported to have subclinical thyroid disease due to inadequate thyroid hormone supplementation (Canaris et al, 2000).

Subclinical hypothyroidism may also result from therapies that destroy thyroid tissue, such as thyroid surgery, radioiodine treatment or external radioiodine therapy. Mild, overt hypothyroidism frequently occurs after external radiotherapy of the head and neck area and develops gradually within the first year, with a risk that appears to be dose-dependent (Biondi & Cooper, 2008). Radioiodine treatment of hyperthyroidism in patients with Graves' disease results in hypothyroidism in at least 50% of patients, depending on the dose administered. Partial thyroidectomy for hyperthyroidism or nodular goiter has been associated with a similar risk for the development of hypothyroidism. Subclinical hypothyroidism soon after radioiodine treatment or partial thyroidectomy may be a transient phenomenon, not always indicative of progressive or permanent hypothyroidism. Even in the absence of ablative thyroid treatment, it has been estimated that 5-20% of patients with Graves' disease will eventually develop hypothyroidism (Boelaert et al, 2009).

Other causes of subclinical hypothyroidism include autoimmune diseases, such as type I diabetes mellitus and Addison's disease. Down and Turner syndromes have also been associated with the development of overt and subclinical hypothyroidism. The risk of subclinical hypothyroidism during pregnancy is considerable in women identified during the first trimester as being positive for antithyroid antibodies (Wilson & Curry, 2005). Non-thyroidal illness may be associated with a transient and modest increase in serum TSH, especially during the recovery phase, although in most of these patients an increase in TSH concentration reflects underlying thyroid disease. Several drugs, including iodine-containing compounds such as radiographic contrast agents, lithium carbonate, cytokines and interferon, may induce subclinical or overt hypothyroidism, particularly in patients with underlying autoimmune thyroiditis (Biondi, 2012).

It is necessary to distinguish subclinical hypothyroidism from other causes of physiological, artificial, or transiently increased serum TSH. Serum TSH concentrations should be measured 3-6 months later to rule out a laboratory error or a transient increase caused, for example, by drugs that interfere with thyroid function, by thyroiditis, and by possible toxic injury to the thyroid gland (Cooper & Biondi, 2012). Serum TSH concentrations are higher in healthy elderly than in healthy young people because of a shift in TSH distribution with age. Rarely, laboratory patterns indistinguishable from subclinical hypothyroidism are observed in patients with TSH-receptor mutations causing mild TSH resistance, mutations that can affect up to 0.6% of Caucasian people. Clues to the presence of this disorder are a family history of increased serum TSH concentrations and an absence of thyroid autoimmunity (Jordan et al, 2003). Serum TSH concentrations are higher in overweight and obese individuals, which may result in a false diagnosis of subclinical hypothyroidism. Mild increases in serum TSH concentration in obese people are usually associated with serum T3 concentrations at the upper limit of the normal range. The latter may be due to increased de-iodinase activity, which acts as a compensatory mechanism during fat accumulation to increase energy expenditure. This altered thyroid hormone pattern can be reversed by weight loss. Table 1 shows the comparison of causes between subclinical hypothyroidism and elevated serum TSH concentrations that are not associated with persistent subclinical hypothyroidism (Biondi & Cooper, 2008) (Cooper & Biondi, 2012).

Causes of subclinical hypothyroidism
1. Chronic autoimmune thyroiditis
: family history of autoimmune thyroid disease, history of associated autoimmune diseases, Down syndrome, Turner's syndrome, etc.
2. Thyroid injury
: partial thyroidectomy, external radiotherapy of head and neck, radioactive iodine therapy, etc.
3. Infiltrative disease of thyroid gland
: Riedel's thyroiditis, amyloidosis, sarcoidosis, hemochromatosis, cystinosis, AIDS, primary thyroid lymphoma
4. Persistent TSH increase after an episode of subacute thyroiditis, post-partum thyroiditis, painless thyroiditis
5. Drugs
: iodine, iodine-containing medications such as amiodarone, radiographic contrast agents, lithium carbonate, carbonate, cytokines (interferon alfa), aminoglutetimide, ethionamide, sulfonamides, sulfonylureas
6. Inadequate replacement theray for overt hypothyroidism
7. Toxic substances, industrial and environmental agents
8. TSH receptor gene mutations
Causes of elevated serum TSH concentrations that are not associated with persistent subclinical hypothyroidism
1. Laboratory analytic problems
: assay variability, abnormal TSH isoform, heterophilic antibodies, etc.
2. Elderly patients with small increases in serum TSH level
3. Obesity
4. Pituitary problem
: pituitary adenoma, isolated pituitary resistance to thyroid hormone, etc.
5. Renal dysfucntion
6. Adrenal insufficiency
7. After withdrawal of thyroid hormone therapy in euthyroid patients
8. Recovery phase of euthyroid sick syndrome

Table 1. Causes of elevated serum TSH concentration

2.3. Prevalence and natural history

The prevalence of subclinical hypothyroidism in adults has been reported to range from 4% to 20% (Cooper & Biondi, 2012). This wide range reflects important differences in race and dietary iodine intake, as well as patient age, gender, body mass index and differences in TSH evaluation methods. Large, population-based screening studies, including the Whickham Survey (Tunbridge et al, 1977), NHANES III (Hollowell et al, 2001), and the Colorado thyroid prevalence study (Canaris et al, 2000), have provided important epidemiological data about subclinical hypothyroidism. According to the Whickham Survey, which defines subclinical hypothyroidism as serum TSH concentrations >6 mU/L, this condition was present in 7.5% of females and 2.8% of males. TSH concentrations did not vary with age in males but increased markedly in females after age 45 years. Serum TSH concentration was not age-related in women negative for antithyroid antibodies. The NHANES III study, which defined subclinical hypothyroidism as serum TSH >4.6 mU/L, reported that 4.3% of individuals had subclinical hypothyroidism. TPO Abs were significantly associated with hypothyroidism, were more prevalent in women than in men, increased with age, and were more prevalent in whites than in blacks. The Colorado study, which defined subclinical hypothyroidism as serum TSH >5.1 mU/L, showed that serum TSH concentrations were elevated in 9.5% of subjects, and that the percentage increased with each decade of age in women but not in men. All of these surveys reported that the prevalence of subclinical hypothyroidism was higher in older populations. This disease is more common in iodine-sufficient than in iodine-deficient countries, suggesting that iodine supplementation may increase its incidence.

The natural history of subclinical hypothyroidism depends on the underlying cause and the characteristics of each patient. However, long-term outcome data on patients with subclinical hypothyroidism are rare, making it difficult to define the definitive course of this disease. Subclinical hypothyroidism may be progressive or reversible. With a progression rate of only 5% per year, it is reasonable to assume that, especially in patients with serum TSH concentrations ≤10 mU/L, subclinical hypothyroidism may not be caused by the progression of any specific disease state (Wilson & Curry, 2005). One large follow up study showed that, of patients with modestly elevated serum TSH concentrations, 60% show a spontaneous return to the reference range during a mean 5 year follow-up period (Meyerovitch et al, 2007). Moreover, many patients with non-autoimmune thyroiditis may develop transient TSH elevation.

In a significant number of patients, especially those who are older, female, and positive for TPO Abs, there is an increased risk of progression to overt hypothyroidism. The Whickham cohort survey, with a 20-year follow-up period, showed that the annual rate of progression from subclinical to overt hypothyroidism was 2.6% in patients negative for thyroid antibodies, but 4.3% if TPO Abs were present. Transient expression of TSH-receptor blocking antibodies may explain the improvements in thyroid function and the progressive TSH normalization that may be observed in some patients with autoimmune hypothyroidism. The annual rate of progression to overt disease was about 4% in women with increased serum TSH and positive for antithyroid antibodies, 2-4% in women with increased serum TSH concentrations alone, and 1-3% in women with only antithyroid antibodies. Serum TSH concentrations tend to return to normal more frequently in people with concentrations of 4-6 mU/L, whereas TSH concentrations of 10-15 mU/L are associated with a reduced rate of normalization of thyroid function. The annual rate of progression to overt hypothyroidism in patients with subclinical hypothyroidism induced by radioiodine or surgery is 2-6%. Pregnant women with Hashimoto thyroiditis also are at high risk of disease progression. High dose iodine intake is also associated with an increased risk of progression to overt hypothyroidism (Biondi & Cooper, 2008).

The risk of progression from subclinical to overt hypothyroidism is less common, whereas the recovery of thyroid function is more common, in children and adolescents than in adults. Progression from mild to overt hypothyroidism may be related to the cause of thyroid hormone deficiency, the basal TSH concentration, and the age of the patient. Transient expression of TSH-receptor blocking antibodies may explain the recovery of thyroid function in some patients (Biondi & Cooper, 2008). Patients previously diagnosed with subclinical hypothyroidism should be reevaluated to determine whether this condition is persistent. This may be accomplished by progressive reduction in LT4 dosage followed by serial TSH testing.

2.4. Consequences of subclinical hypothyroidism

Subclinical hypothyroidism may be associated with adverse cardiovascular events, cardiac dysfunction, lipid metabolism, and neuropsychiatric symptoms. To date, however, there is insufficient evidence regarding the association between long-term subclinical hypothyroidism and systemic sequelae.

2.4.1. The cardiovascular system and the risk of heart failure

Cardiovascular diseases are the most common causes of death worldwide, primarily affecting older adults. Abnormal TSH concentrations may be a novel cardiac risk factor. Even mildly altered thyroid status has been reported to affect serum cholesterol concentrations, heart rhythm and rate, ventricular function, risk of coronary artery disease, and cardiovascular mortality. Patients with subclinical hypothyroidism may have depressed systolic function at rest, and left ventricular diastolic dysfunction at rest and during exercise. Vascular function may also be impaired by thyroid hormone deficiency. However, the risks of cardiovascular and heart failure in patients with subclinical hypothyroidism remain unclear. Several large scale meta-analyses have assessed the risks of cardiovascular and all-cause mortality in patients with subclinical hypothyroidism. In one meta-analysis, cardiovascular mortality was higher in patients <65 years old with subclinical hypothyroidism, but not in older people (Razvi et al, 2008). A second meta-analysis confirmed that subclinical hypothyroidism was associated with modestly increased cardiovascular risks of coronary heart disease and total mortality (Ochs et al, 2008). In addition, reanalysis of the data from the Whickham Survey cohort showed that systolic and diastolic blood pressures and total cholesterol concentrations were higher in patients with subclinical hypothyroidism than in controls in a euthyroid state (Razvi et al, 2010). However, a large prospective cohort study of 559 subjects aged 85 year, including subclinical hypothyroidism was present in 30 patients and 21 individuals monitored for 4 years, provided opposite evidences. This study found that raised serum TSH concentrations was associated with decreased mortality in individuals older than 85 years, and this might be attributed to a lower metabolic rate. In this study, individuals with subclinial hypothyroidism had lower all-causes and cardiovascular mortality than clinically euthyroid individuals, although serum cholesterol levels were higher

(Gussekloo et al, 2004). Similarly, other studies reported that subclinical hypothyroidism was not associated with increased overall mortality risk in elderly subjects. Crucially, a meta-analysis of individual participant data from 11 prospective cohort studies has shown no overall association of subclinical hypothyroidism with coronary heart disease events, mortality or total mortality (Rodondi et al, 2010). However, significant associations were observed when the degree of serum TSH elevation was stratified, in that coronary heart disease events and mortality risks were significantly increased in individuals with serum TSH >10 mU/L. This correlation with greater biochemical abnormality was consistent with studies in patients with heart failure, in that incident heart failure risk was evident, or of greater magnitude, when serum TSH was > 10 mU/L. By contrast with studies suggesting that the risk of coronary heart disease decreased with patient age, findings of this meta-analysis showed no interaction between mortality due to coronary heart disease and age.

In summary, several prospective, population-based cohort studies found that subclinical hypothyroidism was associated with increased risks of cardiovascular disease and mortality, whereas other, similar studies showed no correlation between subclinical hypothyroidism and the incidence of and mortality due to coronary heart disease.

2.4.2. *Lipid profiles*

Thyroid hormones have varied effects on lipid metabolism, because thyroid function regulates cholesterol synthesis and degradation and mediates the activity of key enzymes in these pathways. Thyroid hormones reduce cholesterol concentration mainly through the increased expression of low-density lipoprotein (LDL)-cholesterol receptors in the liver and peripheral organs (Duntas & Brenta, 2012). Overt hypothyroidism increases the serum concentrations of total and LDL-cholesterol, as well as altering the concentrations of other lipoproteins and apolipoproteins. In contrast, lipid changes in individuals with subclinical hypothyroidism are considerably less marked, with studies showing inconsistent results. For example, studies comparing lipid profiles in subclinical hypothyroid patients and euthyroid controls have found that subclinical hypothyroidism was associated with lipid abnormalities, especially increases in total and LDL cholesterol, but its effects on the concentrations of high-density lipoprotein (HDL)-cholesterol, triglycerides and lipoprotein(a) were unclear (Cappola & Ladenson, 2003) (Duntas & Wartofsky, 2007).

The United States Colorado study, with a population sample of 25,862 subjects, showed that patients with subclinical hypothyroidism had higher total cholesterol concentrations than euthyroid individuals (Canaris et al, 2000). In the NHANES III cohort, cholesterol and triglyceride concentrations were higher in patients with subclinical hypothyroidism than in euthyroid subjects, but these effects were no longer observed after adjusting for variables such as sex, race, age, and treatment with lipid lowering drugs (Hollowell et al, 2001). In contrast, recent studies that distributed patients into groups based on the severity of dyslipidemia found that the incidence of subclinical hypothyroidism was highest in the group with the highest serum cholesterol concentrations (Bindels et al, 1999). Lipid patterns were particularly altered in patients with subclinical hypothyroidism and a serum TSH concentration >10 mU/L, especially in older patients. The discrepancy between these study results may be due to the heterogeneity of the populations studied, including differences in TSH concentrations used to define subclinical hypothyroidism and selection criteria based on age, sex, race, smoking history, and insulin resistance. Although hyperinsulinemia may increase the hepatic output of very low-density lipoprotein (VLDL) particles, hypothyroidism may suppress their removal, resulting in a net accumulation of modified lipoproteins. Moreover, LDL particles in subjects with subclinical hypothyroidism have an impaired composition, becoming triglyceride-rich lipoproteins (Duntas & Brenta, 2012). VLDL remnants and intermediate-density lipoproteins (IDL) tend to accumulate in the circulation. However, the fractional clearance rates of triglycerides and cholesteryl esters have been reported equal in patients with subclinical hypothyroidism and controls, indicating that lipolysis and the removal of remnant triglyceride rich lipoproteins were normal. Nevertheless, transfer of triglycerides to HDL was lower in subjects with subclinical hypothyroidism than in controls.

In summary, the association between lipid patterns and subclinical hypothyroidism remains unclear. This may reflect differences in population-based studies, as well as differences in age, gender, and ethnicity of the subjects examined. Taken together, these findings have resulted in the formulation of a hypothesis, that there is no TSH cutoff threshold associated with lipids. However, smoking and insulin resistance may play important roles in mediating the effects of subclinical hypothyroidism on serum lipids.

2.4.3. *Mood and cognitive changes*

The relationships between overt thyroid disease and mood impairment and cognitive dysfunction have been described. Overt hypothyroidism is a frequent cause of major depressive disorder, including melancholia, and may lead to reversible dementia. Several relatively small-volume studies found more hypothyroid associated signs and symptoms of mood disorders in individuals with subclinical hyperthyroidism than in euthyroid individuals. Subclinical hypothyroidism may be associated with current depressive symptoms, current major depression and a lifetime history of major depression (Joffe et al, 2012) (Chueire et al, 2007). These studies have reported a higher frequency and/or severity of current depressive symptoms in young or middle-aged adults with subclinical hypothyroidism than in matched euthyroid controls. Moreover, the lifetime prevalence of major depressive disorder has been reported higher in individuals with subclinical hypothyroidism than in euthyroid subjects. These findings suggest an association, but not necessarily a direct causal relationship, between subclinical hypothyroidism and mood disturbance or disorders. Recent studies, however, have suggested that patients with primary major depressive illness have a reduced rate of response to antidepressants and are at greater risk of chronicity of depression if they have comorbid subclinical hypothyroidism.

Although many studies have assessed the relationship between mild hypothyroidism and cognitive dysfunction, these studies have produced somewhat conflicting findings. A recent cross-sectional study of 5865 patients in England aged ≥65 years with no known thyroid disease (168 with subclinical hypothyroidism defined by TSH >5.5 mIU/L) was performed in primary care practices to evaluate the association with mood and cognitive changes. This study found no associations between mild hypothyroidism and cognitive function, depres-

http://dx.doi.org/10.5772/53688

sion, and anxiety (Roberts et al, 2006). In contrast, evaluation of brain function by functional magnetic resonance imaging (MRI) in patients with overt and subclinical hypothyroidism and euthyroid subjects suggested that working memory, but not other memory functions, was impaired by subclinical hypothyroidism, with impairment more severe in patients with overt hypothyroidism (Zhu et al, 2006). Whereas some studies included only older subjects, other studies include broad ranges of age groups, limiting the conclusions that can be drawn from these data. Perhaps, the most problematic methodological issue in these studies is their reliance on limited measures of cognitive function, especially the Mini Mental State Examination, which provides a very limited assessment of cognition and is likely relatively insensitive to potentially subtle, although clinically meaningful, neuropsychological impairments. This may explain the discrepancy among studies, with some finding and others not finding an association between cognitive alterations and subclinical hypothyroidism (Joffe et al, 2012). Nonetheless, these studies have shown that younger adults with subclinical hypothyroidism may experience mild cognitive abnormalities, generally difficulties with selective attention and new learning. Studies in older adults have found that subclinical hypothyroidism may be associated with deficits in attention, in some aspects of executive functioning, verbal and visual recall, and in reaction time, but these deficits may differ in older and younger individuals, and in men women (Samuels et al, 2008).

The relationship between subclinical hypothyroidism and vulnerability to dementia, especially Alzheimer's disease, has been evaluated in older adults. Although high TSH concentrations were associated with an increased risk of developing Alzheimer's disease or dementia, the association between subclinical hypothyroidism and dementia is unclear. Moreover, the brains of older adults may show differential sensitivity, manifesting as cognitive changes, to small perturbations of the thyroid axis.

In summary, the pattern and severity of mood and cognitive symptoms in patients with subclinical hypothyroidism have not been fully delineated, although both depressive symptoms and depressive syndromes may occur with increased frequency. It is difficult to distinguish euthyroid subjects from patients with subclinical hypothyroidism based on these symptoms. Subclinical hypothyroidism may also be associated with current cognitive impairment and the further risk of cognitive decline. In addition, these symptoms are probably related to disease severity, disease duration, and individual sensitivity to thyroid hormone deficiency. Age may also affect the correlations between subclinical hypothyroidism and mood, cognition, and Alzheimer's disease. Larger randomized controlled studies are necessary to assess the importance of mood and cognitive function in both younger and older age groups, especially in individuals with minimally elevated TSH.

2.5. Treatment

There has been much discussion about the screening and treatment of patients with subclinical hypothyroidism. Because of the difficulties in interpreting data from many different sources, the AACE, the US Endocrine Society and the ATA convened a panel in 2002 to formulate evidence-based guidelines for the diagnosis, screening, and treatment of subclinical hypothyroidism (Surks et al, 2004). The consensus panel recommended that patients with elevated serum TSH undergo repeat testing, along with a serum fT4 measurement, from 2 weeks to 3 months later. If these tests confirm subclinical hypothyroidism, further evaluation is required, including clinical assessment of signs and symptoms; history taking to determine if the patient had been previously treated for hyperthyroidism (e.g., with radioiodine therapy or partial thyroidectomy), or if there is a family history of thyroid disease; and determination of the occurrence of thyroid enlargement. These patients should also be screened for hyperlipidemia. Although the presence of TPO Ab increases the risk of progression to overt hypothyroidism, the panel found insufficient evidence to recommend for or against obtaining titers because determining the presence of antibodies does not change patient management.

The panel found good evidence that subclinical hypothyroidism is associated with progression to overt hypothyroidism, and fair evidence that serum TSH concentrations >10 mU/L are associated with elevated total and LDL cholesterol concentrations. The panel recommended that patients with serum TSH concentrations >10 mU/L be treated with levothyroxine sodium (LT4). There is no conclusive evidence that treatment will improve symptoms or associated clinical conditions such as hyperlipidemia; however, because 2-10% of patients progress to overt hypothyroidism, treatment may prevent symptom development in patients with low fT4 concentrations. Most other guidelines and expert views also recommend treatment of subclinical hypothyroid patients with TSH concentrations >10 mU/L (Biondi & Cooper, 2008) (Gharib et al, 2005) (Khandelwal & Tandon, 2012) (Vaidya & Pearce, 2008).

Treatment of asymptomatic patients with serum TSH concentrations between 4.5 and 10 mU/L remains unclear. The panel recommended that only pregnant women and women contemplating pregnancy be treated for subclinical hypothyroidism and TSH concentrations ≤10 mU/L, based on a possible association between high TSH and subsequent neuropsychological complications in offspring. According to recent ATA guidelines, if a woman is hypothyroid prior to pregnancy, it recommended that her dosage be adjusted so that TSH is below 2.5 mU/L prior to conception (Stagnaro-Green et al, 2011). This lowers the risk of the TSH elevating in the first trimester. If a woman is diagnosed as hypothyroid during pregnancy, she should be treated without delay, with the goal of restoring her thyroid levels to normal as quickly as possible. In pregnancy, overt hypothyroidism is defined as a TSH above 2.5 mU/L, along with a decreased fT4 level. Even if a woman has normal fT4, if TSH is above 10.0 mU/L during pregnancy, it is also considered to be overt hypothyroidism. Subclinical hypothyroidism is defined as TSH between 2.5 and 10 mU/L, with a normal fT4 level. During the first trimester, the TSH level should be maintained at a level of between 0.1 and 2.5 mIU/L, 0.2 to 3.0 mIU/L during the second trimester, and 0.3 to 3.0 mIU/L in the third trimester. By the time a woman is four to six weeks pregnant, her dose of thyroid medication will usually need to be increased, potentially by as much as 50 percent. A woman with thyroid autoimmunity with positive thyroid antibodies who has normal TSH levels in the early stages of her pregnancy is still at increased risk of becoming hypothyroid at any point in the pregnancy. She should be monitored regularly through the pregnancy for elevated TSH (Stagnaro-Green et al, 2011).

The panel recommended against routine treatment of patients with subclinical hypothyroidism and serum TSH ≤10 mU/L, as available data do not support a clear-cut benefit for early treatment of these patients. However, in a separate consensus statement, these societies recommended that most subclinical hypothyroid patients be considered for treatment, with the key determinant being the clinical judgment of the provider (Gharib et al, 2005). Recently some experts further consolidated the available evidence and recommended LT4 therapy in women who are pregnant, planning pregnancy, have ovulatory dysfunction, or are infertile; as well as in patients with symptoms, goiter, anti-TPO antibodies, and high background cardiovascular risk, including those with hypertension, hypercholesterolemia, insulin resistance or diabetes, isolated diastolic dysfunction, or evidence of impaired endothelial function (Biondi & Cooper, 2008) (Khandelwal & Tandon, 2012). Current evidence suggests that middle-aged individuals are more likely to benefit from treatment than elderly individuals. Asymptomatic individuals should undergo repeat thyroid function tests every 6 to 12 months. There is also insufficient evidence to support therapeutic intervention in patients with symptoms of hypothyroidism and serum TSH concentrations between 4.5 and 10 mU/L. The panel suggested, however, that these patients be started on LT4, with treatment continued only in those experiencing symptomatic benefit (Woeber, 2005).

Thyroid hormone preparations available for treatment of hypothyroidism include levothyroxine sodium (L-thyroxine; LT4) and liothyronine sodium (L-triiodothyronine; LT3). LT4 is synthetically produced but identical to T4 secreted by the thyroid. LT4 is the preferred drug because its administration closely mimics glandular secretion and its conversion to T3 is appropriately regulated by tissues, which maintain a steady and adequate supply. Its long half-life of 7 days allows single daily dose administration and results in only small fluctuations in serum concentrations between daily doses (Khandelwal & Tandon, 2012) (Woeber, 2005). Serum T4 concentrations peak 2-4 hours after an oral dose and remain above normal for approximately 6 hours in patients receiving daily replacement therapy. LT4 is also recognized to have a narrow toxic to therapeutic ratio, with excess amounts having significant clinical consequences. Adverse effects of over-replacement include the risk of bone loss, especially in postmenopausal women, and increased risk of atrial fibrillation. Transient scalp hair loss can also take place during the first few weeks of LT4 treatment. Allergic reactions have been rarely reported, but these were almost always reactions to dye or other inactive constituents. LT3 is a synthetic form of natural T3 hormone with the same actions as the natural product. It has a half-life of 1 day, thus requiring multiple doses daily. Another disadvantage of LT3 is the increase in serum T3 concentration to supranormal values, up to 250-600%, in the absorption phase, during which many patients report adverse effects, especially palpitations (Wiersinga, 2001) (Woeber, 2005). Treatment with LT3 should therefore be considered only in patients with LT4 maldigestion or malabsorption, as well as in patients who cannot convert T4 to T3 (Celi et al, 2011). Otherwise, it is not intended as sole maintenance therapy in patients with hypothyroidism. Combined treatment with LT4 and LT3 has been attempted to more closely mimic the thyroid secretion patterns of T4 and T3. However, there is no currently available preparation containing both LT4 and LT3 in combination that adequately reproduces the relative quantities of these hormones produced by the human thyroid gland. Furthermore, no preparation results in a pattern of sustained release of thyroid hormones similar to that of the human thyroid (Woeber, 2005).

The goal of treatment is to restore the individual to a euthyroid state, with resolution of signs and symptoms of hypothyroidism. Chronic under- or over- replacement is common in clinical practice, with over-treatment occurring in about 20% of LT4-treated patients (Canaris et al, 2000) (Parle et al, 1993). The rapidity with which the euthyroid state should be attained is dictated by several factors, notably the age of the patient, the duration and severity of hypothyroidism and the presence of other co-morbid conditions, specifically cardiac disease. It has been recommended that LT4 be taken as a single daily dose on an empty stomach at least 30 minutes before breakfast. Individual LT4 requirements are greatly dependent on an individual's lean body mass, rather than on total body weight. Patients with subclinical hypothyroidism and minimal thyroid hormone deficiency may be controlled with daily LT4 dosages as low as 25-50 μg. After initiation of thyroid hormone therapy, the symptoms and signs of hypothyroidism should be assessed at each follow-up visit. The earliest clinical response to LT4 replacement is usually diuresis and weight loss, leading to mobilization of interstitial fluid as glycosaminoglycans are degraded. Weight loss is predominantly due to fluid loss, and is unlikely to exceed 5 kg, even in obese patients, especially if pre-treatment TSH concentrations were only modestly elevated. Two months after initiating therapy, the minimum time required for the pituitary-thyroid axis to re-set, the dose should be monitored by measuring serum TSH, with or without serum T4. Serum TSH should be maintained in the lower half of the normal range (0.5-2.0 mU/L) (McDermott, 2009).

An important cause of persistently elevated TSH despite an adequate replacement dose of LT4 is patient non-compliance. These patients may have elevated TSH with high normal or elevated fT4, as they may not take LT4 for days and then take several pills a few days before testing. These patients do not require changes in LT4 dose; rather, emphasis should be placed on compliance with therapy and thyroid function tests should be repeated in 3-4 weeks. Other causes of persistently elevated TSH despite an apparently adequate dose of LT4 include malabsorption and interference by drugs. Coeliac disease should be excluded, as it may be present in patients with hypothyroidism because of its autoimmune nature. The presence of heterophilic antibodies in a patient's serum can also result in an artificial elevation of TSH (Khandelwal & Tandon, 2012).

3. Conclusion

Subclinical hypothyroidism is a frequent clinical problem, readily diagnosed by laboratory methods. Since most patients with this condition are asymptomatic, screening is required to detect the condition in most cases. As there is insufficient evidence to support population-based data, the associations between subclinical hypothyroidism and adverse clinical outcomes remain unclear. Subclinical hypothyroidism was recently reported to be associated with increased risks of cardiovascular disease and heart failure. Subclinical hypothyroidism may or may not be correlated with other systemic conditions, such as changes in lipid metabolism, mood and cognition, with the clinical significance of these systemic effects after long-term subclinical hypothyroidism being unclear. Findings suggest that these systemic sequelae of subclinical hypothyroidism are associated with increased disease severity, disease duration, age, and individual sensitivity to thyroid hormone deficiency.

The benefits of treatment of subclinical hypothyroidism remain unclear, despite the potential risk of progression to overt disease, and there is no definite consensus on thyroid hormone and TSH cutoff values at which treatment should be contemplated. It has been recommended that all patients with subclinical hypothyroidism with TSH >10 mU/L or showing symptoms be treated, as should all pregnant women with any degree of subclinical hypothyroidism. The benefits of treatment of asymptomatic patients with subclinical hypothyroidism and serum TSH ≤ 10 mU/L remain unclear. Most expert groups have recommended LT4 therapy for patients with a mild degree of subclinical hypothyroidism (TSH ≤ 10 mU/L) only if they have symptoms, goiter, anti-TPO antibodies or infertility. Adequacy of treatment is monitored by measuring serum TSH and fT4 concentrations. Special considerations are needed in pregnant women, children, elderly patients and patients with cardiac disease. Under- and over- treatment are common in clinical practice and should be avoided.

Acknowledgment

All authors including Drs. Lee, and Chung have no conflicts of interest or financial ties to disclose.

Author details

Jandee Lee[1] and Woong Youn Chung[2]

1 Department of Surgery, Eulji University College of Medicine, Seoul, South Korea

2 Department of Surgery, Yonsei Univeristy College of Medicine, Seoul, South Korea

References

[1] Bindels, A., Westendorp, R. G., & Frölich, M. (1999). The prevalence of subclinical hypothyroidism at different total plasma cholesterol levels in middle aged men and women: a need for case-finding? Clin Endocrinol (Oxf), , 50(2), 217-220.

[2] Biondi, B. (2010). Thyroid and obesity: an intriguing relationship. J Clin Endocrinol Metab , 95(8), 3614-3617.

[3] Biondi, B. (2012). Natural history, diagnosis and management of subclinical thyroid dysfunction. Best Pract Res Clin Endocrinol Metab, , 26(4), 431-446.

[4] Biondi, B., & Cooper, . (2008). The clinical significance of subclinical thyroid dysfunction. Endocr Rev, , 29(1), 76-131.

[5] Biondi, B., Palmieri, E. A., & Klain, M. (2005). Subclinical hyperthyroidism: clinical features and treatment options. Eur J Endocrinol, , 152(1), 1-9.

[6] Boelaert, K., Syed, , & Manji, N. (2009). Prediction of cure and risk of hypothyroidism in patients receiving 131I for hyperthyroidism. Clin Endocrinol (Oxf), , 70(1), 129-138.

[7] Canaris, G. J., Manowitz, N. R., & Mayor, G. (2000). The Colorado thyroid disease prevalence study. Arch Intern Med, , 160(4), 526-534.

[8] Cappola, A. R., & Ladenson, P. W. (2003). Hypothyroidism and atherosclerosis. J Clin Endocrinol Metab, , 88(6), 2438-2444.

[9] Celi, F. S., Zemskova, M., & Linderman, . (2011). Metabolic effects of liothyronine therapy in hypothyroidism: a randomized, double-blind, crossover trial of liothyronine versus levothyroxine. J Clin Endocrinol Metab, , 96(11), 3466-3474.

[10] Chueire, V. B., Romaldini, J. H., & Ward, L. S. (2007). Subclinical hypothyroidism increase the risk for depression in the elderly. Arch Gerontol Geriatr, , 44(1), 21-28.

[11] Cooper, D., & Biondi, B. (2012). Subclinical thyroid disease. Lancet, 379 9821. , 1142-1154.

[12] Duntas, L. H., & Brenta, G. (2012). The effect of thyroid disorders on lipid levels and metabolism. Med Clin North Am, , 96(2), 269-281.

[13] Duntas, L. H., & Wartofsky, L. (2007). Cardiovascular risk and subclinical hypothyroidism: focus on lipids and new emerging risk factors. What is the evidence? *DuntasL. H.WartofskyL. (2007) Cardiovascular risk and subclinical hypothyroidism: focus on lipids and new emerging risk factors. What is the evidence? Thyroid, Vol.17, No.11, pp. 1075-1084*, 17(11), 1075-1084.

[14] Gharib, H., Tuttle, R. M., & Baskin, H. J. (2005). Subclinical thyroid dysfunction: a joint statement on management from the American Association of Clinical Endocrinologists, the American Thyroid Association, and the Endocrine Society. J Clin Endocrinol Metab, , 90(1), 581-587.

[15] Gussekloo, J., van Exel, E., & de Craen, A. J. (2004). Thyroid status, disability and cognitive function, and survival in old age. JAMA, , 292(21), 2591-2599.

[16] Hollowell, J. G., Staehling, N. W., & Flanders, W. D. (2001). Serum TSH, T(4), and thyroid antibodies in the United States population (1988 to 1944): National Health and Nutrition Examination Survey (NHANES III). J Clin Endocrinol Metab, , 87(2), 489-499.

[17] Joffe, R. T., Pearce, E. N., & Hennessey, J. V. (2012). Subclinical hypo*thyroid*ism, mood and cognition in older adults: a review. Int J Geriatr. Psychiatry, Epub ahead of print. DOIgps.3796

[18] Jordan, N., Williams, N., & Gregory, J. W. (2003). The W546X mutation of the thyrotropin receptor gene: potential major contributor to thyroid dysfunction in a Caucasian population. J Clin Endocrinol Metab, , 88(3), 1002-1005.

[19] Khandelwal, D., & Tandon, N. (2012). Overt and subclinical hypothyroidism: who to treat and how. *Drugs*, 72(1), 17-33.

[20] Kratzsch, J., Fiedler, G. M., & Leichtle, A. (2005). New reference intervals for thyrotropin and thyroid hormones based on National Academy of Clinical Biochemistry criteria and regular ultrasonography of the thyroid. Clin Chem, , 51(8), 1480-1486.

[21] Mc Dermott, M. T. (2009). In the clinic. Hypothyroidism. Ann Intern Med, pp.ITC 61, 151(11)

[22] Meyerovitch, J., Rotman-Pikielny, P., & Sherf, M. (2007). Serum thyrotropin measurements in the community: five-year follow-up in a large network of primary care physicians. Arch Intern Med, , 167(14), 1533-1538.

[23] Ochs, N., Auer, R., & Bauer, D. C. (2008). Meta-analysis: subclinical thyroid dysfunction and the risk for coronary heart disease and mortality. Ann Intern Med, , 148(11), 832-845.

[24] Parle, J. V., Franklyn, J. A., & Cross, K. W. (1993). Thyroxine prescription in the community: serum thyroid stimulating hormone level assays as an indicator of undertreatment or overtreatment. Br J Gen Pract, , 43(368), 107-109.

[25] Razvi, S., Shakoor, A., & Vanderpump, M. (2008). The influence of age on the relationship between subclinical hypothyroidism and ischemic heart disease: a metaanalysis. J Clin Endocrinol Metab, , 93(8), 2998-3007.

[26] Razvi, S., Weaver, J. U., & Vanderpump, M. P. (2010). The incidence of ischemic heart disease and mortality in people with subclinical hypothyroidism: reanalysis of the Whickham Survey cohort. J Clin Endocrinol Metab, , 95(4), 1734-1740.

[27] Roberts, L. M., Pattison, H., & Roalfe, A. (2006). Is subclinical thyroid dysfunction in the elderly associated with depression or cognitive dysfunction? Ann Intern Med, , 145(8), 573-581.

[28] Rodondi, N., den, Elzen. W. P., & Bauer, D. C. (2010). Subclinical hypothyroidism and the risk of coronary heart disease and mortality. JAMA, , 304(12), 1365-1374.

[29] Samuels, M. H. (2008). Cognitive function in untreated hypothyroidism and hyperthyroidism. Curr Opin Endocrinol Diabetes Obes, , 15(5), 429-433.

[30] Stagnaro-Green, A., Abalovich, M., & Alexander, E. (2011). Guidelines of the American Thyroid Association for the diagnosis and management of thyroid disease during pregnancy and postpartum. Thyroid, , 21(10), 1081-1125.

[31] Surks, M. I., Ortiz, E., & Daniels, G. H. (2004). Subclinical thyroid disease: scientific review and guidelines for diagnosis and management. JAMA, , 292(2), 228-238.

[32] Tunbridge, W. M., Evered, D. C., & Hall, R. (1977). The spectrum of thyroid disease in a community: the Whickham survey. Clin Endocrinol (Oxf), , 7(6), 481-493.

[33] Vaidya, B., & Pearce, S. H. (2008). Management of hypothyroidism in adults. BMJ, doi:bmj.a801., 337, a801.

[34] Vejbjerg, P., Knudsen, N., & Perrild, H. (2006). The association between hypoechogenicity or irregular echo pattern at thyroid ultrasonography and thyroid function in the general population. Eur J Endocrinol, , 155(4), 547-552.

[35] Wiersinga, W. M. (2001). Thyroid hormone replacement therapy. Horm Res, Suppl1, , 56, 74-81.

[36] Wilson, G., Curry, R. W., & Jr , . (2005). Subclinical thyroid disease. Am Fam Physician, , 72(8), 1517-1524.

[37] Woeber, K. A. (2005). Treatment of hypothyroidism. In: Braverman, LE. & Utiger, RD. (eds). Werner and Ingabar's the thyroid: a fundamental and clinical text. Philadelphia (PA): Lippincott Williams & Wilkins, , 864-869.

[38] Zhu, D. F., Wang, Z. X., & Zhang, D. R. (2006). fMRI revealed neural substrate for reversible working memory dysfunction in subclinical hypothyroidism. Brain, , 129(11), 2923-2930.

Chapter 8

Non-Thyroidal Illness: Physiopathology and Clinical Implications

Antonio Mancini, Sebastiano Raimondo,
Chantal Di Segni, Mariasara Persano and
Alfredo Pontecorvi

Additional information is available at the end of the chapter

http://dx.doi.org/10.5772/55644

1. Introduction

In critical illness, several abnormalities in thyroid hormone (TH) secretion, metabolism and action have been described in patients without previous diagnosis of intrinsic thyroid disease and are collectively called "Non thyroidal syndrome" (NTIS) [1]; this term is now largely employed, in the place of "euthyroid sick syndrome" [2-4] or "low-T_3 syndrome", due to the most common abnormality, a decreased level of serum total triiodothyronine (T_3), which can be detected very early, within 2 hours after the onset of severe physical stress [5-7]. However, T_3 lowering is only one of the endocrine picture described is such a situation; therefore the term NTIS seems to be more appropriate, also strengthening its extrathyroidal source.

NTIS has been depicted in about 70% of hospitalized patients for different diseases [8-10]. Moreover, the severity of morbidity and outcome in patients studied in intensive care unit (ICU) has been correlated with the alteration in thyroid function [11,12]. The hormonal response exhibits different pattern in acute and chronic phase, since in the first phase the alteration predominate in peripheral metabolism of TH, while in the latter central mechanisms controlling thyroid secretion progressively arise [13,14].

Since there is no clear evidence of tissue hypothyroidism, such a condition seems to be an adaptative response, and thyroid replacement therapy is not usually required, but this topic is still debated, since indirect signs of true hypothyroidism at tissue levels have been showed [15]. The question is open and different reviews have been published on this topic [1, 16-20]; but, very recently different molecular mechanisms have been shown to gain insight the complex situation of NTIS. The role of intracellular oxidative stress (OS) has been underlined. Therefore we present a review of these recent results and some personal data in patients affected by chronic obstructive pulmonary disease and patients studied after major cardiovascular surgery.

2. Clinical observations

A low T_3 state has been described in a variety of clinical situations, such as starvation [21], sepsis [22], surgery [23], trauma [24], myocardial infarction and heart failure [25,26], cardiopulmonary bypass [27], respiratory failure [28], bone marrow transplantation [29], other severe illness [30]. In a very recent paper in unselected ICU patients, free T_3 (fT_3) was the most powerful and the only independent predictor of ICU mortality, with a prognostic improving value when added to APACHE II score [31]. A retrospective study in a large group of patients treated with mechanical ventilation (MV) confirmed that NTIS represents a risk factor for prolonged MV [32].

Due to the importance of TH in **cardiac function**, it is not surprising that cardiac patients have been extensively studied under this profile. TH influence cardiac function with different mechanisms: inotropic and chronotropic positive effect via nuclear and non-nuclear pathways in cardiomyocytes, increase in cardiac contractility through augmented tissue oxygen delivery and consumption; decrease in systemic vascular resistance, through direct TH action on vascular smooth muscle cells; other endocrine effects are exerted on renin-angiotensin-aldosterone axis and on erythropoietin secretion [19, 33].

One of the early studies was performed in patients serially followed after acute myocardial infarction; a sustained and prolonged decrease of total T_3 (TT_3) and fT_3 was described, while TT_4 but not fT_4 showed a transient decrease; thyroxine binding globulin (TBG) levels remained unchanged, while thyroxine binding prealbumin (TBPA) and albumin exhibited a prolonged fall. TSH, despite low T_3, did not increase, remaining inappropriately low [34]. In this sense, the increase of TSH was shown to be correlated with a good prognosis [35].

It has been reported that patients with heart failure have low T_3 serum concentrations, which correlate with cardiac function [36]. In advanced heart failure, a low fT_3 index/reverse T_3 ratio was associated with higher right atrial pulmonary artery and pulmonary capillary wedge and lower ejection fraction [26].

Low T_3 syndrome has been considered a strong predictor of death and directly implicated in poor prognosis of cardiac patients in a large group of patients admitted in a cardiology department [37].

TH are implicated in metabolic function of myocardial cells; they have been shown to inversely correlate with Coenzyme Q_{10} (CoQ_{10}), a component of mitochondrial respiratory chain, also endowed with powerful antioxidant properties [38]. Preliminary data of our group in patients studied after major heart surgery showed low T_3 levels concurrently with signs of tissue hypothyroidism (elevated CoQ_{10} levels) [39]. In fact we found CoQ_{10} levels, evaluated by high performance liquid chromatography (HPLC), in the hypothyroid range, despite the fact cardiac diseases are well known to be associated with low CoQ_{10}.

The studies in **pulmonary disorders** have not been so extensively investigated [40-42]. In the just cited paper, low T_3 state was again considered a predictor of outcome in respiratory failure [28]. Among chronic conditions, no conclusive data are reported on chronic obstructive pulmonary disease (COPD), as reported in a recent review [43]. No clear evidence of thyroid function alteration has been reported in such a condition [44], although in patients with severe hypoxemia a strong positive correlation between total T_3/total T_4 ratio (TT_3/TT_4) and PaO_2 has been described [45]. Increased fT_3 concentrations have been reported in stable COPD, with a positive association to $PaCO_2$ [46], while others reported lower total T_3, fT_3 and TT_3/TT_4 ratios in patients with severe hypoxemia [47]. Low Forced Expiratory Volume at 1st second (FEV_1) is associated with low basal and stimulated levels of thyroid stimulating hormone (TSH) [48]; however the impact of hypoxemia on TSH response to exogenous thyrotropin releasing hormone (TRH) is controversial [45,46].

We have recently studied patients with COPD, evaluating lung parameters and antioxidant parameters, due to a possible involvement of OS in NTIS (see below). COPD is a complex condition, which cannot be considered a lung-related disorder, but rather a systemic disease also associated to increased oxidative stress. We evaluated thyroid hormones and antioxidant systems, the lipophilic CoQ_{10} and total antioxidant capacity (TAC) in COPD patients to reveal the presence of a low-T_3 syndrome in COPD and investigate the correlation between thyroid hormones, lung function parameters and antioxidants. The evaluation of CoQ_{10} was particularly interesting, also for the energetic role of this molecule, which is a component of the mitochondrial respiratory chain, as above stated; its concentrations were also corrected for cholesterol, due to its lipophilic nature. We studied 32 COPD patients and 45 controls; CoQ_{10} was assayed by HPLC; TAC by the metmyoglobin-ABTS method and expressed as latency time (LAG) in radical species appearance. We found significantly lower LAG values, fT_3 and fT_4 levels and significantly higher TSH in COPD patients vs controls. LAG values significantly correlated with fT_3 concentration. Twelve out of 32 patients exhibited fT_3 levels lower than normal range. When dividing COPD patients in two groups on the basis of the fT_3 concentration (normal fT_3 COPD and low fT_3 COPD), we observed lower LAG values in normal fT_3-COPD, compared to healthy subjects, with a further significant reduction in low fT_3-COPD patients. Moreover higher TSH concentrations were present in normal fT_3-COPD, compared to healthy subjects, with a further significant increase in low fT_3-COPD patients. CoQ_{10}/cholesterol ratio was higher in low fT_3-COPD vs normal fT_3-COPD, with a nearly significant difference.These data seem to indicate an increased oxidative stress in low fT_3-COPD and a role of fT_3 in modulating antioxidant systems. However low fT_3 levels are joined to metabolic indexes of true hypothyroidism, suggesting that elevated CoQ_{10} expresses a reduced tissue utilization. Interestingly, there was no significant difference in lung parameters when comparing normal- or low-fT_3 COPD patients, according to the definition of COPD as a systemic disease, with respiratory parameters unable to define the severity of disease. In fact metabolic dysfunctions (i.e. osteoporosis, vascular and cardiac involvement, muscle impairment) play a role in the natural history of disease but were found poorly related to respiratory impairment, underlying the need of indexes related to a real tissue condition; the pattern of fT_3 could indicate such a situation, as reinforced by the pattern of CoQ_{10} levels; decreased plasma antioxidant capacity and increased CoQ_{10} levels in low fT_3-COPD again suggested a possible condition of hypothyroidism at tissue levels [49].

The thyroid function has been investigated in patients with acute **kidney injury**. TSH levels inversely correlated with urea concentrations. 82.9% of patients exhibited alteration in thyroid function, especially low-T_3. This picture was ameliorated by improvement of renal function. No prognostic role was attributed to this dysfunction [50].

Primary hypothyroidism (non-autoimmune) is often observed in patients with chronic kidney disease (CKD); in particular the prevalence of subclinical hypothyroidism is related to GRF decline [51]. The earliest and the most common thyroid function abnormality in CKD patients is a low T_3 level (especially TT_3 than fT_3) [52]. The mechanisms for T_3 decrease in this condition are: fasting, chronic metabolic acidosis and chronic protein malnutrition, influencing T_4 deiodination, as well as protein binding of T_3. Moreover, inflammatory cytokines such as tumor necrosis factor (TNF)-α and interleukin (IL)-1 inhibit the expression of type 1 5'-deiodinase (see below), which is responsible for peripheral conversion of T_4 to T_3 [53]. Alteration of renal handling of iodine can increase serum iodine levels, causing a prolonged Wolff – Chaikoff effect [54]. A prognostic role has been attributed to the hormonal marker: the low fT_3 levels in CKD patients have been correlated with higher levels of markers of inflammation [highly sensitive C-reactive protein (hsCRP), IL-6, etc.], malnutrition (lower prealbumin, IGF-1), increased endothelial dysfunction, poorer cardiac function, poor survival, and higher all-cause as well as cardiovascular mortality in some studies [53, 55].

Little is known in TH alterations in acute **liver failure** (ALF) [56]. An animal model was investigated (pigs subjected to surgical liver devascularisation). In this case serum T_4 and T_3 levels were markedly decreased, but fT_3 and TSH did not change. The downregulation of T_4 and T_3 levels during ALF seems to correlate well with the severity of disease and was also related to alteration in parameters of inflammation, oxidative stress and myocardial thyroid receptors; thus the mechanisms in this case seem to be very complex. In humans acute liver failure (ALF) is accompanied by hormonal implications, as has been recently shown for the hepatoadrenal syndrome [57], since an unexpected incidence of adrenal failure was discovered in ALF and post-transplantation patients; a glucocorticoid treatment can influence outcome. Thyroid function alterations have been described during chronic liver failure [58-60]; a low T_4-variant of NTIS has been described in a subgroup of patients with cirrhosis at risk for decreased survival [58]; serum levels of fT_3 and TT_4 (but not TT_3 and fT_4) were significantly lower in patients with hepatic encephalopathy compared to decompensated cirrhotic patients without encephalopathy [60]. Much less clear data are available for ALF [61, 62]. In cirrhotic and also in acutely ill patients from various etiologies, derangements of thyroid hormones are common (up to 79% in the latter group, as reported from autoptic observations) [63].

Finally, during **starvation** (especially carbohydrate deprivation) deiodination of T_4 to T_3 is rapidly inhibited, causing the low-T_3 syndrome [1, 21, 64]. Interestingly, caloric deprivation can be also a major factor influencing TH in severe illness, as demonstrated in bacterial sepsis [65].

A particular model is that of eating disorders, especially anorexia nervosa, in which low-T_3 is accompanied by a constellation of hormone alteration, index of hypothalamic derangement [66]. Other psychiatric models should be considered with caution when evaluating thyroid alterations, due to other interfering factors, such as the underlying psychiatric disorder, substance abuse or other medications [67].

On the basis of the reported studies and other reviews [68, 69] we can summarized the main variations in the pituitary-thyroid axis as reported in Fig. 1, according to the severity of NTIS.

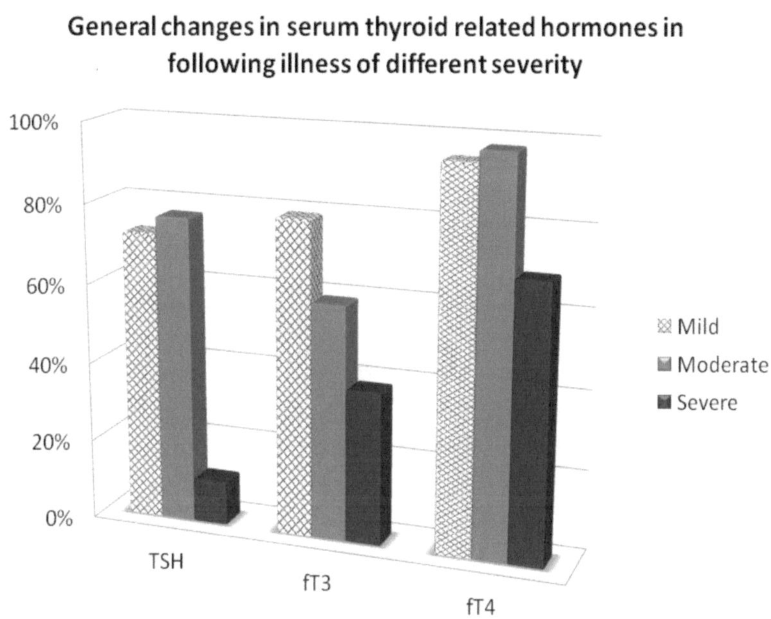

Figure 1.

3. Physiopathological mechanisms

Various mechanisms are responsible for the TH pattern observed in different situations, keeping in mind the difference between "acute" and "chronic" phases and possible differences related to the underlying diseases. They can summarize in four categories: central TSH regulation, TH blood transportation, peripheral metabolism by deiodinases, actions at receptorial and post-receptorial levels.

a. Central regulation of TSH

Basal TSH levels are usually normal or low, but not extremely inhibited [1, 70, 71]; in most cases they are inadequate in respect to thyroid hormone levels. The response to TRH is variable, ranging from blunted to normal response [72, 73]; the response to TRH, even in presence of low basal level, can be interpreted as a sign of hypothalamic dysfunction, according to data concerning other hormones (gonadotropins, ACTH-cortisol axis) [13, 74]. Absence of circadian rhythm has been reported [75]. The variation of glicosilation is responsible for reduced bioactivity [76]. The finding that TH alterations are partially reversed by the combined infusion of TRH and GH secretagogues [77] reinforces the role of central component of NTIS.

b. Transportation

Also transportation of thyroid hormones is altered; Thyroxine binding globulin (TBG) has been shown to be reduced, probably for increased cleavage by proteases. The binding to transport protein is also negatively influenced by inhibitors (not only in serum, but also in tissues), therefore influencing the metabolism of TH [1]. Recently, decrease of TBG, determined by RIA or radioimmunodiffusion, albumin and transthyretin (TTR) have been described in septic patients [78]; therefore the total binding power of serum is low, in the view of authors, without the need to postulate the effects of additional factors, such as binding inhibitors or modification of binding affinity.

c. Deiodinase

A lot of studies concern the activity of deiodinases, the main group of enzymes, which by removal of iodine, catalyze activation or inactivation of TH. They are selenoproteins, members of the thioredoxin family, and require a thiol cofactor for their activity [20,79]. The activation of prohormone T_4 into the biologically active hormone T_3 is catalyzed by type 1 (D1, encoded by DIO1) and type 2 (D2, encoded by DIO2) via deiodination of the outer ring; on the contrary, the removal of inner ring iodine is catalyzed by type 3 (D3, encoded by DIO3), causing inactivation of both T_4 and T_3 [80]. In humans, 80% of circulating T_3 comes from deiodination by D1 and D2, while the other 20% comes directly from thyroid secretion. The most common alteration in NTIS patients is a decrease in T_3, caused by reduced conversion of T_4 to T_3 [81]. The Deiodinase 1 is down regulated, as demonstrated in liver, causing reduced T_3 generation [1]. Deiodinase 3 is instead increased, as observed in liver and muscle, especially in the case of low tissue perfusion, and the conversion of T_3 to reverse-T_3 (rT_3) is a mechanism reinforcing the low T_3 levels [80]. However, central and peripheral deiodinases are differently regulated; T_3 in the pituitary are normal since local deiodinaton is enhanced, thus the pituitary is actually euthyroid and therefore TSH circulating levels inappropriate to other tissue fT_3 levels [1]. The role of D3 has recently been reviewed [82]. Moreover more recent studies focused on modulation of deiodinases activity, rather than their levels (see below).

d. Thyroid receptors and Postreceptorial mechanisms

It has been shown that thyroid hormone receptors (TR) are down-regulated in skeletal muscle of patients with non-septic shock; in particular they showed lower expression of TR-β, TR-α_1 and their nuclear partner retinoid X receptor γ (RXRG) [83]. The RXRA gene expression was higher, even if its protein was lower, suggesting the existence of post-transcriptional mechanisms that down-regulate protein levels. Nuclear factor of kappa light chain enhancer of activated B cells (NkFB), a transcriptional factor involved in immune and inflammatory response, attenuates the induction of DIO1 by T_3 [84]; however NkFB1 activation was not different in comparison to control subjects. However the results are not unequivocal, since there results were not reproducible in cultures of human smooth muscle cells (HSkMC) incubated with the patients' serum [83].

Molecular mechanisms of thyroid action in NTIS have been recently investigated in other models, studying, other than TR, also the transporters, which allow TH to be transported across the plasma membrane in order to be metabolized and interact with their receptors. Monocarboxylate transporter 8 (MCT8) has been shown to be a very active and specific transporter [85]. Moreover, other proteins modulate the transcription function of TR, acting as coactivators or corepressors; among the latter the silencing mediator of retinoid and TR (SMRT) via histone deacetylation [86]. In patients with septic shock, skeletal muscle expression of TR-β1, RXRG and D2 was lower than in control group and RXRA was higher. In subcutaneous adipose tissue, the authors found lower MCT8, TRHB1, THRA1, RXRG and SMRT and higher UCP3 expression, suggesting decreased thyroid hormone action [87].

Interestingly, the reduced expression of TH transporters has been considered a compensatory mechanism (rather than a cause of low- T_3), strongly suggesting a real hypothyroidism at tissue levels in such a condition [88].

4. The role of cytokines

The role of cytokines, as key molecules involved in coordinating the hormone, immune and inflammatory response to a variety of stressful stimuli, has been largely investigated [1].

In a series of septic patients studied shortly after admission to an ICU, TT_4, fT_4, TT_3 and TSH were depressed, and IL-1B, sIL-2R and TNFα were elevated [89] suggesting central suppression of TSH, even if the relationship with cytokines was not so clear. The hypothalamic-pituitary-adrenal axis was activated as expected. It has been shown that continuous infusion of IL-1 in rats cause suppression of TSH, T_3 and fT_4; higher doses of IL-1 were accompanied by a febrile reaction and suppression of food intake, with a cascade of events altering thyroid hormone economy [90], but IL-1 did not reproduce the decrease in hepatic 5′-deiodinase activity believed to be characteristic of NTIS.

TNF is another proinflammatory cytokine that is thought to be involved in many of the illnesses associated with NTI. Infusion of rTNF in man produced a decrease in serum T_3 and TSH and increase in r T_3 [91]. These studies suggest that TNF could be involved in the IL-6-mediated activation of hypothalamic-pituitary axis. Also in this case other data did not confirm the role of TNF, since the effects of endotoxin of TH in humans were not counteracted by the TNFα blockade by specific IgG fusion proteins [92]. TNFα was found during in vitro studies to activate NkFB [93], which in turn inhibits the T_3-induced expression of D1 as above reported.

On the contrary, an important role has been attributed to IL-6, which is often elevated in serum of NTIS patients [94] and its level is inversely related to T_3 levels [95]. Short term infusion of rIL-6 to human volunteers [96] caused a suppression of TSH, but daily injections over 42 days cause only a modest decrease in T_3 and a transient increase in r T_3 and in fT_4 concentrations.

More recent evidences on the role of IL-6 have been reported by studies in human cell lines: the effects of IL-6 on both endogenous cofactor-mediated and dithiotreitol-stimulated cell sonicate deiodinase activity have been studied [80]. In this model T_3 generation by D1 and D2 was suppressed by IL-6, despite an increase in sonicate dediodinases (and mRNAs): this inhibitory action was prevented by addition of N-acetyl-cysteine (NAC), an antioxidant that restores intracellular glutathione (GSH) concentrations. The interest of the paper is also the link of deiodinase activity and OS (see below).

Finally, the potential interaction between the complex network of cytokines and the hypothalamic pituitary thyroid axis, even if is not possible to build a simplistic model, probably plays a pathogenetic role in NTIS [1]. The role of cytokines in eating disorders and related TH alterations has also been reviewed [97].

5. Oxidative stress in NTIS

Previous studies have shown that both hyperthyroidism and hypothyroidism are associated with enhanced oxidative stress involving enzymatic and non-enzymatic antioxidants [98]. Besides, some complications of hyperthyroidism are due just to the oxidative stress in target tissues [99]. Thyroid hormones *per se* can act as oxidants and produce DNA-damage (contrasted by catalase), probably through the phenolic group, similar to that of steroidal estrogens [100]. Many other mechanisms, reviewed by Venditti & Di Meo [101], can be involved, with a specificity in tissue response. We recently reviewed the relationships between thyroid hormone, OS and reproduction [102].

At a systemic level, also in humans, hyperthyroidism has been associated with reduced circulating levels of alpha-tocopherol [103, 104] and Coenzyme Q_{10} [38, 104]. Coenzyme Q_{10} showed a trend to increase in hypothyroidism [38]; it appeared to be a sensitive index of tissue effect of thyroid hormones, in situations in which drug interference, such as amiodarone [105] or systemic illness inducing a low-T_3 conditions [106] complicate the interpretation of thyroid hormone levels. However, data on hypothyroidism in humans are conflicting [102]. Baskol et al showed in a group of 33 patients with primary hypothyroidism elevated malondialdehyde (MDA) and nitric oxide (NO) levels and low paraoxonase (PON1) activity, while superoxide dismutase (SOD) was not different from controls. Interestingly, thyroid treatment decreased MDA and increased PON1, without reaching levels observed in controls [107]. They concluded that a prooxidant environment in hypothyroidism could play a role in the pathogenesis of atherosclerosis in such patients. Elevated MDA levels were also shown in subclinical hypothyroidism [108]; the increased in OX was attributed to lack of antioxidants but also to altered lipid metabolism, since MDA showed a correlation with LDL-cholesterol, total cholesterol and triglycerides. Total antioxidant status (TAS) was similar in overt hypothyroidism, subclinical hypothyroidism and controls.

Another study [109] showed increased levels of thiobarbituric acid reactive substances (TBARS), but also of antioxidants, such as SOD, catalase (CAT) and Vitamin E. All these parameters correlated with T_3; moreover the correlation between T_3 and CAT remained significant also when corrected with total cholesterol. This datum was not confirmed by other authors [110, 111]. We showed low Total Antioxidant Capacity (TAC) levels in hypothyroid patients and increased CoQ_{10} levels also in secondary hypothyroidism (mainly due to its metabolic role in mitochondrial respiratory chain and therefore underutilized in hypothyroid tissue). In the last case, hypothyroidism has a predominant effect on the possible decreasing effect of OS [112].

Different conditions with NTIS are associated to OS, due to augmented production of radical oxygen species (ROS) or nitrogen species [113]; since thyroid hormones, as above stated, can increase ROS generation, OS could be viewed as a compensatory mechanism since, decreasing metabolic rate, could protect against further radical generation. A reducing environment is maintained in the cytosol by intracellular thiols, especially GSH and Thioredoxin (TRX), which, as we have seen, are cofactors for deiodinases. Therefore their depletion, due to buffering effect against radical propagation, could interfere with the conversion of T_4 to T_3 [79]. Moreover, another reported mechanism is the nuclear sequestration of the SECIS binding protein 2 (SPB2), which reduces incorporation of selenocysteine residues in the selenoproteins [114]. IL-6 is known to induce OS, therefore an unifying hypothesis is cytokine-induced OS and a secondary alteration of expression and activity of deiodinases [79]. However further studies can clarify these complex interaction and especially the potential role of antioxidant in protecting against OS in NTIS.

On the basis of the physiopathological studies above reported, we can conclude that the alterations of pituitary-thyroid axes do not only depend from the severity of the disease, but also from the nutritional status of the patients and their inflammatory response, also related to oxidative stress (see fig. 2).

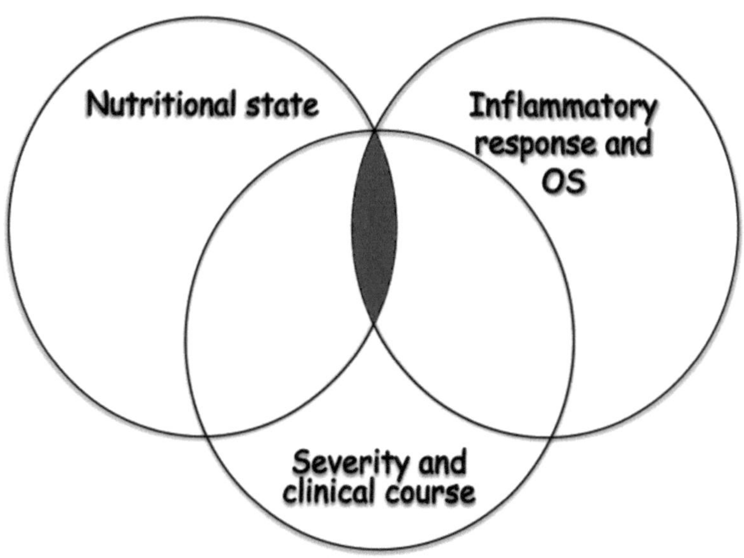

Figure 2. Interaction of factors influencing pituitary-thyroid axis

6. Treatment

Controversial results have been reported on the topic of replacement therapy. The replacement therapy with 1.5 μg/Kg BW L-thyroxine iv was able to restore normal T_4 levels, but not T_3 levels, without effect on mortality, which remained at 80% both in treated patients and control groups [115]. Similarly, another study in burns, using 200 μg T_3/daily, did not show significant benefits [116].

Despite studies in animals were in favour of a positive effect in experimental renal failure [1], in humans an increased mortality was showed in a group of acute renal failure treated with L-thyroxine and no beneficial effect of T_3 was observed in transplanted patients [117,118].

Studies in humans showed a slight cardiovascular benefit in patients with shock, respiratory disease, coronary artery bypass draft, premature infants [1, 119].

The discrepancies in the reported study, however, can be attributed to different severity of low-T_3, different schedule of treatment, clinical situations with very different physiopathology, so that it is difficult to obtain a definitive conclusion.

Other interventional studies are reviewed by Bello et al. [19], showing in their complex a beneficial effects on cardiovascular parameters, but not unequivocal benefit of patients' outcome. In fact, in patients with dilated cardiomyopathy, the administration of TH significantly increased left ventricular end-diastolic volume and stroke volume while decreased heart rate [120]. In patients studied after coronary artery bypass surgery, the administration of intravenous T_3 or placebo produced an increase in cardiac output and lowered systemic vascular resistance, without influencing the patients' outcome and therapeutic schedules [121]. In contrast, another study [122] performed after elective coronary artery bypass grafting showed a beneficial effect of intravenous T_3 administration on incidence of postoperative myocardial ischemia and on need for pacemakers or mechanical cardiac support devices. It must be reminded that the administration of TH can directly influence myocardial oxygen supply and demand, causing myocardial ischemic events, even in the absence of coronary artery stenosis or spasms, as reported in some cases [123].

Similar conclusions, biochemical rather than clinical advantage, were drawn in a group of patients after acute burn injuries [124].

7. Conclusion

In conclusion, we cannot answer the dilemma, just poned by eminent authors [125,126], about the treatment of low T_3 in NTIS. Some data argue in favour of a real hypothyroidism at tissue level in NTIS; therefore this condition cannot be simply considered an adaptive response. Probably, a full understanding of molecular mechanisms, which cause or are a consequence of low T_3 levels, will allow choosing patients who can really have a benefit from replacement therapy and the appropriate schedule of treatment.

Author details

Antonio Mancini, Sebastiano Raimondo, Chantal Di Segni, Mariasara Persano and Alfredo Pontecorvi

Dept of Internal Medicine, Division of Endocrinology, Catholic University School of Medicine, Rome, Italy

References

[1] De Groot LJ. Non-thyroidal illness syndrome is a manifestation of hypothalamic-pituitary dysfunction, and in view of current evidence, should be treated with appropriate replacement therapies. Crit Care Clin. 2006;22(1) 57-86, vi.

[2] Rubenfeld S. Euthyroid sick syndrome. N Engl J Med 1978;299 1414.

[3] Wartofsky L, Burman KD. Alterations in thyroid function in patients with systemic illness: the "Euthyroid sick syndrome". Endocr Rev 1982;3 164-217.

[4] Chopra IJ. Euthyroid sick syndrome: abnormalities in circulating thyroid hormones and thyroid hormone physiology in illness (NTI). Med Grand Rounds 1982;1 201–212.

[5] Chopra IJ, Chopra U, Smith SR, Reza M, Solomon DH. Reciprocal changes in serum concentrations of 3,3',5-triiodothyronine (T3) in systemic illnesses. J Clin Endocrinol Metab 1975;41 1043–1049.

[6] Umpierrez GE. Euthyroid Sick Syndrome, South Med J 2002;95(5) 506-513.

[7] Michalaki M, Vagenakis AG, Makri M, Kalfarentzos F, Kyriazopoulou V. Dissociation of the early decline in serum T(3)concentration and serum IL-6 rise and TNF-alpha in illness syndrome induced by abdominal surgery. J Clin Endocrinol Metab 2001;86 4198–4205.

[8] Chopra IJ. Clinical review 86: Euthyroid sick syndrome: is it a misnomer? J Clin Endocrinol Metab 1997;82 329–334.

[9] Bermudez F, Surks MI, Oppenheimer JH. High incidence of decreased serum triiodothyronine concentration in patients with non thyroidal disease. J Clin Endocrinol Metab 1975; 41 27–40.

[10] Kaplan MM, Larsen PR, Crantz FR, Dzau VJ, Rossing TH, Haddow JE. Prevalence of abnormal thyroid function test results in patients with acute medical illnesses. Am J Med 1982;72 9–16.

[11] Marx C, Petros S, Bornstein SR, Weise M, Wendt M, Menschikowski M, Engelmann L, Hoffken G. Adrenocortical hormones in survivors and nonsurvivors of severe sepsis: diverse time course of dehydroepiandrosterone, dehydroepiandrosterone-sulfate, and cortisol. Crit Care Med 2003;31 1382–1388.

[12] Schuetz P, Muller B, Nusbaumer C, Wieland M, Christ-Crain M. Circulating levels of GH predict mortality and complement prognostic scores in critically ill medical patients. Eur J Endocrinol 2009;160 157-163.

[13] Van den Berghe G, De Zegher F, Bouillon R. Acute and prolonged critical illness as different neuroendocrine paradigms. J Clin Endocrinol Metab 1998;83 1827-1834.

[14] Van den Berghe G. Dynamic neuroendocrine responses to critical illness. Frontiers Neuroendocrinol 2002;23 370-391.

[15] Mancini A, Corbo GM, Gaballo A, Valente S, Gigliotti P, Cimino V, De Marinis L, Principi F, Littarru GP. Relationships between plasma CoQ10 levels and thyroid hormones in chronic obstructive pulmonary disease. Biofactors 2005;25 (1-4) 201-204.

[16] Peeters RP, Wouters PJ, Kaptein E, van Toor H, Visser TJ, Van den Berghe G. Reduced activation and increased inactivation of thyroid hormone in tissues of critically ill patients. J Clin Endocrinol Metab. 2003; 88 (7) 3202-3211.

[17] Luca F, Goichot B, Brue T. Non thyroidal illnesses (NTIS). Ann Endocrinol (Paris) 2010;71 (Suppl 1) S 13- 24.

[18] Economidou F, Douka E, Tzanela M, Nanas S, Kotanidou A. Thyroid function during critical illness. Hormones 2011;10 (2) 117-124.

[19] Bello G, Ceaichisciuc I, Silva S, Antonelli M. The role of thyroid dysfunction in the critically ill: a review of literature. Minerva Anestesiol 2010;76 (11) 919-928.

[20] Magagnin Wajner S, Maia AL. New insights toward the acute non thyroidal illness syndrome. Front Endocrinol 2012;3 (8) 1-7 Epub 26 Jan 2012

[21] Henneman G, Docter R, Krenning EP. Causes and effects of the low T3 syndrome during caloric deprivation and non-thyroidal illness: an overview. Acta Med Austriaca 1988;15 42-45.

[22] Monig H, Arendt T, Meyer M, Kloehn S, Bewig B. Activation of the hypothalamo-pituitary-adrenal axis in response to septic or non-septic diseases- implications for the euthyroid sick syndrome. Intensive Care Med 1999;25 1402-1406.

[23] Cherem HJ, Nellen HH, Barabejski FG, Chong MBA, Lifshits GA. Thyroid function and abdominal surgery. A longitudinal study. Arch Med Res 1992;23 143-147.

[24] Ilias I, Stamoulis K, Armaganidis A, Lyberopoulos P, Tzanela M, Orfanos S, Theodorakopoulou M, Tsagarakis S, Dimopoulou I. Contribution of endocrine parameters in predicting outcome of multiple trauma patients in an intensive care unit. Hormones 2007;6 218-226.

[25] Vardarli I, Schmidt R, Wdowinski JM, Teuber J, Schwedes U, Usadel KH. The hypothalamo-hypophyseal thyroid axis, plasma protein concentration and the hypophyseogonadal axis in low T3 syndrome following acute myocardial infarct. Klinische Wochenschrift 1987;65 129-133.

[26] Hamilton MA, Stevenson LW, Lun M, Walden JA. Altered thyroid hormone metabolism in advanced heart failure. J Am Coll Cardiol. 1990;16 (1) 91-95.

[27] Holland FW, Brown PS, Weintraub BD, Clark RE. Cardiopulmonary bypass and thyroid function: an "euthyroid sick syndrome". Ann Thorac Surg 1991;52 46-50.

[28] Scoscia E, Baglioni S, Eslami A, Iervasi G, Monti S, Todisco T. Clinical study "Low triiodothyronine (T3) state: a predictor of outcome in respiratory failure? Results of a clinical pilot study. Eur J Endocrinol 2004;151 557-560.

[29] Vexiau P, Perez- Castiglioni P, Socie G, Devergie A, Toubert ME, Aractingi S, Gluckmann E. The " Euthyroid sick syndrome": incidence, risk factors and prognostic value soon after allogenic bone marrow transplantation. Br J Hematol 1993;85 778-782.

[30] Kaptein EM. Clinical relevance of thyroid hormone alterations in non-thyroidal illness. Thyroid International 1997;4 22-25.

[31] Wang F, Pan W, Wang H, Wang S, Pan S,Ge J. Relationship between thyroid function and ICU mortality: a prospective observation study. Crit Care 2012;16 (1) R11.

[32] Bello G, Pennisi MA, Montini L, Silva S, Maviglia R, Cavallaro F, Bianchi A, De Marinis L, Antonelli M. Nonthyroidal illness syndrome and prolonged mechanical ventilation in patients admitted to the ICU. Chest 2009;135 (6) 1448-1454.

[33] Klein I, Ojamaa K. Thyroid hormone and the cardiovascular system. N Engl J Med 2001;344 501-509.

[34] Franklyn JA, Gammage MD, Ramsden DB, Sheppard MC. Thyroid status in patients after acute myocardial infarction. Clin Sci (Lond) 1984;67 585-590.

[35] De Marinis L, Mancini A, Masala R, Torlontano M, Sandric S, Barbarino A. Evaluation of pituitary-thyroid axis response to acute myocardial infarction. J Endocrinol Invest 1985;8 507-511.

[36] Opasich C, Pacini F, Ambrosino N. Sick euthyroid syndrome in patients with moderate to severe chronic heart failure. Eur Heart J 1996;17 1860–1866.

[37] Iervasi G, Pingitore A, Landi P, Raciti M, Ripoli A, Scarlattini M, L'Abbate A, Donato L. Low- T3 syndrome: a strong prognostic predictor of death in patients with heart disease. Circulation 2003;107 (5) 708-713.

[38] Mancini A, Festa R, Di Donna V, Leone E, Littarru GP, Silvestrini A, Meucci E, Pontecorvi A. Hormones and antioxidant systems: role of pituitary and pituitary-dependent axes. J Endocrinol Invest 2010;33 (6) 422-433.

[39] Mancini A, Corbo GM, Scapigliati A, Leone E, Conti M, Littarru GP, Meucci E, De Marinis L, Pontecorvi A. Low-T3 syndrome in chronic obstructive pulmonary disease and heart surgery patients: evaluation of plasma antioxidant systems. Endocrine Abstracts 2008;16 752.

[40] Chow CC, Mak TW, Chan CH & Cockram CS. Euthyroid sick syndrome in pulmonary tuberculosis before and after treatment. Ann Clin Biochem 1995;32 385-391.

[41] Kawakami M, Usami I, Kuroki H & Goto M. Thyroid hormones in patients with clinical stable pneumoconiosis. Nihon Kyobu Shikkan Gakkai Zasshi 1993;31 1215-1219.

[42] Wawrzynska L, Sakowicz A & Filipecki S. Euthyroid sick syndrome in patients with respiratory failure. Pneumol Alergol Pol 1996;64 (Suppl 2) 193-199.

[43] Laghi F, Adiguzel N, Tobin MJ. Endocrinological derangements in COPD. Eur Respir J 2009;34 975-996.

[44] Creutzberg EC, Casaburi R. Endocrinological disturbances in chronic obstructive pulmonary disease. Eur Respir J 2003;22 (Suppl 46) 76s-80s.

[45] Dimopolou I, Ilias I, Mastorakos G, Mantzos E, Roussos C, Koutras DA. Effects of severity of chronic obstructive pulmonary disease on thyroid function. Metabolism Clin Exper 2001;50 1397-1401.

[46] Okutan O, Kartaloglu Z, Onde ME, Bozkanat E, Kunter E. Pulmonary function tests and thyroid hormone concentrations in patients with chronic obstructive pulmonary disease. Med Princ Pract 2004;13 126-128.

[47] Karadag F, Ozcan H, Karul AB, Yilmaz M, Cildag O. Correlates of non-thyroidal illness syndrome in chronic obstructive pulmonary disease. Respir Med 2007;101 1439-1446.

[48] Bratel T, Wennlund A, Carlstrom K. Impact of hypoxaemia on neuroendocrine function and catecholamine secretion in chronic obstructive pulmonary disease (COPD): Effects of long-term oxygen treatment. Respir Med 2000;94 1221-1228.

[49] Mancini A, Corbo GM, Gaballo A, Raimondo S, Di Segni C, Gigliotti P, Silvestrini A, Valente S, Littarru GP, Pontecorvi A, Meucci E. Relationship between plasma antioxidants and thyroid hormones in chronic obstructive pulmonary disease. Exp Clin Endocrinol Diab 2012;120 623-628.

[50] Iglesias P, Olea T, Vega-Cabrera C, Heras M, Bajo MA, Del Peso G, Arias MJ, Selgas R, Díez JJ. Thyroid function tests in acute kidney injury. J Nephrol. 2012;0. doi: 10.5301/jn.5000106.

[51] Lo JC, Chertow GM, Go AS, Hsu CY. Increased prevalence of subclinical and clinical hypothyroidism in persons with chronic kidney disease. Kidney Int 2005;67 1047-1052.

[52] Wiederkehr MR, Kalogiros J, Krapf R. Correction of metabolic acidosis improves thyroid and growth hormone axes in haemodialysis patients. Nephrol Dial Transplant 2004;19 1190-1197.

[53] Zoccali C, Tripepi G, Cutrupi S, Pizzini P, Mallamaci F. Low triiodothyronine: A new facet of inflammation in end-stage renal disease. J Am Soc Nephrol 2005;16 2789-2795.

[54] Bando Y, Ushiogi Y, Okafuji K, Toya D, Tanaka N, Miura S. Non-autoimmune primary hypothyroidism in diabetic and non-diabetic chronic renal dysfunction. Exp Clin Endocrinol Diabetes 2002;110 408-415.

[55] Carrero JJ, Qureshi AR, Axelsson J, Yilmaz MI, Rehnmark S, Witt MR, Barany P, Heimburger O, Suliman ME, Alvestand A, Lindholm B, Stenvinkel P. Clinical and biochemical implications of low thyroid hormone levels (total and free forms) in euthyroid patients with chronic kidney disease. J Intern Med 2007;262 690-701

[56] Kostopanagiotou G, Kalimeris K, Mourouzis I, Costopanagiotou C, Arkadopoulos N, Panagopoulos D, Papoutsidakis N, Chranioti A, Pafiti A, Spanou D, Smyrniotis V, Pantos C. Thyroid hormones alterations during acute liver failure: possible underlying mechanisms and consequences. Endocrine 2009;36 (2) 198-204.

[57] Marik PE, Gayowski T, Starzl TE. The hepatoadrenal syndrome: a common yet unrecognized clinical condition. Crit Care Med 2005;33 1254-1259

[58] Caregaro L, Alberino F, Amodio P, Merkel C, Angeli P, Plebani M, Gatta A. Nutritional and prognostic significance of serum hypothyroxinemia in hospitalized patients with liver cirrhosis. J Hepatol 1998;28 115-121

[59] Zietz B, Lock G, Plach B, Drobnik W, Grossmann J, Scholmercih J, Straub RH. Dysfunction of the hypothalamic-pituitary-glandular axes and relation to Child-Pugh classification in male patients with alcoholic and virus-related cirrhosis. Eur J Gastroenterol Hepatol 2003;15 495-501.

[60] Kayacetin E, Kisakol G, Kaya A. Low serum total thyroxine and free triiodothyronine in patients with hepatic encephalopathy due to non-alcoholic cirrhosis. Swiss Med Wkly 2003;133 210-213.

[61] Bratusch-Marrain P, Vierhapper H, Grubeck-Loebenstein B, Waldhausl W, Kleinberger G. Pituitary-thyroid dysfunction in severe non-thyroidal disease: "low-T4 syndrome". Endokrinologie 1982;80 207-212.

[62] Kaptein EM, Robinson WJ, Grieb DA. Peripheral serum thyroxine, triiodothyronine and reverse triiodothyronine kinetics in the low state of acute nonthyroidal illnesses. J Clin Invest 1982;69 526-535.

[63] Arem R, Wiener GJ, Kaplan SG, Kim HS, Reichlin S, Kaplan MM. Reduced tissue thyroid hormone levels in fatal illness. Metabolism 1993;42 1102-1108.

[64] Hennemann G, Docter R, Krenning EP. Causes and effects of the low-T3 syndrome during caloric deprivation and non-thyroidal illness: an overview. Acta Med Austriaca 1988;15 (suppl 1) 42-45.

[65] Richmand DA, Molitch ME, O'Donnell TF. Altered thyroid hormone levels in bacterial sepsis: the role of nutritional adequacy. Metabolism 1980;29 936-942.

[66] Mancini A, Di Donna V, Leone E, Giacchi E. Endocrine alterations in anorexia nervosa. In: Mancini A, Daini S, Caruana L (eds) Anorexia nervosa: a multidisciplinary approach. New York: Nova Science Pub Inc; 2010. p3-30.

[67] Dickerman AL, Barnhill JW. Abormal thyroid function tests in psychiatric patients: a red herring? Am J Psychiatry 2012;169 (2) 127-133.

[68] Salvatore D, Davies TF, Schumberger M, Hay ID, Larsen PR. Thyroid physiology and diagnostic evaluation of patients with thyroid disorders. In: Melmed S, Polonsky KS, Larsen PR, Kronenberg HM (Eds) Williams Textbook of Endocrinology 12th Ed. Philadelphia: Elsevier Saunders; 2011. p 327-361.

[69] Warner MH, Beckett GJ. Mechanisms behind the non-thyroidal illness syndrome: an update. J Endocrinol 2010;205 1-13

[70] Melmed S, Geola FL, Reed AW, Pekary AE, Park J, Hershman JM. A comparison of methods for assessing thyroid function in illness. J Clin Endocrinol Metab 1982;54 300-306.

[71] Docter R, Krenning EP, de Jong M, Hennemann G. The sick euthyroid syndrome: changes in thyroid hormone serum parameters and hormone metabolism. Clin Endocrinol 1993;39 499-518.

[72] Vierhapper H, Laggner A, Waldhausl W, Grubeck-Loebenstein B, Kleinberger G. Impaired secretion of TSH in critically ill patients with 'low T4-syndrome'. Acta Endocrinol 1982;101 542-549.

[73] Faber J, Kirkegaard C, Rasmussen B, Westh H, Busch-Sorensen M, Jensen IW. Pituitary-thyroid axis in critical illness. J Clin Endocrinol Metab 1987;65 315-320.

[74] Van den Berghe G, Weekers F, Baxter RC, Wouters P, Iranmanesh A, Bouillon R, Veldhuis JD. Five-day pulsatile gonadotropin-releasing hormone administration unveils combined hypothalamic-pituitary-gonadal defects underlying profound hypoandrogenism in man with prolonged critical illness. J Clin Endocrinol Metab 2001;86 3217-3226.

[75] Arem R, Deppe S. Fatal nonthyroidal illness may impair nocturnal thyrotropin levels. Am J Med 1990;88 258-262.

[76] Lee H- Y, Suhl J, Pekary AE, Hershman JM. Secretion of thyrotropin with reduced concanavalin-A-binding activity in patients with severe nonthyroid illness. J Clin Endocrinol Metab 1987;65 942.

[77] Van den Berghe G, De Zegher F, Baxter RC, Veldhuis JD, Wouters P, Schetz M, Verwaest C, Van der Vorst E, Lauwers P, Bouillon R, Bowers CY. Neuroendocrinology of prolonged critical illness: effects of exogenous thyrotropin-releasing hormone and its combination with growth hormone secretagogues. J Clin Endocrinol Metab 1998;83 309–319.

[78] Afandi B, Vera R, Schussler GC, Yap MG. Concordant decreases of thyroxine and thyroxine binding protein concentrations during sepsis. Metabolism 2000;49 (6) 753-754.

[79] Maia AL, Kim BW, Huang SA, Harney JW, Larsen PR. Type 2 iodothyronine deiodinase is the major source of plasma T3 in euthyroid humans. J Clin Invest 2005;115 (9) 2524-2533.

[80] Wajner SM, Goemann IM, Bueno AL, Larsen PR, Maia AL. IL-6 promotes nonthyroidal illness syndrome by blocking thyroxine activation while promoting thyroid hormone inactivation in human cells. J Clin Invest. 2011;121 (5) 1834-1845.

[81] Chopra IJ. Clinical review 86: Euthyroid sick syndrome: is it a misnomer? J Clin Endocrinol Metab 1997;82 (2) 329–334.

[82] Dentice M, Domenico S. Deiodinases: the balance of thyroidal hormone. Local impact of thyroid hormone inactivation. J Endocrinol 2011;209 273-282.

[83] Lado-Abeal J, Romero A, Castro-Piedras I, Rodriguez-Perez A, Alvarez-Escudero J. Thyroid hormone receptors are down-regulated in skeletal muscle of patients with non-thyroidal illness syndrome secondary to non-septic shock. Eur J Endocrinol 2010;163 (5) 765-73.

[84] Nagaya T, Fujieda M, Otsuka G, Yang JP, Okamoto T & Seo H. A potential role of activated NF-kB in the pathogenesis of euthyroid sick syndrome. J Clin Invest 2000;106 393-402.

[85] Friesema EC, Ganguly S, Abdalla A, Manning Fox JE, Halestrap AP & Visser TJ. Identification of monocarboxylate transporter 8 as a specific thyroid hormone transporter. J Biol Chem 2003;278 40128-40135.

[86] Goodson M, Jonas BA, Privalsky MA. Corepressors: custom tailoring and alterations while you wait. Nucl Recept Signal 2005;3 e003.

[87] Rodriguez-Perez A, Palos-Paz F, Kaptein E, Visser TJ, Dominguez-Gerpe L, Alvarez-Escudero J, Lado-Abeal J. Identification of molecular mechanisms related to nonthyroidal illness syndrome in skeletal muscle and adipose tissue from patients with septic shock. Clin Endocrinol (Oxf) 2008;68 (5) 821-827.

[88] Mebis L, Paletta D, Debaveye Y, Ellger B, Langouche L, D'Hoore A, Darras VM, Visser TJ, Van den Berghe G. Expression of thyroid hormone transporters during critical illness. Eur J Endocrinol 2009;161 (2) 243-250.

[89] Monig H, Arendt T, Meyer M, Kloehn S, Bewig B. Activation of the hypothalamic-pituitary-adrenal axis in response to septic or non-septic disease-implications for the euthyroid sick syndrome. Intensive Care Med 1999;25 1402-1406.

[90] Hermus RM, Sweep CGJ, Van Der Meer MJM, Ross HA, Smals AGH, Benraad TJ, Kloppenborg PWC. Continuous infusion of interleukin-1 induces a nonthyroidal illness syndrome in the rat. Endocrinology 1992;131 2139-2146.

[91] Van der Poll T, Romijn JA, Wiersinga WM, Saurwein HP. Tumor necrosis factor: a putative mediator of the sick euthyroid syndrome in man. J Clin Endocrinol Metab 1990;71 1567-1572.

[92] Van der Poll T, Endert E, Coyle SM, Agosti JM, Lowry SF. Neutralization of TNF does not influence endotoxin induced changes in thyroid hormone metabolism in humans. Am J Physiol 1999;276 R357-362.

[93] Nagaya T, Fujieda M, Otsuka G, Yang JP, Okamoto T, Seo H. A potential role of activated NF-kappa B in the pathogenesis of euthyroid sick syndrome. J Clin Invest 2000;106 393-402.

[94] Bartalena L, Brogioni S, Grasso L, Velluzzi F, Martino E. Relationship of the increased serum interleukin-6 concentration to changes of thyroid function in nonthyroidal illness. J Endocrinol Invest 1994;17 269-274.

[95] Boelen A, Platvoet-ter Schiphorst MC, Wiersinga WM. Association between serum interleukin-6 and serum 3,5,3′-triiodothyronine in nonthyroidal illness. J Clin Endocrinol Metab 1993;77 1695-1699.

[96] Stouthard JML, Van Der Poll T, Endert E, Bakker PJM, Veenhof CHN, Sauerwein HP, Romijn JA. Effects of acute and chronic interleukin-6 administration on thyroid hormone metabolism in humans. J Clin Endocrinol Metab 1994;79 1342-1346.

[97] Mancini A, Leone E, Di Donna V, Festa R. Anorexia nervosa and cytokines. In: Mancini A, Daini S, Caruana L (eds) Anorexia nervosa: a multidisciplinary approach. New York: Nova Science Pub Inc; 2010. p 31-49.

[98] Resch U, Helsel G, Tatzber F & Sinzinger H. Antioxidant status in thyroid dysfunction. Clin Chem Lab Med 2002;40 1132-1134.

[99] Asayama K, Kato K. Oxidative muscular injury and its relevance to hyperthyroidism. Free Radic Biol Med 1990;8 293-303.

[100] Dobrzynska MM, Baumgartner A & Andersin D. Antioxidants modulate thyroid hormone- and noradrenaline-induced DNA damage in human sperm. Mutagenesis 2004;19 (49) 325-330.

[101] Venditti P, Di Meo S. Thyroid hormone-induced oxidative stress. Cell Mol Life Sci 2006;63 (4) 414-434.

[102] Mancini A, Giacchi E, Raimondo S, Di Segni C, Silvestrini A, Meucci E. Hypothyroidism, oxidative stress and reproduction. In: Springer D (ed) Hypothyroidism-Influencess and treatments. Rijeka: InTech; 2012. p 117-134.

[103] Ademoglou E, Gokkusu C, Yarman S & Azizlerli H. The effect of Methimazol on oxidant and antioxidant system in patients with hyperthyroidism. Pharmacol Res 1998;3 93-96.

[104] Bianchi G, Solaroli E, Zaccheroni V, Grossi G, Bargossi AM & Melchionda N. Oxidative stress and anti-oxidant metabolites in patients with hyperthyroidism: effect of treatment. Horm metab res 1990;31 620-624.

[105] Mancini A, De Marinis L, Calabrò F, Sciuto R, Oradei A, Lippa S, Sandric S, Littaru GP, Barbarino A. Evaluation of metabolic status in amiodarone-induced thyroid disorders: plasma Coenzyme Q10 determination. J Endocrinol Invest 1989;12 511-516.

[106] Mancini A, Corbo GM, Gaballo A, Valente S, Gigliotti P, Cimino V, De Marinis L, Principi F, Littarru GP. Relationships between plasma Coenzyme Q10 levels and thyroid hormones in chronic obstructive pulmonary disease. Biofactors 2005;25 (1-4) 201-204.

[107] Baskol G, Atmaca H, Tanriverdi F, Baskol M, Kocer D & Bayram F. Oxidative stress and enzymatic antioxidant status in patients with hypothyroidism before and after treatment. Exp Clin Endocrinol Diab 2007;115 (8) 522-526.

[108] Torun AN, Kulaksizoglu S, Kulaksizoglu M, Pamuk BO, Isbilen E & Tutuncu NB. Serum total antioxidant status and lipid peroxidation marker malondialdehyde levels in overt and subclinical hypothyroidism. Clin Endocrinol (Oxf) 2009;70 (3) 469-474.

[109] Santi A, Duarte MM, Moresco RN, Menezes C, Bagatini MD, Schetinger MR & Loro VL. Association beetwen thyroid hormones, lipids and oxidative stress biomarkers in overt hypothyroidism. Clin Chem Lab Med 2010;48 (11) 1635- 1639.

[110] Coria MJ, Pastràn AI, Gimenez MS. Serum oxidative stress parameters of women with hypothyroidism. Acta Biomed 2009;80 135-139.

[111] Kebapcilar L, Akinci B, Bayraktar F, Comlekci A, Solak A, Demir T, Yener S, Küme T, Yesil S. Plasma thiobarbituric acid-reactive substance levels in subclinical hypothyroidism. Med princ pract 2007;16 432-436.

[112] Mancini A, Leone E, Silvestrini A, Festa R, Di Donna V, De Marinis L, Pontecorvi A, Littarru GP, Meucci E. Evaluation of antioxidant systems in pituitary-adrenal axis diseases. Pituitary 2010;13 (2) 138-145.

[113] Abilés J, de la Cruz AP, Castaño J, Rodríguez-Elvira M, Aguayo E, Moreno-Torres R, Llopis J, Aranda P, Argüelles S, Ayala A, de la Quintana AM, Planells EM. Oxidative stress is increased in critically ill patients according to antioxidant vitamins intake, independent of severity: a cohort study. Crit Care 2006;10 (5) R146.

[114] Papp LV, Lu J, Striebel F, Kennedy D, Holmgren A, Khanna KK. The redox state of SECIS binding protein 2 controls its localization and selenocysteine incorporation function. Mol Cell Biol 2006;26 (13) 4895-910.

[115] Brent GA, Hershman JM Thyroxine therapy in patients with severe illnesses and lower serum thyroxine concentration. J Clin Endocrinol Metab 1986;63 1-8.

[116] Becker RA, Vaughan GM, Ziegler MG, Seraile LG, Goldfarb W, Mansour EH, McManus WF, Pruitt BA, Mason AD. Hypermetabolic low triiodothyronine syndrome of burn injury. Crit Care Med 1982;10 870-875.

[117] Acker CG, Singh AR, Flick RP, Bernardini J, Greenberg A, Johnson JP. A trial of thyroxine in acute renal failure. Kidney Int 2000;57 293-298.

[118] Acker CG, Flick R, Shapiro R, Scantlebury VP, Jordan ML, Vivas C, Greenberg A, Johnson JP. Thyroid hormone in the treatment of post-transplant acute tubular necrosis (ATN). Am J Transplant 2002;2 57-61.

[119] Schoenberger W, Grimm W, Emmrich P, Gempp W. Thyroid administration lowers mortality in premature infants. Lancet 1979;2 1181.

[120] Pingitore A, Galli E, Barison A, Iervasi A, Scarlattini M, Nucci D, L'Abbate A, Mariotti R, Iervasi G. Acute effects of triiothyronine (T3) replacement therapy in patients with chronic heart failure and low-T3 syndrome: a randomized, placebo-controlled study. J Clin Endocrinol Metab 2008;93 1351-1358.

[121] Klemperer JD, Klein I, Gomez M, Helm RE, Ojamaa K, Thomas SJ, Isom OW, Krieger K. Thyroid hormone treatment after coronary-artery bypass surgery. N Engl J Med 1995;333 1522-1527.

[122] Mullis-Jansson SL, Argenziano M, Corwin S, Homma S, Weinberg AD, Williams M, Rose EA, Smith CR. A randomized double-blind study of the effect of triodothyronine on cardiac function and morbidity after coronary bypass surgery. J Thorac Cardiovasc Surg 1999;117 1128-1134.

[123] Bergeron GA, Goldsmith R, Schiller NB. Myocardial infarction, severe reversible ischemia, and shock following excess thyroid administration in a woman with normal coronary arteries. Arch Intern Med 1988;148 1450-1453.

[124] Becker RA, Vaughan GM, Zeigler MG, et al. Hypermetabolic low triiodothyronine syndrome of burn injury. Crit Care Med 1982;10 870-875.

[125] De Groot LJ. Dangerous dogmas in medicine: the nonthyroidal illness syndrome. J Clin Endocrinol Metab 1999;84 151-164.

[126] Chopra IJ. Nonthyroidal illness syndrome or euthyroid sick syndrome? Endocr Pract 1996;2 45-52.

Section 4

Imaging Techniques

Chapter 9

The Role of Ultrasound in the Differential Diagnosis of Hypothyroidism

Jan Kratky, Jan Jiskra and Eliška Potluková

Additional information is available at the end of the chapter

http://dx.doi.org/10.5772/54678

1. Introduction

Over the last decades, ultrasound has become the leading imaging technique used in the diagnostic workout of thyroid diseases. Thanks to rapid technical improvement, we are now able to differentiate precisely even very small lesions in the thyroid tissue, which previously would have stayed unrecognised. Similarly, the Doppler techniques are able to visualise blood perfusion in the thyroid parenchyma, thyroid nodules and lymphatic nodes with an excellent precision. Due to its availability, low financial cost, noninvasivity and a lacking radiation load, ultrasound is widely used as the imaging method of choice in the diagnosis of thyroid pathologies. In many countries, it has replaced radionuclide techniques, which are now being used only in specific diagnostic questions or in the treatment of selected thyroid disorders.

In this Chapter, we are going to review the role of thyroid ultrasound in the diagnostic workout of thyroid diseases with focus on hypothyroidism. We are going to discuss ultrasound appearance of the thyroid tissue in various thyroid diseases leading to thyroid dysfunction, including thyroid disease in pregnancy and postpartum thyroiditis. We are also going to present interesting cases from our experience.

1.1. Basic principles of ultrasound

As many other important inventions, ultrasound was originally developed for military purposes. It was used in World War I and II in the location of submarines. Sonar was able not only to precisely measure the depth of a reflecting surface under water, but it could also identify an object in motion. In 1950, ultrasound was introduced into medicine as a research tool in the USA; and in 1965, the Jutendo Medical Ultrasound Research Centre in Japan was founded [1].

Basically, an ultrasound probe acts as a transmitter and a receiver of ultrasound waves at the same time. Visualisation of a structure of an organ is made possible by an analysis of the received altered ultrasound waves that were reflected and refracted at the interfaces of various tissues. Ultrasound is a longitudinal sound wave of frequency higher than 20 kHz. For medical purposes, the usually used frequency varies between 2-18 MHz, depending on the examined tissue (for thyroid ultrasound typically 7.5-10 MHz). The source of these waves is a quartz crystal placed in a transducer probe. It generates and receives waves using piezoelectric effect, which is based on rapid deformation of a piezoelectric crystal by an applied electrical charge. Accordingly, when the piezoelectric crystal absorbs the mechanical energy of ultrasound waves, it produces an electric current. This ability is used for the detection and display of the reflected waves. The wave reflection occurs at the interface of tissues with different acoustic impedance. The greater the difference in impedance of each tissue, the greater the amount of energy reflected back.

Tissues with frequent interfaces such as normal thyroid gland display as hyperechogenic area; in contrast, structures with no interfaces such as cysts full of liquid are anechogenic. Two-dimensional map of the layout of echogenicity is called B-mode and it is used as the basic display mode in thyroid sonography. Another mode used for displaying the vascularisation of tissue is the Doppler mode. It is based on Doppler's effect: the shift in frequency and wavelength of reflecting waves caused by reflection from moving objects (red blood cells circulating in vessels). This frequency shift displays as a colour-coded overlay on top of a B-mode image (colour Doppler) [2].

1.2. The use of thyroid ultrasound in the world

The indications for thyroid ultrasound (TUS) vary considerably across the world, as well as the availability of ultrasound devices and physicians´ competences. According to the guidelines of the American Thyroid Association (ATA) for management of hypothyroidism, the "uncomplicated hypothyroid patients are usually observed by primary care physicians and there is no recommendation to do TUS in these patients" [3]. In Europe, the situation is different: many hypothyroid patients with Hashimoto thyroiditis are followed by an endocrinologist during their whole life. For example, in our country (the Czech Republic), TUS belongs to the elementary diagnostic methods in the diagnostic process (together with the laboratory assessment of the thyroid stimulating hormone /TSH/, free thyroxine /FT4/and autoantibodies against thyroid autoantigens).

While in the United States the TUS is usually performed by a radiologist and it is used primarily in the management of thyroid nodules and thyroid carcinoma, the European endocrinologists do the ultrasound often themselves in their outpatients departments. In Europe, thyroid ultrasound is used much more frequently than in the USA, e.g. if the cause of hypothyroidism is unclear; in the differential diagnosis of hyperthyroidism, in amiodarone-induced thyroid disease etc. (Kahaly et al. 2011).

http://dx.doi.org/10.5772/54678

1.3. The ultrasound image of a normal thyroid gland

In order to interpret the ultrasound findings correctly, it is important to be familiar with the anatomy of the thyroid gland. The thyroid is situated in the anterior region of the neck, below the thyroid cartilage with the isthmus located inferior to the cricoid cartilage. In the transversal plane, thyroid lobes are bounded by infrahyoid muscles (anteriorly), trachea (medially), carotid arteries (laterally) and oesophagus (usually on the left) and prevertebral fascia (posteriorly) (Fig. 1). In the elderly, the thyroid gland shifts caudally and often partially retrosternally. In general, the right thyroid lobe is larger than the left one. Rarely, we may visualise the processus pyramidalis as a thin finger-like structure emerging from the isthmus. It is important to check the presence of absence of the lobus pyramidalis especially in patients planned for total thyroidectomy – we have encountered a relapse of Graves′ disease in a forgotten lobus pyramidalis after total thyroidectomy. Anteriorly, the lobes are covered by the infrahyoid and laterally by the sternocleidomastoid muscles. These muscles are important for the evaluation of the echogenicity of the thyroid parenchyma: a healthy thyroid is relatively hyperechogenic as compared to the echogenicity of the muscles.

The size of the thyroid is calculated in millilitres as the sum of the volumes of both lobes (isthmus is neglected). The volume of one thyroid lobe is calculated as:

V (ml) = width x depth x length x 0.479 (cm)

Normal thyroid volume in females is less than 18 ml and in males less than 22 ml. In our experience – in an iodine-sufficient country – the thyroid volumes are generally much smaller (irrespective of the thyroid function) [4]; and true goitres are rare. The lower threshold of normal thyroid volume has not been determined.

The blood is supplied to the thyroid abundantly by the superior and inferior thyroid arteries. Thyroid veins form a thick plexus around the gland. Sometimes, relatively strong vessels occur also inside the parenchyma and it is important to differentiate them from pseudocysts or small hypoechogenic nodules by the Doppler or by the movement of the probe. Perfusion of the thyroid increases on several occasions: in the settings of an increased cardiac output (a stressed patient), in gravidity, during an active autoimmune inflammation – active Graves′ disease or Hashimoto′s thyroiditis and in untreated primary hypothyroidism because of TSH stimulation. In Graves′ disease, the perfusion is very high (typically of the image of a so called "thyroid inferno"). Doppler imaging of the thyroid perfusion is crucial in the differential diagnosis of thyrotoxicosis: increased in Graves′ disease and hyperfunctioning nodules, decreased in breakdown of the thyroid tissue – as is the case of postpartum thyroiditis, De Quervain thyroiditis or amiodarone-induced thyrotoxicosis type 2.

2. The use of TUS in the differential diagnosis of hypothyroidism

Thyroid ultrasound is crucial in the differential diagnosis of hypothyroidism, particularly, if thyroid antibodies are negative. It allows us to determine whether the thyroid is present and

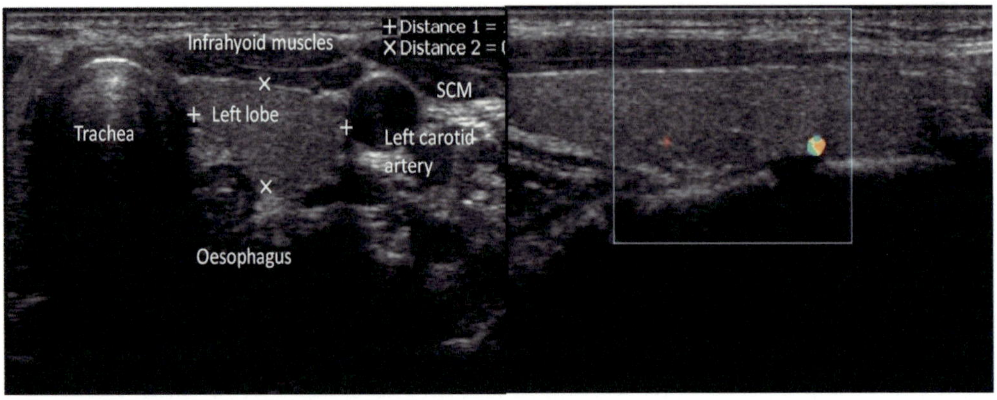

Figure 1. Normal TUS image of left thyroid lobe (euthyroid patient with negative thyroid autoantibodies). Note the low perfusion on the Doppler imaging (right).

to visualise the parenchyma. In this part of the Chapter, we will summarise the ultrasound findings in individual causes of hypothyroidism.

2.1. Rare causes of hypothyroidism

Inborn developmental defects belong among the very rare causes of hypothyroidism: most often hypoplasia, less frequently agenesis or hemiagenesis of the thyroid gland; and ectopic thyroid tissue. These defects are generally diagnosed in early childhood. In children, TUS is performed in cases of positive screening for congenital hypothyroidism. Moreover, scintigraphy may provide the best information on developmental thyroid defects.

2.2. Postoperative states

Hypothyroidism may also develop in patients after total thyroidectomy without an adequate levothyroxine substitution. TUS is important especially in elderly patients with a cognitive deficit and without an obvious scar on the neck. Moreover, TUS should be performed in all patients after total thyroidectomy in order to evaluate a possible presence of a residual thyroid tissue. After thyroidectomy, TUS shouldn´t be performed earlier than two or three months after operations due to the tissue oedema. Patients with thyroid residue should be substituted with higher doses of levothyroxine in order to achieve serum TSH levels in the lower part of the normal reference range (due to an increased risk of thyroid carcinoma in remnant thyroid tissue). Ultrasound image of a patient after total thyroidectomy is shown in Fig. 2.

2.3. Iodine deficiency

From the global point of view, iodine deficiency constitutes a major epidemiological problem. According to the WHO statistics, approximately 13% of the world population has a goitre caused by iodine deficiency [5]. In the developed countries, severe iodine deficiency contributes to the manifest hypothyroidism only to a small extent, although even a milder deficiency may predispose to thyroid dysfunction, e.g. in pregnancy. The typical ultrasound finding in

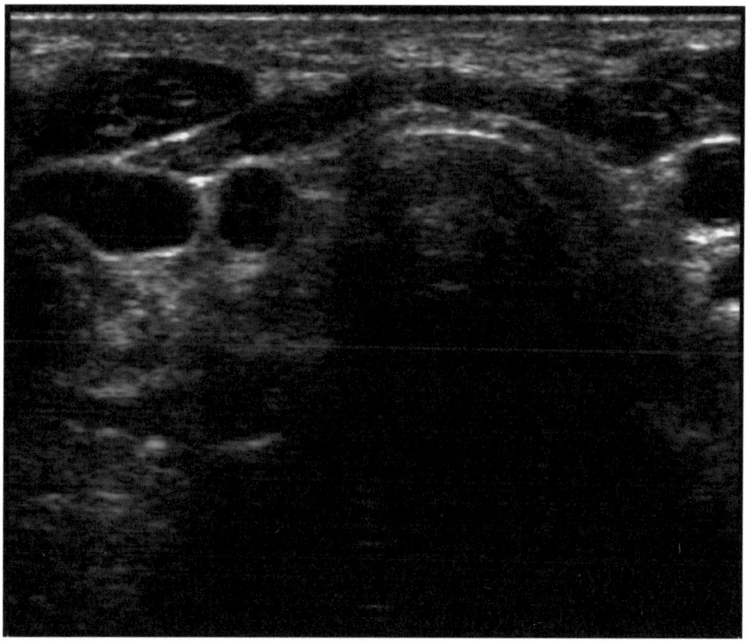

Figure 2. Absent thyroid gland in a patient after total thyroidectomy due to papillary thyroid carcinoma. Note fibrous tissue without residual thyroid parenchyma in the thyroid beds.

iodine deficient patients is a diffuse goitre which often becomes nodular (Fig.3). The perfusion is normal. Enlargement of the thyroid gland is an adaptive process in low iodine intake and it can sometimes lead to dysphagia or dyspnoe due the compression of oesophagus and trachea, respectively. Narrowing of the trachea may be visualised on TUS, but the goitre often reaches below the sternum and it is thus inaccessible for TUS examination. In these cases, we indicate CT scan in order to describe the size of the gland and the extent of trachea compression. Such information are crucial for the decision whether to operate and from which surgical access (classical or through sternotomy).

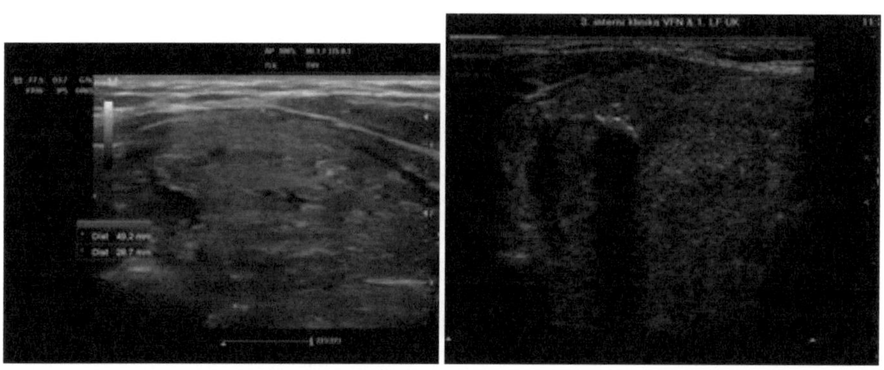

Figure 3. TUS of a diffuse goitre in a euthyroid patient (on the left) and multinodular goitre (on the right).

2.4. Hashimoto's thyroiditis (autoimmune thyroiditis)

The most common cause of hypothyroidism in iodine sufficient areas is the Hashimoto's thyroiditis - HT (autoimmune thyroiditis, chronic lymphocytic thyroiditis). HT with the presence of goitre may be more frequently observed in iodine-deficient areas, whereas the majority of patients with HT in iodine- sufficient areas have a normal thyroid volume. In Greek children, the thyroid volume was associated with the degree of hypothyroidism, it positively correlated with serum TSH concentrations, and it decreased after treatment with levothyroxine [6], [7]. The typical TUS appearance of autoimmune (Hashimoto's) thyroiditis includes an inhomogenous, hypoechogenic pattern (as compared to the echogenicity of the neck muscles). Vascularisation of the thyroid gland may be diffusely increased (Fig. 4). In cases with severe hypothyroidism with TSH up to 100 mIU/l and more, which may occur e.g. after delivery, the thyroid gland increases dramatically its volume and the ultrasound image may be one of a very hypoechogenic goitre with fibrotic septae (honeycomb-like) (Fig. 5).

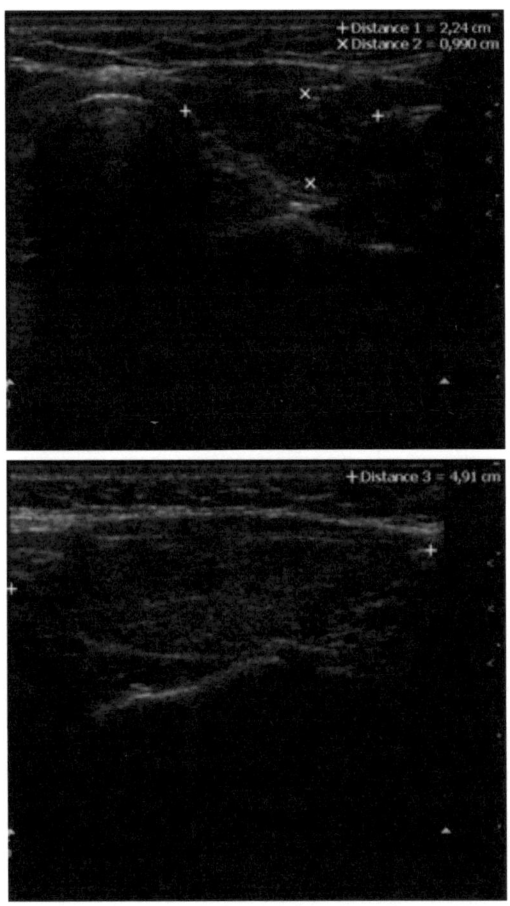

Figure 4. Typical TUS image of Hashimoto's thyroiditis (TSH 17 mIU/l, highly positive thyroid autoantibodies). Note the inhomogenous and hypoechogenic thyroid texture.

http://dx.doi.org/10.5772/54678

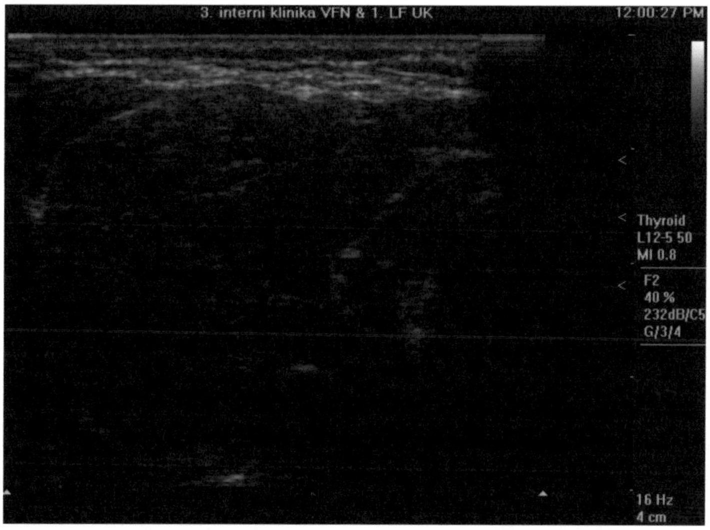

Figure 5. TUS image of the right thyroid lobe in a patient with Hashimoto´s thyroiditis with a large goitre.

It is important to mention that Hashimoto´s thyroiditis may also have a different appearance on the ultrasound. Atrophic thyroiditis is a common variant of HT, especially in a long-term active disease. A progressive fibrotisation in the inflammatorily changed tissue may lead to an atrophy of the parenchyma with a significant reduction in the thyroid volume. This corresponds to the ultrasound finding of a very small and inhomogeneous thyroid gland, which may be both hypo- and hyperechogenic (in case of an advanced fibrotisation) (Fig. 6).

Moreover, some patients with positive antithyroid antibodies and thyroid dysfunction may have a normal echogenicity of the parenchyma, which is filled with small sharply circumscribed hypoechogenic lesions, which look like moth-eaten (Fig. 7). It is unknown what mechanism predisposes individual patients to which ultrasound image of thyroiditis.

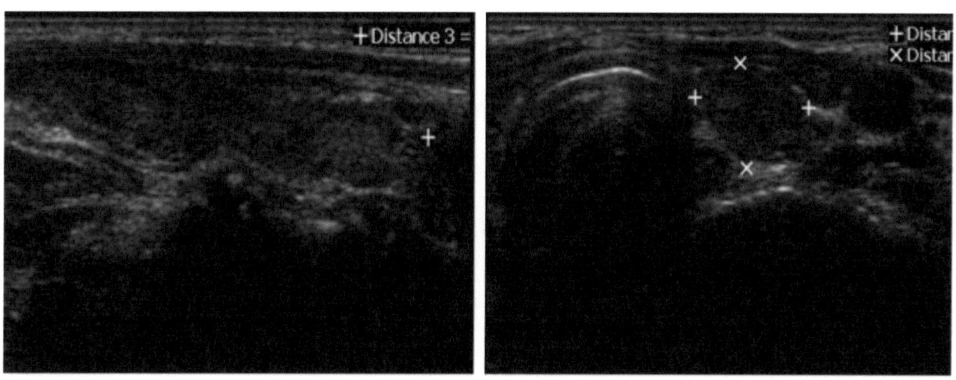

Figure 6. TUS of atrophic thyroiditis (a patient with mild hypothyroidism: TSH 9.43 mIU/l, highly positive anti-TPO antibodies).

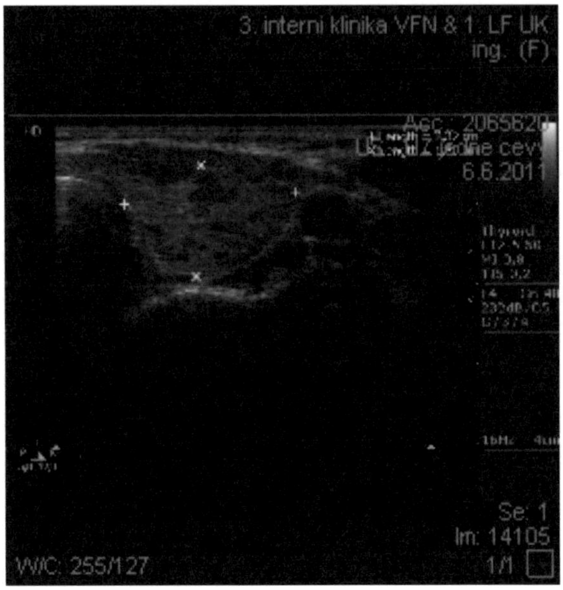

Figure 7. TUS picture of a "moth-eaten thyroid" in patient with HT.

TUS does not always correspond to the laboratory results. As we discuss later, the discrepancy between TUS image and the degree of antithyroid antibodies-positivity may be particularly striking during pregnancy.

Usually, upon the diagnosis of hypothyroidism, a positivity of thyroid antibodies is regarded as an evidence of an autoimmune thyroid disease. However, according to some studies, autoimmune pattern in TUS is more specific for the diagnosis of autoimmune thyroid disease (AITD) than the positivity of antibodies. In the study of Rago et al., during three years of follow-up none of the TPOAb-positive patients with negative TUS developed hypothyroidism, in contrast to 58 % of the TPOAb-positive euthyroid patients with positive TUS who became hypothyroid[8]. Moreover, thyroid dysfunction was found in 13.7% of patients with thyroid hypoechogenicity with negative antibodies in comparison to none of the antibody-negative subjects with normal TUS [8]. This suggests that TUS is a useful diagnostic method in the evaluation of the risk of developing hypothyroidism.

2.5. Subacute (De Quervein's) thyroiditis

Subacute (De Quervein's) thyroiditis is an inflammatory disease of the thyroid gland, which usually occurs after a respiratory (viral, bacterial) infection. The initial phase of the disease is characterised by hyperthyroidism accompanied by local migrating neck pain, increased temperature and constitutional symptoms (myalgias, arthralgias, fatigue), and elevation of serum acute phase proteins (C-reactive protein) and blood-sedimentation rate. Although it is primarily not an autoimmune disease, approximately 15% of cases can transform into Hashimoto´s thyroiditis and develop a permanent hypothyroidism with positive anti-thyroid antibodies[9]. Typical TUS of subacute thyroiditis consists of irregularly shaped hypoechogenic areas (Fig. 8) which may contrast with areas of normal thyroid parenchyma in the in initial phase. Hypervascularisation is not present. The extent of hypoechogenic areas within the thyroid tissue is a positive predictor of subsequent long-term hypothyroidism – patients with bilateral hypoechogenic areas at presentation had a six times higher risk of developing permanent hypothyroidism than patients with unilateral hypoechogenic areas[10].

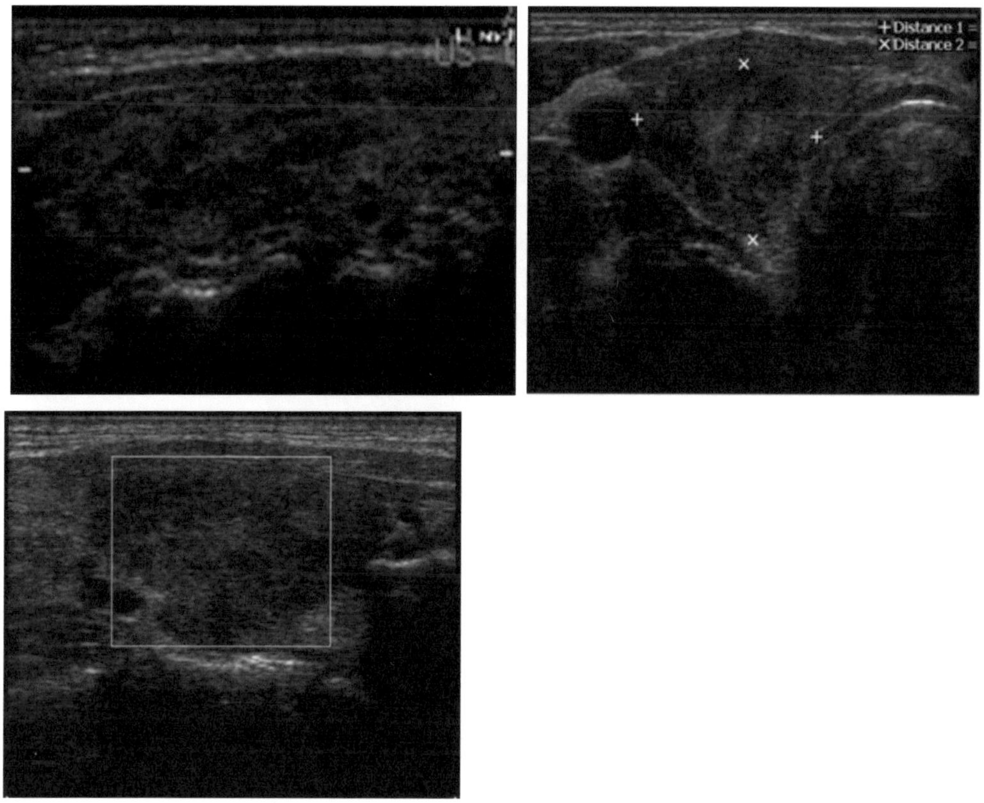

Figure 8. TUS image of subacute thyroiditis in the hyperthyroid phase (FT3: 10.7 pmol/l, FT4: 33.1 pmol/l, TSH: 0.039 mIU/l, antibodies negative). Note the low perfusion as shown by the Doppler imaging (right).

2.6. Amiodarone-induced hypothyroidism

Amiodarone is an antiarrhythmic drug often used in treatment of ventricular and supraventricular tachyarrhythmias. Each tablet contains about 37% (i.e. 75 mg) of organic iodide; 8-17% of which is released as free iodide. Thus, a 100-mg tablet contains an amount of iodine that is 250-times higher than the recommended daily iodine requirement [11].

Autoimmune thyroid dysfunction occurs in up to 22% patients treated with amiodarone, depending on the iodine saturation in the geographical area [12]. Amiodarone can cause both hyper- and hypofunction of the thyroid gland, which may develop both in a normal thyroid gland or in settings of a preexisting thyroid disease. Excessive iodine intake inhibits the synthesis of thyroid hormones in patients with Hashimoto's thyroiditis and it may worsen the hypothyroidism. High doses of iodine can damage the thyroid follicles and they may accelerate the natural trend of Hashimoto's thyroiditis toward hypothyroidism [13]. The ultrasound image of amiodarone-induced hypothyroidism may be similar to the typical findings in an autoimmune inflammatory thyroid process – an inhomogeneous hypoechogenic pattern (Fig. 9) ; or the thyroid gland may even have a normal texture.

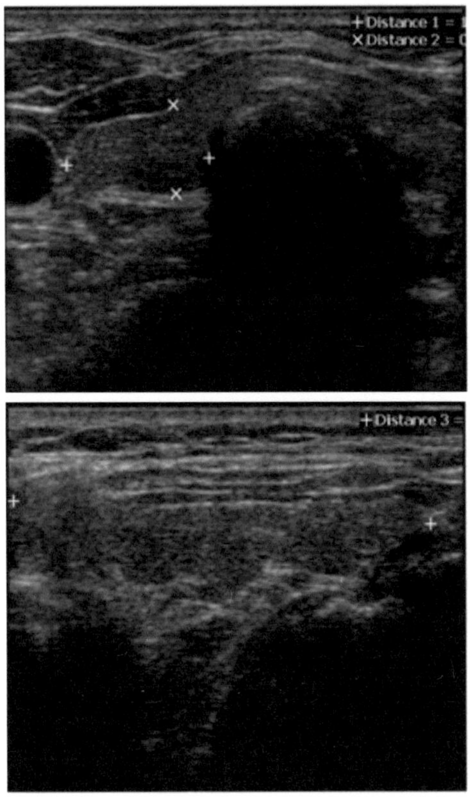

Figure 9. TUS image in a 69-year-old patient who developed hypothyroidism after treatment by amiodarone.

3. TUS during pregnancy and postpartum

3.1. Changes of TUS image in pregnancy

The relationship between antithyroid antibodies-positivity and the TUS image may change in the settings of altered hormonal state, e.g. in pregnancy. According to our findings, nearly a half (42.5%) of the TPOAb-positive pregnant women do not have an autoimmune pattern in thyroid ultrasound, while in the non-pregnant controls, it was only 22.4% [14]. In our study, we have also shown that the occurrence of hypothyroidism in pregnancy and the rate of preterm delivery were linked to an autoimmune pattern in TUS. Thus, a normal TUS image in a TPOAb-positive euthyroid pregnant woman might be a favourable predictive parameter[14].

3.2. Postpartum thyroiditis

The incidence of PPT is reported between 5-10% [15]. Postpartum thyroiditis (PPT) is a disease that occurs in the relationship to pregnancy and it manifests itself by a transient thyrotoxicosis with a following hypothyroidism. Usually, it occurs 2-6 months after delivery and it presents with a few (4-8) weeks lasting hyperthyroidism, which may spontaneously resolve to a euthyroid state or switch to hypothyroidism. Approximately one half of patients do not develop temporary hyperthyroidism and the disease manifests itself by postpartum hypothyroidism [15]. Persistent hypothyroidism develops in 50 % of women with PPT[16]. Moreover, TPOAb-positivity in the first trimester of pregnancy is associated with a higher risk of developing PPT: almost 60% of TPOAb-positive women develop PPT [17], [18].

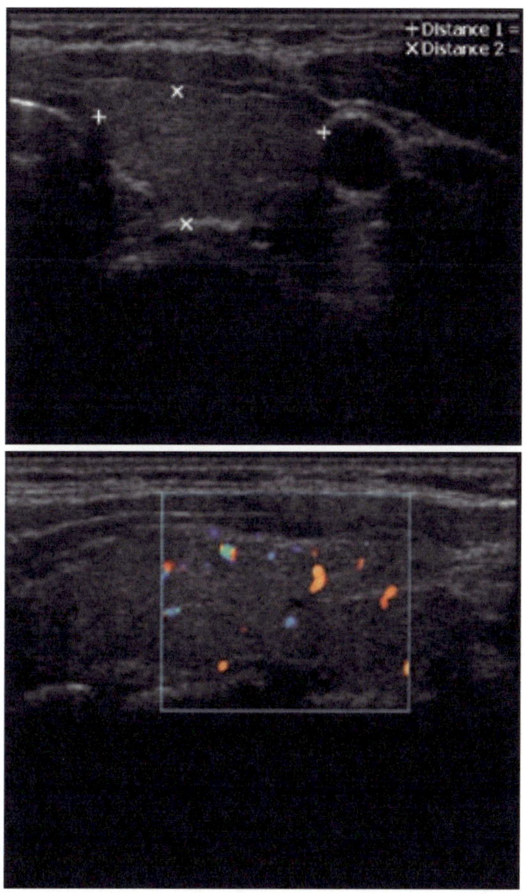

Figure 10. TUS of the left thyroid lobe of patient with PPT which occurred two months after delivery (TSH 0.024 mIU/l, fT4 28.9 pmol/l, TPOAb 746 kIU/l). Four months after delivery, the patient developed hypothyroidism.

The TUS image in PPT in both hyper- and hypothyroid phases includes typical autoimmune pattern (enlargement, inhomogeneous hypoechogenic parenchyma with an increased vascularisation) (Fig. 10). There are no significant differences in the TUS image between these two phases; probably because the transient hyperthyroidism is caused by disintegration of follicles during the inflammation processes in thyroid gland. Higher levels of TPOAb in pregnancy are associated with a higher prevalence of ultrasound changes [19].

4. Interesting cases from our experience

4.1. Healthy women with autoimmune pattern in TUS

A 35-year-old healthy woman with no clinical signs and symptoms of hypothyroidism and a negative history of thyroid disease was examined as a member of a control group in a clinical study. Her thyroid laboratory tests were all normal (Table 1). Surprisingly, the ultrasound examination revealed a typical image of Hashimoto´s thyroiditis: the thyroid parenchyma was inhomogenous and hypoechogenic with an increased vascularisation. After three months, her TUS findings remained unchanged and her TSH was again in the normal range. Next control is scheduled in six months – these results are not yet available at the time of publication of this Chapter.

	First visit	**After 3 months**	**Normal Ranges**
TSH (mIU/l)	0.800	1.967	0.5 – 4.9
free T3 (pmol/l)	5.1	-	3.4 – 6.3
free T4 (pmol/l)	14.6	-	11.5 – 22.7
TPOAb (kU/l)	45	-	0 – 60
TgAb (kU/l)	52.5	-	0 – 60

Table 1. Laboratory findings in a healthy woman with a typical autoimmune pattern on thyroid ultrasound (Fig. 11).

It remains unclear whether thyroid dysfunction and/or antithyroid antibodies-positivity will develop at a later stage or whether it is a variant of HT with negative antithyroid antibodies and without progression to hypothyroidism. According to the results of an Italian prospective study, euthyroid patients with autoimmune pattern in TUS are in a significantly higher risk of developing hypothyroidism than those with positive antibodies but normal TUS. Correspondingly, individuals with both positive TUS and antibodies are in a higher risk than those with positive antibodies but normal TUS[8]. It remains unclear how often and how long these patients should be followed.

http://dx.doi.org/10.5772/54678

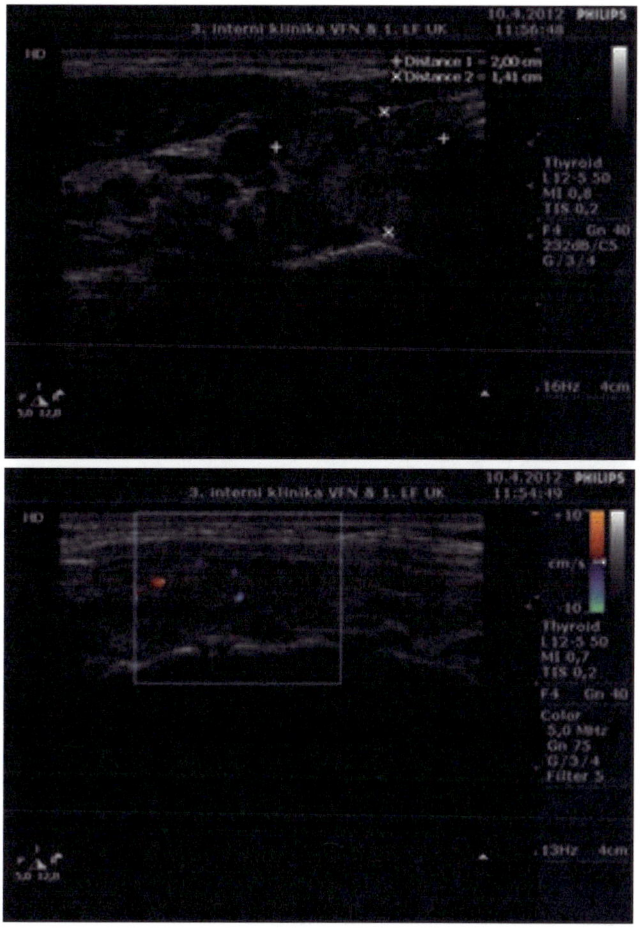

Figure 11. TUS image in a young euthyroid woman with negative antithyroid antibodies.

4.2. Thyroid carcinoma in a pregnant woman

A 33-year-old pregnant woman was referred to our Outpatient department due to a small nodule in the right lobe of her thyroid gland. Her laboratory findings were normal (TSH 1.606 mIU/l, FT4: 11.7 pmol/l, negative antibodies). In the third trimester of pregnancy, TUS and fine needle aspiration biopsy (FNAB) were performed. On the TUS, two nodules (one hypoechogenic and one isoechogenic) in the right lobe were visible. The rest of the thyroid tissue had a normal ultrasound pattern. FNAB of the hypoechogenic one (Fig. 12) yielded a diagnostic conclusion of Bethesda V (suspicion of malignancy).

A suppression therapy with 100 ug of levothyroxine per day was initiated. One month after the delivery patient underwent total thyroidectomy with a histological finding of thyroid papillary carcinoma. The tumour was clinically and histopathologically evaluated as low-risk, thus radioiodine ablation was not performed. During one year of follow-up, no thyroid tissue was found on the neck sonography and serum thyroglobulin remained undetectable.

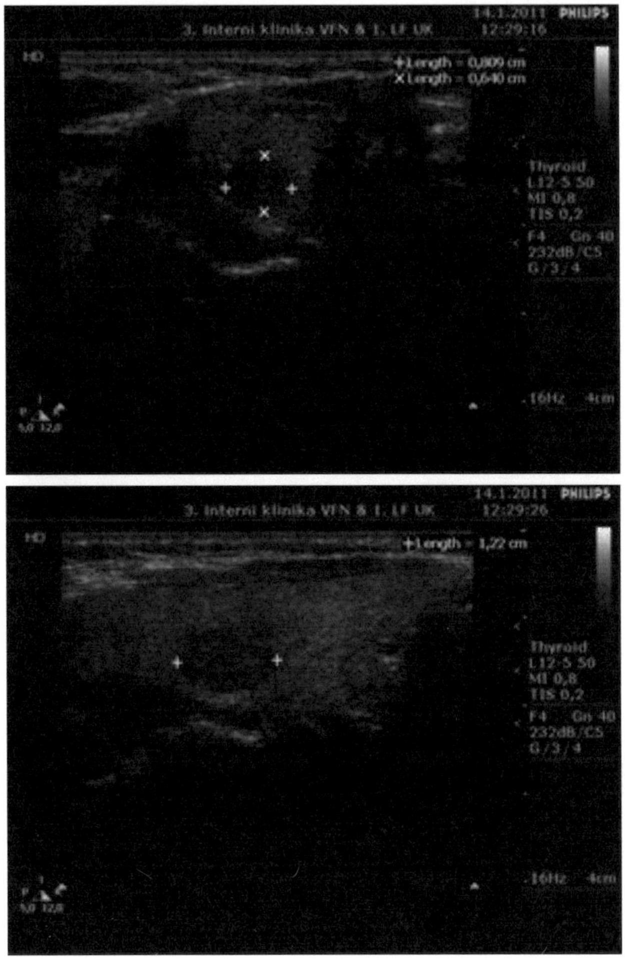

Figure 12. TUS image of a thyroid papillary carcinoma (8x6x12 mm) in a pregnant euthyroid TPOAb-negative woman.

4.3. Hypothyroid patient with AL amyloidosis

A 32-year-old woman with AL amyloidosis affecting the kidneys, liver, spleen, bone marrow and intestine was referred to our Outpatient department in order to evaluate her TSH elevation. The diagnosis of AL amyloidosis was made in 2006 through a kidney biopsy, which was indicated because of a renal insufficiency (creatinine 180 umol/l) and proteinuria (15 g/24h). The affection of other organs was subsequently confirmed by biopsies. At presentation, the patient´s TSH was 8.073 mIU/l, fT4 16.7 pmol/l and antithyroid antibodies were negative. The TUS yielded an image of a mildly inhomogeneous and hypoechogenic thyroid gland with a normal vascularisation (Fig. 13). Cytological specimen obtained by FNAB proved an infiltration of the thyroid tissue by amyloid. It confirmed thus the diagnosis of thyroid amyloidosis. Substitution therapy with 50 ug of levothyroxine was started and the patient is now euthyroid.

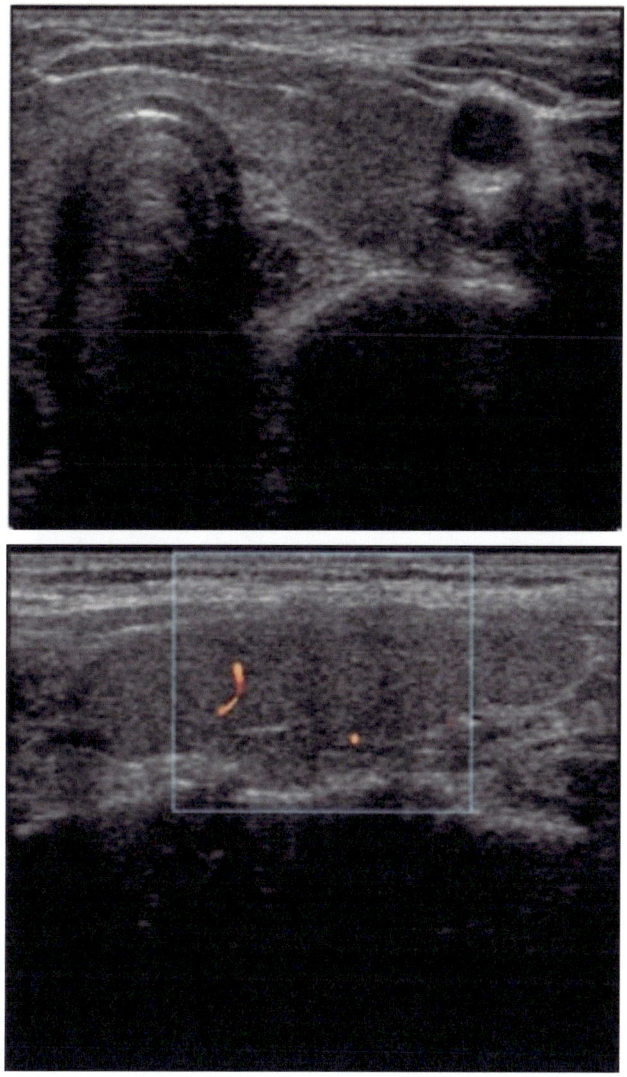

Figure 13. TUS image of thyroid amyloidosis confirmed by cytology.

5. Conclusion

Thyroid ultrasound is an optimal initial imaging method in the evaluation of thyroid disorders thanks to its noninvasivity, availability and no radiation load. It is widely used not only in the management of thyroid nodules, but also in the diagnostic workup of thyroid dysfunction. In a hypothyroid patient, the TUS may lead to cost savings: if a typical autoimmune pattern is present on TUS, the measurement of antithyroid antibodies is not necessary for the diagnosis of Hashimoto´s thyroiditis. Moreover, the ultrasound image contributes to the decision process whether to treat patients with positive antithyroid antibodies who are euthyroid or have only a mild subclinical hypothyroidism. TUS in this setting is especially valuable in case of women who wish to conceive or are pregnant.

In our opinion, TUS should be performed in all patients with thyroid dysfunction and, in case of young women and pregnant women, also in those who are euthyroid but are positive for antithyroid antibodies. Moreover, we believe that if we, the treating endocrinologists, perform TUS by ourselves, we may improve the care of our patients.

Author details

Jan Kratky, Jan Jiskra and Eliška Potluková*

Third Department of Internal Medicine, General University Hospital and First Faculty of Medicine, Charles University in Prague, Czech Republic

References

[1] Hassani, S. Principles of ultrasonography. *J Natl Med Assoc* , 1974 - 66 .

[2] Støylen, A. Basic ultrasound, echocardiography and Doppler for clinicians. http://folk.ntnu.no/stoylen/strainrate/Ultrasound/. (2010).

[3] Singer, P. A, Cooper, D. S, Levy, E. G, Ladenson, P. W, Braverman, L. E, Daniels, G, & Greenspan, F. S. McDougall IR & Nikolai TF. Treatment guidelines for patients with hyperthyroidism and hypothyroidism. Standards of Care Committee, American Thyroid Association. *JAMA* , 1995 - 273 .

[4] Dvorakova, M, Bilek, R, Cerovska, J, Hill, M, Novak, Z, Vavrejnova, V, & Vlcek, P. Vrbikova J & Zamrazil V. [The volumes of the thyroid gland in adults aged years in the Czech Republic--determination of the norms]. *Vnitr Lek* (2006 5). , 18-65.

[5] World Health Organization UNCsFInternational Council for Control of Iodine Deficiency Disorders. *Assessment of the iodine deficiency disorders and monitoring their elimination. WHO document WHO/NHD/01.1.*: Geneva: World Health Organization, (2001).

[6] Skarpa, V, Kappaousta, E, Tertipi, A, Anyfandakis, K, Vakaki, M, & Dolianiti, M. Fotinou A & Papathanasiou A. Epidemiological characteristics of children with autoimmune thyroid disease. *Hormones (Athens)* , 2011 - 10 .

[7] Scarpa, V, Kousta, E, Tertipi, A, Vakaki, M, Fotinou, A, & Petrou, V. Hadjiathanasiou C & Papathanasiou A. Treatment with thyroxine reduces thyroid volume in euthyroid children and adolescents with chronic autoimmune thyroiditis. *Horm Res Paediatr* , 2010 - 73 .

[8] Rago, T, Chiovato, L, & Grasso, L. Pinchera A & Vitti P. Thyroid ultrasonography as a tool for detecting thyroid autoimmune diseases and predicting thyroid dsfunction in apparently healthy subjects. *J Endocrinol Invest* , 2001 - 24 .

[9] Fatourechi, V, Aniszewski, J. P, & Fatourechi, G. Z. Atkinson EJ & Jacobsen SJ. Clinical features and outcome of subacute thyroiditis in an incidence cohort: Olmsted County, Minnesota, study. *J Clin Endocrinol Metab* , 2003 - 88 .

[10] Nishihara, E, Amino, N, Ohye, H, Ota, H, Ito, M, & Kubota, S. Fukata S & Miyauchi A. Extent of hypoechogenic area in the thyroid is related with thyroid dysfunction after subacute thyroiditis. *J Endocrinol Invest* , 2009 - 32 .

[11] Basaria S & Cooper DSAmiodarone and the thyroid. *Am J Med* , 2005 - 118 .

[12] Martino, E, & Bartalena, L. Bogazzi F & Braverman LE. The effects of amiodarone on the thyroid. *Endocr Rev* , 2001 - 22 .

[13] Gopalan M & Griffing GTThyroid Dysfunction Induced by Amiodarone Therapy. http://emedicine.medscape.com/article/overview#a0101. (2012).

[14] Jiskra, J, Bartakova, J, Holinka, S, Limanova, Z, Springer, D, Fait, T, & Antosova, M. Telicka Z & Potlukova E. Low concordance between positive antibodies to thyroperoxidase and thyroid ultrasound autoimmune pattern in pregnant women. *Endocr J* , 2011 - 58 .

[15] Lazarus, J. H. Postpartum thyroid disease. In *The thyroid and reproduction.*, Eds JH Lazarus, V Pirags & S Butz. Stuttgart: Georg Thieme Verlag, (2008). , 105-113.

[16] Premawardhana, L. D, Parkes, A. B, Ammari, F, John, R, & Darke, C. Adams H & Lazarus JH. Postpartum thyroiditis and long-term thyroid status: prognostic influence of thyroid peroxidase antibodies and ultrasound echogenicity. *J Clin Endocrinol Metab* , 2000 - 85 .

[17] Hidaka, Y, Tamaki, H, Iwatani, Y, & Tada, H. Mitsuda N & Amino N. Prediction of post-partum Graves' thyrotoxicosis by measurement of thyroid stimulating antibody in early pregnancy. *Clin Endocrinol (Oxf)* , 1994 - 41 .

[18] Premawardhana, L. D, Parkes, A. B, & John, R. Harris B & Lazarus JH. Thyroid peroxidase antibodies in early pregnancy: utility for prediction of postpartum thyroid dysfunction and implications for screening. *Thyroid* , 2004 - 14 .

[19] Parkes, A. B, Adams, H, Othman, S, & Hall, R. John R & Lazarus JH. The role of complement in the pathogenesis of postpartum thyroiditis: ultrasound echogenicity and the degree of complement-induced thyroid damage. *Thyroid* , 1996 - 6 .